CHINESE MEDICINE AND HEALING

CHINESE MEDICINE

AND HEALING

An Illustrated History

EDITED BY TJ Hinrichs and Linda L. Barnes

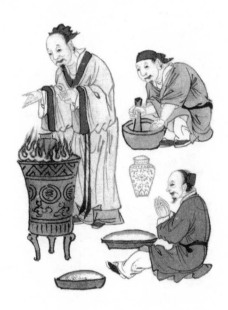

The Belknap Press of Harvard University Press

CAMBRIDGE, MASSACHUSETTS · LONDON, ENGLAND · 2013

Library of Congress Cataloging-in-Publication Data

Chinese medicine and healing : an illustrated history / edited by TJ
Hinrichs and Linda L. Barnes.

   p.   cm.

   Includes bibliographical references and index.

   ISBN 978-0-674-04737-2 (alk. paper)

 1. Medicine, Chinese.   I. Hinrichs, T. J.   II. Barnes, Linda L.

   R601.C48273 2013

610—dc23

2012010749

*To the memory of the inimitable Peter Cairo, musician
and automobile mechanic, and dedicated student of martial
arts and of Chinese herbal medicine.*

*To teachers Arthur Kleinman, Tu Weiming, Peter Bol, and
John Carman, each of whom has gifted generations of students
with their insights, guidance, and exceptional contributions
to their fields.*

Contents

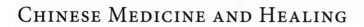

CHINESE MEDICINE AND HEALING

INTRODUCTION

Linda L. Barnes and TJ Hinrichs

Editors' note: Because we shared equally in the conceptualizing, development, writing, and editing related to this book, we have listed our names in alternating order on the cover and here in the Introduction, to reflect the parity of our involvement.

. . .

STUDIES OF MEDICINE AND HEALING in China have exploded in the last two decades, producing an interdisciplinary and rapidly changing field. This book, rather than being a single author's synthesis, collects the work of leading scholars from around the world, all writing on the periods and topics of their research expertise.

Why, for our title, did we choose *Chinese Medicine and Healing* and not just *Chinese Medicine*? This book aspires to integrate the contributions of medical historians and anthropologists who have long cast their nets beyond the narrow confines of "medicine," salient as a specialized form of healing because of its accessibility through written literature and privileged orthodox status. Healing, however, is shaped not only by the clean lines of theory but also by the messy contingencies of practice; not only by doctors but also by complex interactions among physicians, patients, and nonphysician caregivers; not only in the exclusive domain of licensed doctors but also in the competition of diverse types of healers; not only in the crisis of illness but also in the day-to-day care of health and in the pursuit of salvation and enlightenment; not only by the exigencies of the sickroom but also by parameters negotiated in complex institutional and economic environments. To foster a fuller understanding, we cast a wider net and included, for example, the roles of *qi* (vital energy) circulation in enhancing health, of divination in diagnosis, and of food and ritual in therapeutics.

Historians have shown that the field of ideas, practices, and practitioners esteemed over others as "medical" has always been in flux and contestation, and the observation is no less true for China's long history. One of the goals of this book is to explore the historical processes that produced shifts in the scope or practice of medicine (in Chinese, *yi*) that changed what was valued as more efficacious or ethical, and that sometimes intensified efforts to establish and reinforce the boundaries of what could be considered properly "medical." The demarcation of medicine, by its very logic, simultaneously delimited what it was not, nonmedical healing. In some periods, physicians became heated in their denigration of healers labeled "shamans" *(wu)* and "adepts" (or "remedy masters," *fangshi*) in such arts as divination—both groups with which physicians were often lumped. In so doing, physicians ignored the therapeutic and conceptual repertoires that they shared with other healers, such as herbal therapies, exorcistic techniques, and Yin-Yang cosmologies, and emphasized differences or simply accused their rivals of charlatanry.

In some periods, status distinctions emerged within the field of medicine. Late imperial scholar-physicians *(ruyi)* saw themselves as epitomizing erudition and subtlety in pulse diagnosis and prescription therapy. During the centuries of their dominance, acupuncture, so prevalent in modern views of what was most unique in "traditional" Chinese medicine, was disparaged as a crude and vulgar technique. In the twentieth century, as "Western medicine" increasingly defined the parameters of best practice, "Chinese medicine" became the embattled "other," and its advocates reinvented it to be simultaneously more modern (rationalized) and more Chinese (elevating the role of such distinctive practices as acupuncture). In Chosŏn Korea (1392–1910), "Eastern medicine" marked Korean indigeneity in contradistinction to "Chinese" styles; in the global context, "oriental medicine" often meant "Chinese medicine," an exotic alternative to cosmopolitan biomedicine.

If the scope of medicine was in flux, so was what we retrospectively label "China" and "Chinese." Political boundaries almost continuously shifted, fragmented, and recombined. The same could be said for the ethnic and linguistic diversity of the region, and as in the case of "medicine," we should consider the arbitrariness and porosity of ethnic and linguistic divisions. If we take shared literate traditions as the basis for what we call "China," we must include those of regions that participated in that literature, known today as Korea, Japan, and Vietnam. If we take certain healing traditions as our defining threads, we must certainly follow their emergence, transmission, and continual reconstitution through time and through their movements around the globe. We have thus treated "China" as a flexible idea rather than as an objectively continuous entity, and where possible have used contemporary terms for political, ethnic, and cultural markers. The maps accompanying each chapter illustrate changing dynastic borders, drawn with dotted lines to remind us that those boundaries were less clearly marked and controlled than those of modern nations.

The global cross-fertilization of practices began well before the nineteenth and twentieth centuries, with influences flowing into, and out of, "China." Historical studies of interactions across different linguistic groups are by their nature difficult and lag behind, but where scholarship permits, the chapters show the ways in which Chinese and other healing traditions adapted techniques, ideas, and materials from each other, revealing "Chinese" medicine and healing to be not simply an artifact of "Chinese culture." The final chapters concentrate entirely on the spread of Chinese healing across the globe, introducing much scholarship that has appeared only in the last decade.

In this book we have avoided certain conceptual frameworks that had traction in earlier scholarship on medicine but which have been found to mask more than they illuminate. Except for very narrow bands of activity at recent points in time, it is hard to fit any variety of Chinese healing into one side or the other of dichotomies between "sacred" and "secular" and between "science" and "religion." The concepts have no precise counterparts in most societies in human history and do not even always work very well for modern biomedicine, often taken as the paradigm of secular scientific medicine. Similarly, from about the nineteenth century, historians heady with the pace of recent technological change tended to write celebrations of the advances of science and medicine. By the middle of the twentieth century, though, it became apparent that it was exceedingly hard to agree on parameters by which progress could be meaningfully measured. Furthermore, scholars came to realize that, in their interest in scientific discovery, they had often projected their own notions of science back in time. They had ignored actors' own understandings of what they were doing, had minimized many things that had been influential in past times but which did not fit modern scientific models, and had overstated the significance of obscure figures whose ideas had been largely disregarded but in some way prefigured modern theories.

To overcome the distortions of modern and outsider perspectives, it helps to pay close attention to the ways in which people understand what they are doing in their own terms: according to their own formulations of knowledge and efficacy, and according to their contextually conditioned assessments of personal and communal good. Therefore, in this book we translate Chinese concepts directly, rather than mapping them against modern biomedical terminology.

In this volume we follow established conventions for English-language writings on China and on Chinese medicine and healing. We render terms according to modern standard pronunciations and prevailing academic transliteration systems: Chinese using *pinyin,* Korean using McCune-Reischauer, Vietnamese using Quốc Ngữ, and Japanese following *Kenkyūsha's New Japanese-English Dictionary,* fourth edition. In the cases of terms such as *qi,* which have become common enough to be included in English dictionaries, we use their transliterated forms throughout; Yin and Yang are familiar enough that we do not bother to italicize them. We give East Asian names in East Asian order, with family names first: Li Shizhen's (1518–1593) family name is Li. When referring to emperors and their courts, we give the dates of the emperor's reign, for example, Emperor Huizong (r. 1101–1125). As part of our effort to minimize presentism, we use contemporary place names with their modern names indicated afterward in parentheses.

To improve the utility of this book as a reference for students and scholars, we have included Chinese characters in the index, with cross-listings under both transliteration and translations. In many cases, translation choices have become standardized, but in others meanings shift with time and context, or remain controversial; we have thus given alternative translations where relevant. In the fields of Daoist and religious studies, for example, scholars prefer to translate *huangdi* as "Yellow Thearch" in order to capture the sense of *di* as a divine or deified ruler. We have chosen nevertheless to stay with the still more common "Yellow Emperor."

We have capitalized certain terms when they are used in a more restricted, technical sense. For example, people might breathe *qi* and bleed blood, but in a certain mode of theorizing, *Qi* stands for the body's Vitalities, or it can stand more specifically for Yang Vitalities and Blood for Yin Vitalities. Similarly, it is possible to dissect and weigh a liver, but in the physiology developed in the *Inner Canon* tradition, the Liver indicated a physiological system that connected the eyesight to changes detectable through the *mo* pulse.

Finally, this collection builds on the magisterial foundations laid by such scholars as Chen Bangxian, Fan Xingzhun, Joseph Needham, Lu Gwei-djen, Nathan Sivin, Paul Unschuld, and Arthur Kleinman. Many of the authors have been their students. Here, we pass along our many teachers' influence through our own scholarship.

ONE

The Pre-Han Period

Constance A. Cook

CONVENTIONALLY, SCHOLARS TRACE CHINESE HISTORY and prehistory back to the middle Yellow River Valley, where we find early versions of the Chinese script appearing around 1200 B.C.E. This strategy is reinforced by China's own historical traditions, which begin with the Shang (~1500?–1046 B.C.E.), Zhou (1046–256 B.C.E.), and Qin (221–206 B.C.E.) regimes that emerged in this region.

These early periods were dominated by the belief that disease was caused by supernatural influences, particularly in the form of curses. Illness could result from daily interaction in the natural world or from discontent among distant or near ancestors, and thus ancient healers had to be experts in local lore, the patient's lineage, and medical techniques. The primary diagnostic tool was divination and the primary method of treatment was exorcism. With the decline in dominance of the Zhou clan system and its corresponding hierarchy of capricious ancestral spirits, a process that became conspicuous in the Spring and Autumn period (ca. 771–481 B.C.E.), explanations for illness gradually shifted away from the supernatural and toward the natural.

A passion for proactively preserving and extending life intensified during the aptly named Warring States period (481–221 B.C.E.), which was marked by the steady conquest of smaller states by larger ones and by the accelerating breakdown of traditional forms of social and political authority and organization. Elites sought health guidance and healing from an increasingly wide array of specialists, including not only shamans, diviners, and exorcists but also adepts who specialized in different life-cultivating "Ways" (Dao) and medical healers (*yi*). These specialists developed cosmologies based on *qi*, a vapor taken to constitute the essence of all matter, patterned according to the complementary and

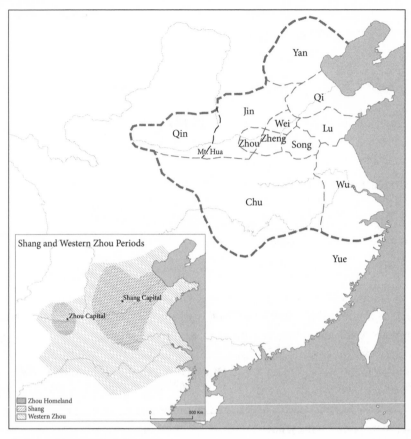

Yan

Jin

Qi

Qin

Wei

Lu

Zhou Zheng Song

Mt. Hua

Chu

Wu

Yue

Shang and Western Zhou Periods

Shang Capital

Zhou Capital

Zhou Homeland
Shang
Western Zhou

0   500 Km

Spring and Autumn Period, ca.
500 B.C.E. Zhou Royal Domain
and Major Fiefs

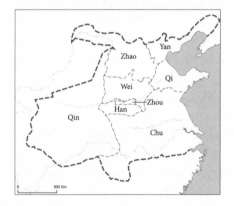

Zhao

Yan

Wei

Qi

Han

Zhou

Qin

Chu

0   500 Km

Warring States, ca. 260 B.C.E.

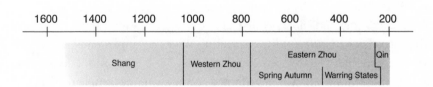

1600   1400   1200   1000   800   600   400   200

Shang

Western Zhou

Eastern Zhou

Qin

Spring Autumn

Warring States

dynamic ideas of Yin and Yang. Yin and Yang originally referred to the movement of shade and sun, respectively, over a hill, and extended to such dualities as dark and light, female and male, and death and life. Yin and Yang also described the directions that organized space (north is Yin compared to south; west is Yin compared to east), and the cycles of days, months, seasons, and years that organized time. The third century B.C.E. saw the elaboration of these systems in terms of various phases, which by the imperial age (inaugurated with the Qin's conquest of the remaining states in 221 B.C.E.) narrowed down to a standard Five Phases *(wuxing)*. These naturalistic cosmologies powerfully reshaped the entire spectrum of health and healing, from diagnostic and prognostic divination to physiological theories, from the disease-producing spiritual and natural realms to ritual and medical treatments.

Our earliest evidence best represents the elite strata of society, who left the richest written and material remains. In these groups, among the many types of spirits who could cause illness, ghosts and ancestors were particular sources of anxiety. Evidence from Neolithic tombs, more than five thousand years ago and long before the appearance of writing, suggest that death was long conceived of as a continuum in which human agency—not always benign—was transferred to the spirit realm. The recently deceased, who still hovered in the liminal postmortem stages between death, burial, and becoming an ancestor, could be especially dangerous to the living, capable of bringing disease and other calamities if not properly transferred to their places in the afterlife. Later texts described an imperative for descendants to perform continuous rituals to assist the transition from human to divine ancestral spirit *(shen)*. Even properly situated ancestral spirits were apt to curse their descendants if dissatisfied with their behavior or with the sacrifices required for them to maintain their rank in the spirit world. The care of the living required care of the dead.

Shang responses to illness began with divination to determine, for example, the cause (perhaps ancestral displeasure), the prognosis, and the appropriate treatment (usually exorcism). To communicate with spirits, diviners working for the royal family used the bones of wild and domesticated animals, as well as tortoise shells imported from the southeast. They posed questions as positive and negative alternatives—Is the toothache caused by X? Is the toothache not caused by X?—and gained their answers by applying hot pokers to the bone in specific places, thus producing cracks. The cracks, like omens, were then "read." Diviners often inscribed the questions and the identities of the questioners on the bone itself to demonstrate to the spirits that efforts had been made and sacrifices performed. The texts and implements were then buried in either caches or tombs, because once their earthly function was finished, they were contaminated and could possess demonic forces themselves, causing even more sickness. (See Figure 1.1.) Only recently, in the early twentieth century, did scholars recognize that the caches of inscribed "dragon bones" that had been dug up and pulverized for medicine for centuries were in fact ancient Shang archives and the earliest examples of writing in Asia.

ORACLE BONES OF THE LATE SHANG DYNASTY (CA. THIRTEENTH–ELEVENTH CENTURIES B.C.E.)

Ken Takashima

The following are transcriptions of the oracle bone inscriptions below into modern Chinese script, with translations into English. Note the pattern in examples 1–3 of testing positive and negative versions of the question. Parentheses indicate words that are implied, unnecessary in the original language but required in English. Square brackets indicate information supplied for context or explanation.

(1A) 告于祖乙 (We) will make a ritual announcement [about the illness of someone not mentioned on this fragment] (to the spirit of) Ancestor Yi.

(1B) 貞小疾勿告于祖乙 Tested [the following proposition to the numen of the turtle]: As for this minor illness, (we) should not make a ritual announcement [about it] (to the spirit of) Ancestor Yi.

(2A) 婦好其延有疾 Fu Hao [a famous consort of King Wuding] might continue to suffer from illness.

(2B) 貞婦好不延有疾 Fu Hao will not continue to suffer from illness.

(3A) [same as 2A]

(3B) [same as 2B with the date and diviner's name, Zheng 爭, added]

(4) 甲戌卜亘貞禦婦好于父乙曹ᴚ Divining on the *jiaxu* day, [diviner] Xuan tested: (We) will conduct the exorcism ritual over Fu Hao [who is suffering from illness] in the presence of the (spirit of the dead) Father Yi with the use of the human captive that we [had previously] pledged [to offer].

(5) 丁卯貞婦凡 (?) 子大疾死 *Dingmao* day tested: Fu Fan's son, being gravely ill, will die.

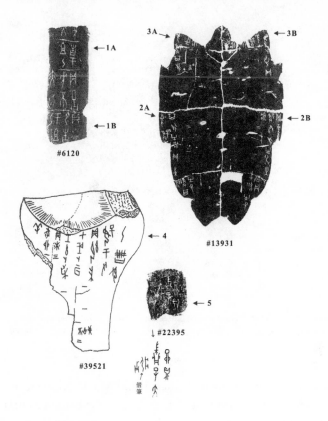

Figure 1.1. Oracle bones of the late Shang Dynasty. The numbers underneath the rubbings and hand drawing (scale reduced from the original) correspond to those in the source: Hu Houxuan, *Jiaguwen heji* (Beijing: Zhonghua shuju, 1978–82), #6120 (vol. 3, p. 898), #13931 (vol. 5, p. 1974), #22395 (vol. 7, p. 2912), #39521 (vol. 13, p. 4908). Courtesy of Zhonghua shuju.

Other evidence comes from bronze vessels used in sacrifices. Both the Shang and Zhou decorated them with a menagerie of dragons, tigers, birds, and other wild animals, which some scholars feel were, like animal bones, used as shamanistic tools for communication, flight, and healing rituals. The metamorphic mask motif, later called the *taotie*, is linked to the part-human, part-animal or -bird imagery associated with healers and spiritual transformation (Chang K. 1983; Childs-Johnson 1987, 1995, 1998; Whitfield 1993). (See Figure 1.2.) The notion of the vessel as a spirit container or transformed body is particularly salient in cases where the entire bronze vessel took on the shape of an animal or an animal symbolically consuming a human tattooed all over with dragon and bird motifs, or when human faces were embedded into the sides of the vessels. This idea is supported by the soul-guiding banner buried in the early Han period

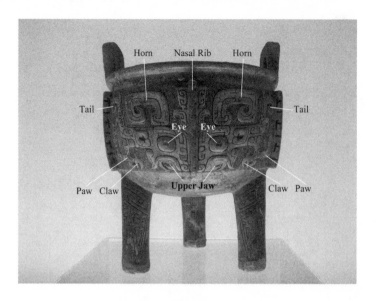

Figure 1.2. Taotie Mask, bronze Ding vessel, late Shang Dynasty, Shanghai Museum, with parts diagrammed. Image licensed under the Creative Commons Attribution-Share Alike 3.0 Unported license.

Mawangdui tomb, which depicts animals forming a vessel shape around pictures of the spirit of the deceased in various stages of evolution from the corpse to a dragon-tailed spirit flying in space (Major 1999, 125–127; Cook 2006a, 119–124; see Chapter 2).

Shang officials in charge of using oracle bones to communicate with the spirit world included diviners *(buren),* invocators *(zhu),* and shamans *(wu).* At the highest social levels, this ritual team diagnosed and treated illness. Perhaps because of their association with the Shang royal dead and Shang earth rituals, after the Zhou people took over as the political hegemons of the Yellow River Valley cultures, shamans became specialists of lower social status.

The Zhou prized bronze vessels and bells over bone and used the former as their sacrificial medium for communication with the ancestors in musical ceremonies. Zhou medical diagnosticians included diviners, minister technicians *(yin,* officers in charge of everything from court business to public works), and scribes or archivists *(shi),* who also divined and read the stars (Harper 1999; Lewis 1999). The esteem felt for these specialists is reflected in a tale from 491 B.C.E. of a southern king, King Zhao of the Chu kingdom. When he became ill, he sent for a Grand Scribe *(taishi)* of Zhou to divine the source of the curse even though Zhou by then had lost all claim to divine authority and power. Naturally, the officer determined that the curse came from the spirit of the Yellow River (to the north of Chu territory where Chu had military aspirations).

Treatment of disease fell to shamans (*xian,* a subcategory of *wu*) and physicians *(yi).* The distinctions between the two groups were not always clear. Shamans *(xian)* were more likely to be linked with oath or prayer incantations (Lin 2008; Poo 2008, 288; Kalinowski 2008, 359). Physicians used needles of stone and bone and perhaps fine jade knives for drawing blood, lancing boils, and excising putrid wounds. Other treatment methods included cauterization, fumigation, and the "sucking" *(shun)* of infected wounds or boils (Han and Wang 1991, 5:83, 196, 206). Both types of healers mixed herbs in mortars, divined with stalks, lived in shrines, and expelled demons (Zhang 2005, 124–127; Lin 2008; Li 2008). Physicians and shamans could not diagnose or cure themselves but required others to exorcise demons on their behalf. Either one might manipulate *qi.* They practiced and instructed others in physical movements and contemplative and macrobiotic disciplines, collectively called "nurturing the divine soul" *(xiushen* or *yangshen),* for conserving and circulating *qi* in order to transcend death (see Harper 1999, 874–883; Roth 1999; Lo 2001b; Puett 2002; Graziani 2008; Lin 2008, 405). Only a shaman, on the other hand, could approach the Earth Altar to beseech gods for protection, a potentially dangerous interaction that physicians did not risk. This may have been due to the shamans' historical connections to earth deities, sacred places, and burials.

While healers during the Shang and Western Zhou periods (1046–771 B.C.E.) lived near the rulers, in later times physicians especially tended to be peripatetic, traveling from patron to patron—to whoever could afford to support them with grain, clothing, or, in at least one case, horses. They worked with state bureaucrats and in teams including "masters" (*shi,* lineage elders with military or ritual expertise), ministers, diviners, invocators, and shamans. Physicians, like scribes, tended to be more educated, and became increasingly specialized. By the Qin period, there were dieticians who prescribed foods and drink according to the season; those who dealt with acute illnesses such as headaches in spring, itchy skin diseases in summer, fever and chills in the fall, and coughing (understood as a condition in which one forces *qi* against its natural downward flow) in winter; and those who dealt with external wounds, such as swellings, suppurating ulcers *(yang),* wounds caused by metal, and breaks. Those who dealt with external wounds had to be skilled in the ancient craft of invoking spirits and prescribing herbs as well as surgical treatments such as lancing boils and excising dead flesh.

By the late Warring States period, healers' negotiations with spirits evolved into a form of litigation, as we see in the case of a third-century B.C.E. Qin prince who became ill in midwinter. According to buried jade tablets recently recovered on Mount Hua (southern Shaanxi Province), a sacred mountain, Prince Qin Yin's prolonged sickness caused him intense physical discomfort in his trunk and upper thigh area, disturbing his sleep. He attributed the illness to offended spirits caused by his ignorance of Zhou statutes and the proper (i.e., Zhou) methods for serving Heaven and Earth, the Four Poles (directions), the Three Radiances (asterisms), mountains and rivers, sky and earth spirits, the Five Annual Sacrificial Sites (Chamber, Stove, Gateway, Door, and Walkway), and the ancestors. Besides animal, jade, and silk sacrifices to the spirits, he also called in an easterner named Shi Jing who was chief of punishments and law to petition the spirits regarding his innocence and to accept the contingency of his upset inner emotional state as an excuse for any inadvertent offense. Shi Jing determined that the curse came from Mount Hua, so he prepared a number of propositions to report to the mountain spirit. These were written in red ink on sets of jades, wrapped in silk, and buried with sacrificial animals on the Yin (north) and Yang (south) sides of the mountain, requesting full recovery of the patient in exchange for the gifts. To guarantee that Mount Hua did not ignore the request, he noted on the jades that the situation was also going to be reported to the higher sky deities of Great Unity *(taiyi)* and Grand General *(da jiangjun)* (a star in Andromeda) (Hou 2005).

The Self and the Corporate Body

Shang and Zhou people did not consider individual human lives separately from their families, polities, or natural and supernatural environments. According to the Shang oracle bones, a foreign attack, damage to fields, famine, and natural disasters were all forms of sickness to be taken as signs and symptoms of breakdown in the king's relationship to the Four Regions, the Sky, the Earth, the (Yellow) River, ancestors, and founder deities. Just as healers treated the aches and pains of the king's body, so too did they treat an ill corporate body (Hsu 2001, 63–67; Lewis 2006a, 13–76). Toward the end of the Western Zhou period, bronze inscriptions, which like special oracle bones displayed in shrines tended up to then to record auspicious events, began to add pleas for the ancestors to intervene with Heaven, who was bringing death to the state, then plagued with enemy incursions, starvation, and possibly epidemics.

From tales about the Spring and Autumn period preserved in *Zuo's Commentary (Zuozhuan),* we know that a political entity required a "spirit throne" *(shenwei)* consisting of an Earth and Grain Spirit Altar *(sheji)* and an Ancestral Shrine *(zongmiao)* in order to survive. The Earth and Grain Altar provided access to nature spirits and was itself treated sometimes as a misbehaving supernatural agent; it was fed blood sacrifices and alcoholic beverages, insulted, consoled, protected, and, when destroyed, called a "corpse" *(shi).*

The notion that one's body or self was a substance shared with and subject to the welfare of the clan—past, present, and future—and to the welfare of the king and the state is evident in Shang oracle bone and Western Zhou period bronze inscriptions. Inscriptions on bronze vessels, like those on oracle bones, were testimonials or reports to the ancestors. Oracle bone inscriptions paid special attention to all of the king's body parts—trunk, lower and upper sections of the leg, eyes, head, arms, elbow, nose, ear, mouth, tongue, belly, bones, and pelvis—and to the health of women who provided the king with heirs. Divination records showed a particular concern with the birthing experiences and suffering in the bones of one such Shang queen, Fu Hao.

The focus on a woman's bones and reproductive health reflected an obsession with mortuary cults as the vehicle for social reproduction and continuity. It was not coincidental that this society used animal bones to communicate with ancestors. Demonic human spirits could be traced to bones that had been incorrectly buried, remained unburied (particularly as a result of drowning or violence), or never received sacrifices (perhaps due to neglect or the lack of descendants). Proper burial of kin remained an important social value and was a key to health.

Since all sorts of demons and ghosts inhabited the landscape, healers were required to know local history as well as the patient's own. In some tales preserved in *Zuo's Commentary* it was not so much a single spiritual agent that might cause illness and death, but the blame directed at an individual by a clan group and their associated spirits. For example, a lord of the state of Chu sickened and died from "blame" because, despite emerging as the winner in a battle, he had lost an extraordinary number of young men from a particular village (Kong 1965, 6:501).

Personal Potency: Practices for Nourishment and Longevity

An individual's life potency *(de)* was also taken to be contingent on the position of his or her progenitors in a hierarchy based on the strength of their connections to the highest source of potency, the High Lord Di *(shangdi)* or Heaven (or Sky, *tian*). The royal line was the most potent, followed by closely related noble lineages and then more distantly related ones. By the sixth century B.C.E. the cosmic scheme that incorporated elite lineages changed dramatically as the old states failed and new groups, particularly from the south, increased their contacts with the peoples of the middle Yellow River Valley. Healers subscribed to an amalgam of old and new etiologies linked to various regional spirit pantheons. Some of these eventually superseded the old Shang and Zhou gods as the primary generators of supernatural influence. In the region of Chu, for example, by the fourth century B.C.E. the supreme celestial power was Grand Unity, a sky deity associated with the North Pole who could also appear in a dark form as Occluded Grand Unity *(shitai)*. This high god did not have a clear relationship to an ancestral hierarchy, as did Heaven or the High Lord *(shangdi)* of old, and its double nature likely reflected the rising popularity of the concepts of Yin and Yang.

Zhou bronze inscriptions, despite their focus on corporate rather than individual health, do record personal rituals for nurturing potency. For the Zhou, potency was earned through ritual and military performances that enhanced the power of the state. Potency derived from Heaven and was accumulated over generations within a lineage connected to a Zhou king. Transition from the role of youth into that of "master" *(shi)* involved a musical ceremony in which the youth ritually "opened up his heart" and "grasped potency" from his ancestral predecessor. These physical embodiments of ancestral potency and the act of blending the self into the corporate body were achieved through the lifetime practice of "following the (ancestral) pattern," a process called "modeling" *(xing)*, the same word used for "molding" a vessel—confirming the notion that the bronze sacrificial vessel likewise represented the embodiment of the ancestor-descendant relationship.

By the Warring States period, the cultivation of potency or *de* took on the sense of nurturing inner moral qualities as well as outer physical "virtue." This traditional cultivation practice, linked to Zhou ritual and the old disintegrated clan hierarchies of founder ancestors, conflicted but eventually melded with new *qi* practices of "nourishing life" *(yangsheng)* in the physical form *(xing)*, the inner nature *(xing)*, the mind *(xin)*, parts of the body, the divine spirit *(shen)*, and awareness *(zhi)*. This practice of nourishing also extended to one's children, one's parents, the elderly, the people *(min)*, animals, all beings *(wanwu)*, and even the abstract concept of potency or virtue itself. Nourishing or self-cultivation was a form of healing. Healers cured *(zhi;* not inconsequently, the word *zhi* also referred to governing a state) the ill through "nourishing" them with herbs *(yao)*; alcoholic brews made of millet, wheat, rice, or other grains combined with fruit and spices *(jiu)*; and meat *(rou)*. Nourishing led to "long life" *(changshou)* and, for those capable of nourishing themselves on *qi*, possibly eternal life *(yongming)*. All bronze inscriptions from the ninth century B.C.E. up through the Warring States period recorded prayers for personal "extended longevity" *(meishou)* as well as lineage fertility. By the end of the Warring States period, the common goal was a permanent state of deathlessness of self and family.

Late Warring States ascetics such as Zhuangzi (ca. 370–286 B.C.E.) advocated nourishing oneself on *qi*. They understood illness and death to be stages of physical metamorphosis, a natural dissolution of self into the greater Dao of *qi;* if controlled through special practices, this would allow them to obtain states of disembodied soul flight and ultimately "release from their corpses" *(shijie)* (Harper 1999, 881–883; Cook 2006a, 22). The sense of a postdeath existence once a powerful person has shed his or her "corpse" was not new and can be extrapolated from mortuary remains since the early Neolithic. Warring States period texts explain that the living had to ritually cut themselves off from the corpse while nurturing the spirit with sacrifices. Bodies of powerful people were bound tightly, wrapped in layers of cloth, sealed in multiple wooden coffins, and buried deep in the earth. Around the sealed inner coffins were chambers for the movement of the spirits, who could at first be quite dangerous to the living (Cook 2006a; Lai 2005).

The movement of *qi* as evident in seasonal change, star movement, or the wind could also be injurious and cause the rise of negative or demonic forces (Li 2008, 1005, 1112–1113). Healing in the late Warring States period required knowledge of the spirits and of the forces and phases of *qi* as they corresponded to time, taste, color, natural material (Earth, Wood, Fire, Metal, and Water) and music (Sivin 1987, 46–80; Allan 1997, 66–70; Harper 1999, 860–866). In the body, fluid circuits of *qi* and blood *(xue)* moved downward and around through the body in a network of channels or vessels *(mo)*. Health required that these circuits be aligned with cosmic movements and not be "weak," move in the wrong direction, or be blocked or stagnant inside any part of the body (Sivin 1987, 117–171; Harper 1998, 69, 77–90; 1999, 876–879; 2001, 99–100, 115–118; Lo 2001b, 27–31; Hsu 2001, 83–85; Li 2008, 1103–1104). Since "rising *qi*" *(shang qi)* was recorded in the fourth century B.C.E. as a symptom of illness, scholars believe that a rudimentary version of this system existed earlier in the Warring States period (Harper 1998, 78; 1999, 877–878; Cook 2006a, 29–32, 71–72, 111–114). The discovery of the third-century B.C.E. Day Books *(rishu)*, which determine the days of "Filling" *(ying)* and "Expelling" *(chu)*, foreshadow the Han preoccupation with filling or emptying Yin and Yang vessels (see Harper 1998, 80–81).

The Inner and Outer Body during the Warring States Period

Texts found in tombs from the fourth century B.C.E. focus on the inner and outer aspects of the body, divided by the body's skin. The inner and outer aspects of the torso were of particular concern. The inner aspect, the "heart and abdomen," was linked to food intake and elimination. Thought *(si)* was located there and needed to "move" *(dong)*, a term later used for the pulsation of blood and *qi* through the body's channels or vessels (Harper 1998, 80 n. 1; Hsu 2001, 75–76). The outer aspect of the torso, along with the patient's "feet and bones," might be discussed in terms of pain (Cook 2006a, 71).

Warring States texts also talk about the interiority of "human nature" *(xing)*, which could be "moved" by physical practices or dance performances accompanying ritual music—activities that can be traced back to the Shang period (McCurley 2005). These movements created emotion, which was an outer expression of the cultivation of one's inner nature and, as such, had to be carefully controlled or illness could result (Li 2008, 1106). While physical practices could fill the body with a divine illumination *(shenming)*, representing the peak of one's vitality and the generation even of supernatural powers, inadequate or poor cultivation methods such as listening to popular music or indulging in food, drink, sex, or cruel behavior would lead to exhaustion and, without treatment, death (Cook 2006a, 19–25).

Approaches to Diagnosis and Treatment

During the Shang period, diviners first had to decide whether the situation was one of sickness, harm, or perhaps *gu* poison (a disease whose early meaning is unclear; for later understandings, see "The Hexagram *Gu*"). If it was sickness, then the question was whether it was serious enough to report to the ancestors. Of particular concern was whether the sickness would last a long time, whether it was due to a curse or to blame, which ancestral spirit was the cause, and whether there might be a heavy rain while the patient was sick (Shang people saw rain as a supernatural agent). Oracle bone divination records noted not only the severity and length of the illness but also whether it had been "corrected" *(zheng)*, been "overcome" *(ke)*, been "cured" *(liao)*, or received spiritual "favor" *(chong)* (Zhang 2005, 95–97).

Symptoms of illness could manifest internally or externally. For example, nightmares, particularly about certain ancestors, required diagnosis and treatment. Diviners and healers had to determine if the dreamer had inadvertently called the spirit and thus required exorcism of the malignant influence. In other cases, dreams might invoke multiple ghosts or omens involving animals—flocks of birds, a stone deer, a white water buffalo, a large tiger—or even sickness itself as a demonic presence. Other recognized symptoms possibly connected to the inner state of the body included headache, dizziness, fever or internal heat, gastric swelling, weakness, abdominal pain, chest pain, abdominal lumps, water retention, yellowness, inflammation of the joints, poisoning, paralysis, breath problems such as hiccups or coughing, elimination problems, goiters, and dwarfism (Zhang 2005, 99–103). Symptoms of demonic influence on the outer body included sores, genital or breast problems, hemorrhoids, burns, wounds, snakebites, and skin diseases (Zhang 2005, 103–104).

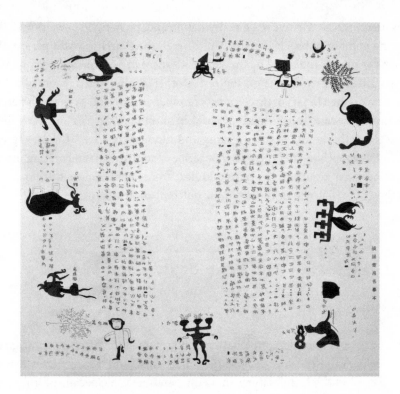

Figure 1.3. Twelve month gods. Corresponding texts describe the creation of the cosmos and time. Fifth to fourth century B.C.E. Manuscript from the state of Chu (Zidankou, Changsha, Hunan). Courtesy of the Arthur M. Sackler Foundation, New York.

Critical to proper diagnosis and to calculating which ancestor might be the source of trouble was not only skill in using oracle bones but also knowledge of the calendar. During the Shang period, every royal ancestor was linked to one of the ten suns or days *(ri)*. The system of ten suns was combined with twelve other signs to form a sixty-day ritual calendar for the performances of regular sacrifices and exorcism (Keightley 1978, 2000; Allan 1991). (See Figure 2.7.) By the third century B.C.E., healers also consulted Day Books to determine the sources of curses and the prognoses of illnesses (Harper 1999; Yang 2000; Cook 2006a, 86–91). These manuals reveal a clear correlation of the influences of the day with directions, colors, and other aspects of the *qi* phases. Every facet of birth, life, and death depended on the influences correlated with particular days. Even the body was mapped as to which stem or sun sign day could affect particular body parts depending on the season and gender (*Shuihudi Qin mu zhujian* 2001, 206).

There is evidence that as early as the Shang period, stalk divination, presumably the casting of dried stalks into patterns that were somehow "read," was used as an alternative to bone divination and, perhaps, in concert with the casting and use of bronze vessels. Up through the Warring States period, the omens or images indicated by the stalk patterns were recorded in sets of numbers written in a stack one on top of the other. By the fourth century B.C.E., diviners divined in sets of three and six number groups, and by the Han period the numbers were transformed into broken and unbroken Yin and Yang lines in sets familiarly known as trigrams and hexagrams. (See "The Hexagram *Gu*.") Eastern Zhou documents tell of scribes and diviners interpreting movement between groups of trigrams and hexagrams upon repeated throws as a method of prediction, including of the outcome of treatments.

The Dreams of the Lord of Jin

Constance A. Cook

The illnesses of the ruler of the Eastern Zhou state of Jin as recounted in *Zuo's Commentary* illustrate the complexities of diagnosis and treatment, along with the roles of multiple divinatory, shamanic, and medical specialists. The story tells how, in 579 B.C.E.,

the Lord of Jin dreamed about a Great Danger [or Pestilence] *(li)* demon with hair down to the ground, beating its breast and leaping about [movements associated with mourning a death], saying: "You murdered my grandson for no reason, so I have requested [justice] from [the High Lord] Di!" It then broke down the main gate [of the Lord of Jin's compound] as well as the door to his private quarters and entered within. The Patriarch [Lord of Jin] was terrified and tried to enter a sanctified chamber, but the door to that was also broken. Then he woke up and summoned a shaman from the Mulberry Fields [a sacred site where divination took place] to explain the dream. The Patriarch said: "What's it about?" and the shaman answered: "You will not eat the new [wheat]!" The Patriarch then suffered illness and sought out a physician from Qin. The Elder of Qin sent him Physician Huan ["Slowness," possibly a pun, as the word *ji* for "sickness" can also mean "quickly" or "acute"].

Yet before [Huan] arrived, the Patriarch dreamed that his sickness took on the forms of two boys who said [to each other]: "That guy is a good healer and we're afraid of his harming us. Where can we escape to?" One of them said: "Reside on top of the *huang* [located between the heart and the diaphragm] and underneath the *gao* [fat above the heart], how about that?" The healer arrived and said: "Nothing can be done about the sickness. It resides on top of the *huang* and beneath the *gao,* so 'beating' *(gong)* would be impossible, 'penetration' *(da)* could not reach, and herbs *(yao)* cannot get to it here. Nothing can be done." The Patriarch said: "You are a good healer," and after rewarding him well according to the proper rites, sent him home.

In the sixth month, on a *bingwu* day [day forty-three of the sexagenary calendar], the Lord of Jin desired some wheat and had one of the agricultural chiefs present some so that the people in charge of food offerings could make it up [into a dish]. He summoned the shaman of the Mulberry Fields, displayed [the offering of new wheat], and killed [the shaman]. But when he tried to eat it, he felt a [sudden] bloating, and went off to the privy, where he fell in and died. A young servant earlier that morning had dreamed of carrying the Patriarch to Heaven on his back and by noon that day was carrying the Lord of Jin out of his privy, so [this boy] followed [the Patriarch's body into the grave] and was buried alive. (Kong 1965, 6:450; Legge and Ming 1972, 5:374; Kalinowski 2008, 361–362)

According to earlier records in *Zuo's Commentary,* the Jin lord had suffered a chronic illness that resulted in vivid dreams and erratic behavior. Many efforts to diagnose the source of his trouble, including interpreting his dreams, resulted in the conclusion that he suffered from curses. However, in one case after he had dreamed of the Li demon, a neighboring official, Zichan of Zheng, a man who could foretell his own death, reinterpreted the visions of demons in terms of newer ideologies, first mythical historical tales and then Yin and Yang. Zichan visited the Jin lord after he had been bedridden for three months with no sign of improvement. The lord had dreamed of the Danger or Pestilence demon *(ligui),* who appeared as a yellow bear entering through the door of his apartments. Generally, the Danger demon can be understood as the embodied idea of a "dangerous condition," one that in the *Classic of Changes* required divination in order to determine whether it was symptomatic of blame. However, Zichan dismissed the identification of the yellow bear as the fearsome demon and explained that it was the spirit of the famous mythical figure Gun, who had turned into a yellow bear when put to death. Gun was the father of Xia Dynasty founder Yu, who by Zichan's time was associated with exorcism rites and protective stepping rituals *(yubu,* performance involving three repeated dance steps to protect against resident demons and resanctify a space, such as a threshold, when crossed) (Harper 1999, 872–873; Lewis 2006b; Poo 2008, 301–309; Li 2008, 1109). Since the Jin occupied the old Xia lands,

Zichan explained, curing the king should require reviving a Xia sacrifice to propitiate this alienated spirit (Kong 1965, 6:762).

When sacrifices failed, another diviner determined that the lord's illness was due to a curse by two obscurely named spirits. So Zichan refined his own prescription for treatment. He explained that the two spirits belonged to two boys from two different sets of sons (by different mothers) of the mythical emperor Di Ku who were punished for fighting with each other. The High Lord, Di, exiled one to Orion's Belt in an area of the sky linked to the fate of Jin (see Pankenier 1999), but since the other boy, a son of Darkness, was hardworking, Di put him in charge of the Fen River. Since the Jin had taken over these ancient lands, these spirits should be considered protective, but they had to be provided sustenance in the form of sacrifices. As deities associated with space, they could not affect the lord's personal body, so Zichan proposed a different diagnosis.

Zichan claimed that the lord's movements around the palace and times chosen for eating meat and drinking were out of sync with the four periods of the day. He had also broken an old taboo by having sex with women of the same clan name as himself. The court summoned a Qin healer named He (meaning "Harmony"), who diagnosed a case analogous to toxic *gu* poisoning, which produced delusions and chaotic behavior, aggravated by listening to music with unconventional rhythms causing extreme emotions (Graziani 2008, 467–479). (See "The Hexagram *Gu*.") Since the passage then proceeds to explain correlative Five Phase theory, there is some suspicion that the tale incorporated later (post-third-century B.C.E.) commentary, which purposely refuted the traditional diagnosis of a spirit curse or demonic influence (Kong 1965, 6:705–709; Legge and Ming 1972, 5:580). Nevertheless, some of the ideas were quite ancient, such as the concept that music affected the heart and that licentious behavior diminished vitality.

THE HEXAGRAM *GU*

Xing Wen

Among the Lord of Jin's various diagnoses was that of the doctor He from Qin, which incorporated hexagram analysis (Kong 1965; Li 2001). There were sixty-four hexagrams, each assembled from two of the eight trigrams, and consisting variously of broken (Yin) and unbroken (Yang) lines. Each trigram and hexagram had a name and associated images, such as the image Heaven for the trigram named *Qian* (see Figure 1.4). These were elaborated into extensive im-age systems for interpreting the dynamic flux of phenomena. How a given situ-ation came to be and could be expected to evolve could be analyzed in relation to its resemblance to one or more of these images. Commonly, the lines of the relevant hexagram might be produced through a procedure involving the cast-ing of milfoil stalks.

The Lord of Jin's diagnosis was not a hard one for He: it was just a bedroom illness similar to *gu*, a kind of mental bewilderment accompanied by abdomi-nal distension. Dr. He explained that the *gu*-like disease of the Lord of Jin was caused by neither demons nor diet, as had previously been diagnosed, but by overindulgence in sexual relations with women. He explained his diagnosis further with the *Gu* hexagram, which consists of the trigrams *Xun* (Wind) at the bottom and *Gen* (Mountain) at the top. He interpreted the mountain at the top blocking as the wind at the bottom. The bottom trigram, *Xun*, also had the image of Elder Daughter, while the top trigram, *Gen*, had the image of Younger Brother. Therefore, the image of hexagram *Gu* is an elder woman seducing a younger man above her. Excessive sexual activities would generate internal Heat and mental bewilderment.

Dr. He's image analysis also extended to the character *gu*, which appeared in oracle bone inscriptions as early as the fourteenth century B.C.E., and de-picted insects or worms inside a vessel. By extension, it could refer to harmful internal heat generated inside a human body as a result of insects or worms. In later centuries, the term *gu* continued to refer more generally to sexual delu-sion, feminine magic, and illnesses involving abdominal pain, but it was in-creasingly associated with demonic magic produced from crawling creatures such as snakes and centipedes (see Feng and Shryock 1935).

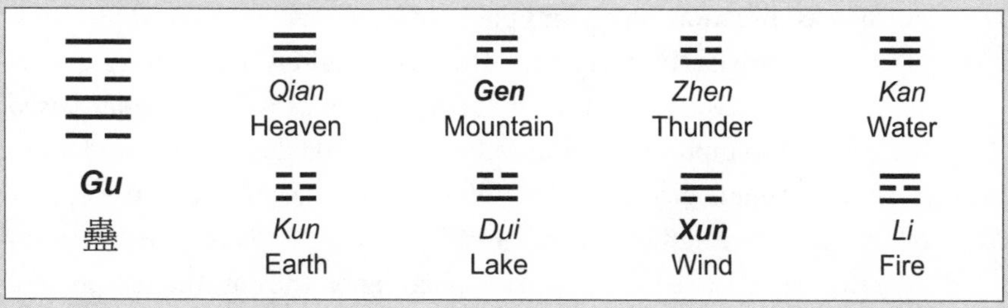

Figure 1.4. The hexagram *Gu*.

Like physicians, diviners became increasingly specialized and their tools more sophisticated. Stalk diviners used a variety of different Change *(yi)* manuals, including the *Zhou Changes (Zhouyi),* also known as the *Classic of Changes (Yijing).* Although excavated versions all include sixty-four named hexagrams (combined from eight possible trigrams) of roughly the same names, the hexagrams had vastly different lines of song or omen texts connected to them, suggesting different traditions. By the Qin period, diviners who worked with numbers also used dice and game boards such as Heaven Plates *(tianpan)* or Model Plates *(shipan)* to determine astrological influences. A ladle-like tool representing the Big Dipper could be spun to point out particular stars within twenty-eight astral "lodges" or spirit-imbued constellations (Harper 1999, 833–843; Yang 2000; Cook 2006a, 33–34, 108). Tortoise bone divination continued to be a specialty, one that, like other methods, may have been handed down in families. A powerful member of the governing elite might have a team of diagnostic diviners, numbering as many as twelve, who worked with ten different types of stalk throwing and bone cracking, alternating the type of divination to refine diagnoses. Diviners could also read signs in body markings, cloud patterns, and spit. Different sets of methods were employed at different seasons, with the summer annual exorcism being the time when the most intense efforts to cure chronic illness occurred, although acute episodes throughout the year also necessitated divination, sacrifice, and exorcism (Cook 2006a, 101–109).

During the Zhou period, auspicious days became less connected to the categories of ancestral spirits than to particular days of the ritual calendar. It is clear, however, that days, and the signs marking them, retained supernatural power despite shifts in the identities of the influences associated with the signs. By the end of the Warring States period, diagnosis and treatment of sickness required complex calculations of day signs and their correlations to other influences, such as direction, color, and phase of *qi,* as well as to astral phenomena and ancestral spirits (Harper 2001). These correlations in turn were understood as affected by rising and falling currents of *qi* as well as gender-based days. If a person's symptoms manifested on a "female day," he or she had to wait for another female day to recover. While patients from the third century B.C.E. on may still have suffered from curses, they were also just as likely influenced by astrological or telluric powers depending on the day, the season, and the position of Year, the planet Jupiter *(sui).*

Sacrifice and Exorcism

As early as the second millennium B.C.E., methods of curing sickness included exorcism of harmful spirits and blood sacrifices offered in payment for the help of the summoned spirit. Both procedures were inexorably linked to the ritual calendar. Specialists chose the ancestors from whom aid would be sought based on the ancestors' sun sign, gender, and rank. Diviners also had to factor in the gender and category of the sacrificial animal (or, occasionally, human captive), the method of its sacrifice and service, and accompanying ceremonies. Healers tried to cure their patrons' chronic illnesses by matching auspicious days of the ritual calendar to particular sacrifices *(sai)* of meat or valuables to specific spirits.

Shang exorcisms included the summoning of ancestral spirits such as the dynastic founder King Tang, male ancestors (and occasionally female ancestors) with particular sun signs, or the parents or various elder brothers and cousins of the afflicted. Animals included various numbers of buffalo, goats, sheep, pigs, dogs, and an unknown lizard-like creature. Different terms specified young, pen-raised, and male or female animals; whether the animals were burned, cut, hacked, or torn apart; and whether they were cooked in cauldrons and served in feasts or with special millet brews. During the feast, the ancestral spirit was summoned in spirit visitation rituals and perhaps given a written or oral pledge (Yao and Ding 1989, 1:143–156).

Although the oracle bone records are too fragmentary to know the details of the rites performed to cure particular ailments or parts of the body, we do know that the exorcism was understood as a type of armed pursuit resulting in either the capture or driving out of the invading force from the sanctified boundaries of a particular physical territory, whether the human body or the political body. The Shang and the Zhou people used the word *yu* to refer not just to "exorcising" harmful influences but also to "chasing" wild animals during a hunt, "driving" war chariots, and "ridding" newly conquered lands of other peoples and spirits. Healing the king's body also healed the corporate political body and vice versa. After Shang queen Fu Hao gave birth, an exorcism was performed. For a healthy family and state, her body and the space in which the pollution of the birthing process occurred had to be resanctified and cleansed of demonic influences.

These connections between exorcising disease or pollution and routing enemies persisted up through the Zhou period. Divination and exorcism remained the primary diagnostic and treatment methods for illness on the micro- and macrocosmic levels of person and state. Birthing and the process of reproduction gave women, already empowered as military, ritual, and political leaders during the Shang period, influence that was not always viewed as positive. Besides concern over the death of the royal woman during childbirth and whether the birth was felicitous (which, in this highly patriarchal society, perhaps meant the birth of a male and heir), there was particular anxiety over malevolent female ancestors.

Implements for warding off demons included staffs made of special woods (peach, mulberry, jujube) or specific objects (shoes, dog feces, mats, hemp cloth) that were applied to sores, buried near the residence, or used to symbolically lash the patient's body. In some cases, the demons could be stabbed, boiled, and eaten—although we have no record of what physical substance if any was in fact consumed. Malevolent spirits could move into and inhabit people and animals, causing them to behave strangely, with sudden bouts of sadness, anger, or hunger or, in the case of animals, talking. Demons could be either visible or invisible. They could cry out, beat drums, call names, and try to command a person to feed them or to let them cross a threshold. They might appear as humans, animals, or insects, or as an invisible force such as the wind. Wind was the probable cause of the "cold" *(han)* ailment mentioned by the late fourth-century to early third-century B.C.E. philosopher Mencius, which required secluding the patient (Kong 1965, 8:72–73). Some visible demons, particularly in the form of children, might walk into one's house uninvited. Adult demons liked to bother people while they slept, having sex with them or just causing bad dreams. Demons were behind rashes on a person's skin, as well as diseases that spread within a family or community (*Shuihudi Qin mu zhujian* 2001, 179–255; Harper 1995; Li 2008, 1112–1113).

Medicines and Potions

Not much is known about pre-Han herbal preparations other than that they were one of several methods of treatment used by physicians and some shamans. Judging from early Han medical manuscripts dating to 168 B.C.E. discovered at Mawangdui (see Chapter 2), we can infer that herbs were used in combination with a variety of other types of ingredients. The 394 ingredients used in the second century B.C.E. derived from a huge range of source types that included 31 minerals, 180 herbs (62 trees, 87 grasses, 19 grains, 12 vegetables), 116 animals (10 human-derived products, 49 mammals, 16 birds, 6 fish, 35 insects), 8 types of clothing, 33 spices or prepared foods, 8 items of daily use, and 30 unidentified items of all categories (Ma 1992, 123–126). Occasional mention of a particular herb in the pre-Han literature suggests a long history for many of these Han recipes. For example, Mencius mentioned the need to have three-year-old mugwort *(ai)* on hand for an illness that a prince had been suffering for seven years (Kong 1965, 8:132; Mengzi and Legge 1972, 2:301). From third-century B.C.E. Day Books, we know that healing potions of worms, stinging insects, hair, feces, afterbirth, ashes, and other substances were mixed with alcohol and ingested, thrown on the body, or hurled at the envisioned demons (Harper 1985, 1998, 1999, 2001).

One living ingredient of potions involved a class of crawling creatures (chong), particularly poisonous ones such as snakes or scorpions. Snakes had an ancient association with curses and likely were used for potions such as gu poison. In the Shang oracle bones, gu represents a state of illness that can persist even if other symptoms have improved. It was possibly perceived as a type of contamination or infestation that could appear in places such as the teeth or could be related to sex (Yao and Ding 2:1025; Zhang 2005, 115). Snakes and their supernatural cousins dragons are a primary artistic motif that originated in the early Neolithic and has descended in one form or another up through to the present. Paintings of shaman-like figures (often wearing animal masks) that have been preserved on funerary architecture from the Warring States and early Han periods depict them controlling dragons with wands, riding in dragon chariots, and handling or eating snakes. These suggest both that snakes were used to quell demons and that they themselves were demons of illness and death (Major 1999, 129–133). Lacquer-painted carved wooden screens, dragon and bird sculptures featuring long tongues and antlers, and staffs with long-tongued heads for catching and controlling snake-like demons were placed in tombs, were used by shamans, and, in the case of the staff, were provided to the ill and infirm (Cook 2006a, 134–143). As a counterimage, birds in Warring States and early Han iconography represented, on the mundane level, catchers of snakes, and on a more metaphorical level represented transcendence over illness and death. (See Figure 1.5) Figures of healers and people capable of deathlessness had been depicted as half bird since at least the Western Zhou period (Childs-Johnson 1995, 1998, 2002; Zhu 1998; Hsu 2001, 51–55).

The use of alcohol as a chaser for medicines and along with meat for nurturing the sick and elderly also had roots in the Neolithic (Zhang 2005, 48–51). For thousands of years, elite tombs featured finely crafted drinking goblets, storage containers, and serving vessels for alcoholic beverages. Shang and Western Zhou period inscriptions record the use in sacrifices to the ancestral spirits of black- or yellow-tinted millet ale (chang, yuchang), possibly brewed with medicinal additives such as hawthorn berries, bee pollen, or other fragrant herbs. (See Figure 1.6.) Gifts of such special brews presented in finely cast lidded bronze buckets were highly valued during the Western Zhou period (Cook 2005, 18–19).

Besides alcohol, meat was also essential to healing and nurturing the elderly and was considered a luxury. Generally, hunting and husbandry were directed

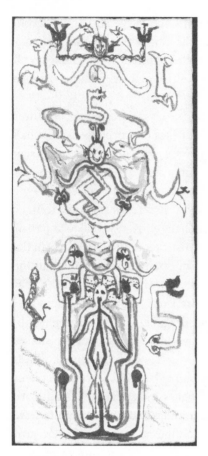

Figure 1.5. Demon quellers, adapted from Zeng Houyi coffin. Drawing courtesy of Constance A. Cook.

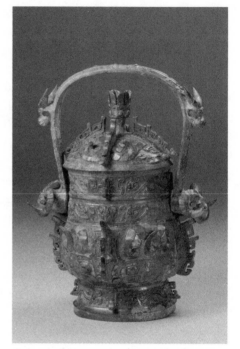

Figure 1.6. Early bronze vessel for ritual ale, the *ge bo you*. Courtesy of the Baoji Bronze Museum, Shaanxi, China.

toward religious feasting. The care taken with different parts of the animal or human sacrifices, the manner of their slaughter, and their preparation all suggest different ritual and healing properties associated with each aspect. For example, in the Shang period, cattle, horses, pigs, sheep, goats, deer, dogs, and fowl were slaughtered in a variety of distinct ways, including drowning and burning. As with the skeletons of powerful humans in Neolithic times, animals in later tombs were often missing certain parts, suggesting their use at another stage of the mortuary ritual. In fourth-century B.C.E. divination and sacrifice healing texts, these same animals (minus the deer and fowl) were divided by age, color, and gender and made into dishes or great soups according to the rank of the spirit being propitiated. Second-century B.C.E. texts specify the uses of animal meat, fur, fat, bones, organs, brains, skin, blood, horns, fetuses, eggs, and human bones, fat, hair, urine, and breast milk. The animals were divided by color and gender and their parts prepared in sauces, dried, burnt, roasted, boiled, blended, or processed in other ways depending on the specific illness and the other ingredients added (Ma 1992; Harper 1998).

While meat was used to satisfy unhappy spirits, some items, such as pepper seeds, were meant to chase them away. Pepper seeds were found not in the "dining rooms" of tombs but among clothing or near items set aside for the worship of the Chamber, Stove, Gateway, Door, and Walkway deities (Chard 1999; Cook 2006a, 20, 60). Valuable items (such as jades, cowries, and precious stones) or clothing items (such as gowns cut certain ways and caps with hanging strings) were also used for protection and to pay spirits for their help in curing the patient. As with animal sacrifices, the shapes and colors were significant.

Treating and Preventing Chronic Illness

For the elite, the treatment of chronic illness required ritual teams who choreographed healing strategies to mitigate a curse. These strategies included divination, magic (using weapons, archery, charms, potions, etc.), exorcism, invocation, sacrifices, drumming, dancing, spitting, and inner and outer purification through meditation and bathing in grain-infused waters. Some specialists were skilled in drumming, singing, and making animal or bird sounds. Others wielded ritual stone and wood weapons (axes, staffs, bows and arrows) or other exorcistic implements in order to release (*jie*) the patient from the curse or to help expel (*chu*) the demonic influence. The procedures mentioned in fourth-century B.C.E. bamboo texts refer to attacking (*gong*), commanding (*ming*), or willing (*shi*) the malevolent influences out of the body—actions that may have involved incantations, drumming, or implements such as staffs or arrows. Arrows, mentioned in the Day Books, could be made out of chicken feathers or thorns and shot from peachwood bows (Cook 2006a, 84). Healers may also have used pointed stones and other shorter pre-acupuncture pointed objects (Harper 1998, 90–94; Lo 2002a, 105–111; Lo 2002b, 208–209).

Other types of therapy, such as massage and exercise, may have been used to prevent as well as treat illness (Zhang 2005, 128–129). By the late Warring States period, the Way or Dao (implying a tradition of sacred knowledge believed to have extended down from antiquity) of Ancestor Peng included seasonal practices for waking and for spending the day performing yoga-like exercises called "pulling" *(yin)*. These exercises often involved using props such as staffs, jade discs, and other items that had earlier associations with healing. Many of the movements were specifically intended to cure certain sets of symptoms or illnesses. By this time, dance performances linked to different ancestral Dao had a long history (McCurley 2005). Musical performances including movement and singing continued into the Warring States period as a method or Dao of achieving transcendence or channeling potency and were included as one of the six essential arts in elite education. By the Qin period, we know that one dance, the Steps of Sage King Yu, was performed as a protective measure when passing across boundaries. Yu, whose first appearance as a founder ancestor occurs perhaps as early as the late ninth century B.C.E., was in Warring States period myth linked to land purification and flood control (Cook 2003; Lewis 2006b). He was also associated with very grand musical events—ones that older youth dared study only after they had learned the tamer dances of the Zhou founders. The early dances and exercises seemed to play multiple roles in healing—exorcism, purification, strength building, transcendence—depending on their associations with particular mythical or founder ancestors, or their Dao (Cook 2003, 2006b, 2009).

By the Qin period, founders were relegated to mythical history and healers manipulated the flow of *qi*. Shamans continued to provide magical protection and the exorcism of demons through spells and propitiation (Harper 1985). The identity of demons varied from representations of generic evil to specific figures from ancient history that were not so much evil as simply misunderstood (see Li 2008, 1111).

Conclusion

The early period was marked by increasing interactions, both collaborative (as in trade and alliance) and conflictual (as in conquest), among peoples from the Yellow River Valley and those of the steppes in the north, the Sichuan basin in the west, and the Yangzi River in the south. From the resulting exchanges (of ideas, material goods, and technologies), instability (produced by war and the breakdown of older traditions) and increasingly complex political institutions and rapidly changing social structures, there emerged great fermentation and such developments as specialized life-cultivating practices, a growing distinction of specialist medical healers from shamanic healers, and naturalistic frameworks for understanding health. These innovations did not displace the world of ancestor-bestowed vitality, diseases caused by curses and demons, divinatory diagnosis, and ritual and exorcistic healing, but they did influence the ways in which those older modalities were understood to operate, and expanded the repertoires available to both patients and healers. With the rise of the Qin and Han empires, cross-cultural interaction and sociopolitical change intensified, but again, rather than erasing the legacies of the Shang and Zhou, tended to develop them in new directions and to integrate them into new syntheses.

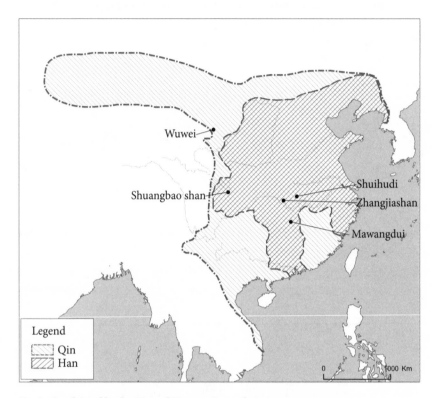

Territories claimed by the Qin and Han empires at their greatest extents

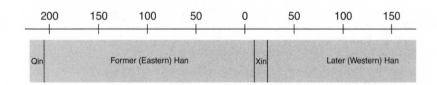

TWO

The Han Period

Vivienne Lo

ALTHOUGH THE QIN (221–206 B.C.E.) inaugurated the imperial era, the longer-lived Han Dynasty (206 B.C.E.–220 C.E.) was a crucial watershed for the development of much that was distinctive to that era. The Han polity and culture built on earlier models but consciously forged new forms in attempts to distance the ruling house from the factionalism of the Warring States and the tyranny of the Qin. Scholars and bureaucrats imagined a prosperous, ordered, unified state with a centralized administration run by career civil servants. This was to operate according to ethics of merit, duty, and respect as embodied in rituals attributed to the Zhou (1045?–256 B.C.E.), retrospectively idealized as a golden era. In fact, by the end of the period, the Han had all the cultural diversity of a population of 58 million spread over an empire that stretched well into Central Asia, commanding the eastern end of the "Silk Roads" (Whitfield 2008) and trade links that reached as far as the Roman Empire.

A sense of transition is found also in the changing attitudes toward medicine and healing. Han practitioners inherited and sustained traditions of health care that fused household remedies, superficial surgery, emergency medicine, demonic and spirit healing, therapeutic exercise, and sexual and breath cultivation. Some passed on their knowledge in rituals that enhanced the prestige of secret knowledge and ancient lore. Throughout the four hundred years of the Han period, parts of these healing traditions became the building blocks for a new medicine framed in terms of *qi* (the essential stuff that powers the universe), Yin and Yang, and the Five Phases *(wuxing)*, the rubrics under which all phenomena came to be categorized.[1] Knowledge about the new medicine was recorded in a growing body of texts written on silk and on bamboo strips.

Through successive compilations and scholarly syntheses, a wide range of practices were gradually worked into a more unified orthodoxy. At the same time, there was a concerted attempt to bring medical knowledge within an all-encompassing belief system that saw divine order in everything—the stars, the spirits, the seasons, the role of the emperor and his government, the human body. The respect for past traditions—enshrined in rituals honoring the ancestors and the legendary culture heroes of antiquity—and a desire for continuity gave the impression of an immutable backdrop to an intellectual consensus about the essential unity of the world. Yet, challenging histories that would hold that the Han intellectual synthesis was universally effective in practice, new archaeological evidence demonstrates to us the wide range of ancient healing practices that were sustained into the imperial period. Under the veneer of a new and systematic medical ideology, there survived remedy literature and textual miscellanies that reveal knowledge and practice of a wide variety of healing arts (Harper 2010).

Imperial Power and Authoritative Medical Writing

The Former (or Western) Han Dynasty emerged from a brief period of chaos that followed the death of the first emperor, Qin Shi Huangdi (256–210 B.C.E.), and the subsequent collapse of the Qin Dynasty. Qin Shi Huangdi's rise had been driven by a ruthless ambition to unify the Warring States under his rule and was marked by a despotism eloquently symbolized in the self-glory of the prodigious terra-cotta army buried with him in his mausoleum. He achieved control of diverse states through the replacement of their various hereditary posts with a comprehensively centralized and bureaucratized government, as well as strict rule through detailed written legal codes. This centralization of power also entailed large-scale projects that aimed at standardization not only in administration but across many aspects of life (such as currency, wheel and track sizes, and scripts), with varying levels of success. In his attempt to monopolize knowledge, Qin Shi Huangdi ordered the burning of the kind of books treasured by scholars, many of whom he distrusted. However, he reprieved certain writings that he deemed to be essential and of practical value, including books on medicine—a measure both of the high regard in which he held medicine and of the value he placed on his own longevity.

The rulers of the new Han Dynasty adopted much of the larger framework and military and legal administration of Qin Shi Huangdi's centralized imperial bureaucratic government. At the same time they distanced themselves from the excesses of his rule, referring instead to loftier ideals of civilization represented by the sage rulers of a utopian world in prehistory. In the same way, writers on medicine attributed the traditional sources of medical knowledge to icons of a legendary past—sages, cultural heroes, and the same mythical rulers. To the Red Emperor or Divine Husbandman (Shennong, traditionally third millennium B.C.E.) was attributed the tradition of trying and testing drugs (and indeed food, which forms part of the same continuum). He was said to have thrashed all plants to extract their essential qualities, tasted them, and then classified them according to their value as foodstuffs and drugs. This tradition was acknowledged in the name of a number of classic *materia medica* (studies of the effects of medicines in the treatment of disease), starting with *The Divine Husbandman's Materia Medica* (*Shennong bencao jing*, ca. first century C.E.). Other mythical or semimythical figures who appear as medical progenitors include Shaman Peng (Wu Peng); a mysterious figure known as Mr. White (Bai Shi); and the learned physician *(yi)* called Bian Que (traditionally sixth to fifth century B.C.E.), who—even more mysteriously—is sometimes depicted as a bird with a human head, as in a Later Han stone relief from present-day Shandong, assumed to depict Bian Que giving treatment with needles. (See Figure 2.1.)

The most celebrated of these ancient sages was the Yellow Emperor (Huangdi; also translated as "Yellow Thearch" to capture the divine resonances of *di*, and as "Yellow Lord"), traditionally ascribed to the prehistorical fifth millennium B.C.E. He was credited with many of the innovations that brought together theories of divine order with approaches to law and punishment, the calendar, ritual, divination, and medicine (Lewis 1990). The logic for medicine was compelling: it revealed a cosmos in which the healthy body had an essential synchrony with the cycles and phases of Heaven and Earth, and in which dissonance produced illness. Physicians, by identifying the specific disharmonies in question, could diagnose, prognosticate, and treat disorders at a more profound level.

Throughout the Han period, a large corpus of medical knowledge was attributed to the Yellow Emperor, largely taking the form of dialogues between the Yellow Emperor and his ministers, such as Lord Thunder (Leigong) and especially Qibo, a specialist in acupuncture and various esoteric matters. There were a number of respected female authorities on the arts of the bedchamber, such as the Plain Girl *(sunü)* and the Dark Girl *(xuannü)*. They imparted information about the strengthening of quintessential generative Essence *(jing)* the finest and most subtle form of *qi*, responsible for reproductive potency and core resistance against illness. Dialogue was a popular form of intellectual exposition in the Han era, designed as a way of exploring contending points of view and unifying diverse opinion.

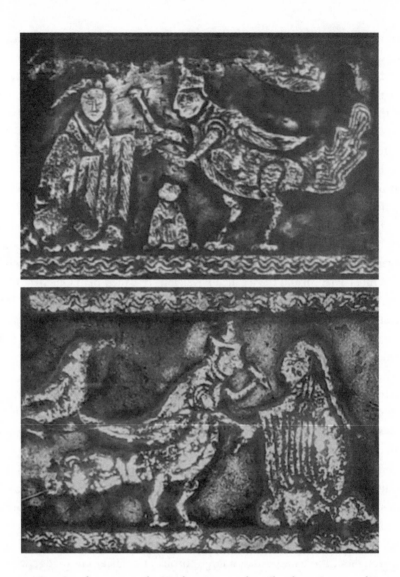

Figure 2.1. Bian Que, from present-day Weishan, Liangyu shan, Shandong. Courtesy of Huang Longxiang.

Books that carry the title *Inner Canon of the Yellow Emperor (Huangdi neijing)* compile the different ways that Han medical theorists began to conceive of the movement of *qi* around the body in twelve channels (*mo,* also transliterated *mai*), and of how the *mo* could be assessed by physicians in places where its pulsation emerged at the surface of the body. In the Han political and intellectual synthesis, Warring States ideas about *qi,* blood, and Yin and Yang were brought to the body in the knowledge and practice of healing the *mo.* Variously translated as "channels," "vessels," or "pulse," at first the *mo* were part of a lineal structuring of the body that connected its inner and outer planes; each channel was designated as one phase of Yin and Yang (Greater Yin or Yang, Lesser Yin or Yang, etc.), a spatiotemporal map that laid the ground for later theorists to imagine a circulation of *qi*. According to the context, the *mo* could mean channels beneath the skin (identifiable by the valleys between the seams of muscles), blood vessels, or streaming pains and other inner bodily sensations experienced as flowing or in response to palpation along a particular plane.

The primary works setting out these classical themes are attributed to the legendary Yellow Emperor and first listed in the imperial bibliography as the *Inner Canon of the Yellow Emperor* and the *Outer Canon of the Yellow Emperor* (*Huangdi neijing* and *Huangdi waijing*). Over time, the *Inner Canon* has been rearranged by editors into three sections, forming separate books: *The Basic Questions (Suwen), The Numinous Pivot (Lingshu),* and *The Grand Basis (Taisu).* Taken together, they discuss acupuncture, the piercing of the body with stones and needles in order to influence the *qi,* and moxibustion, heat treatment to the same end, often performed by burning the plant called mugwort. This chapter describes what we know about the four hundred years of medical society and cultures within which the anonymous authors of the *Inner Canon* reflected on the nature of the body, sickness, and treatment.

When They Are Dead You Can Cut Them Up and Take a Look

It has become a commonplace to state that knowledge and practice of medicine during the Han period came to be derived not from observation of the tissues, bones, and viscera of the physical body but from an imagination of its inner workings as homologous with the order of the external worlds, its natural rhythms as observed in the movements of heaven and earth, and its sociopolitical realities. Yet we must look beyond and through the testimony of classical medical treatises. The *Inner Canon of the Yellow Emperor,* for example, does contain details of the dimensions of the organs of the digestive tract, and states that measurements of the internal organs of humans, their firmness and fragility, and their ability to receive grains are easy to know. While the cutting up of live bodies for medical purposes was not a customary practice anywhere in the ancient world, in the turbulent interregnum between the Former and Later Han, the so-called usurper (or, from other points of view, reformer) Wang Mang (r. 9–23 C.E.) ordered the dissection of the executed rebel leader Wang Sunqing (d. 16 C.E.), with anatomical investigations, including careful measurement and weighing of his internal organs. Although deep surgery, as all over the ancient world, received little attention elsewhere in the historical records, the biography of the legendary physician Hua Tuo (second century C.E.) tells us that he practiced it using a numbing concoction *(mafeisan)* to render his patients "as if drunk or dead or unconscious." It is likely, if these accounts have some basis in actual practice, that he or physicians like him were working on the abdominal wounds of battle victims. Deep surgery was, of course, a very risky practice prior to the introduction of effective antiseptics in the nineteenth century. The perception of very real danger, as well as the lower social class of those employed on the battlefield, would have rendered this kind of intervention crude and unsophisticated when other, less invasive means with scholarly pedigrees, such as medicinal remedies and early forms of moxibustion and acupuncture, were available. Superficial surgery was, of course, to be found everywhere.

Medical Manuscripts

Throughout most of the Han period, medical texts carried a high status, and mere possession of a manuscript could enhance one's personal power and influence. This applied not just to the scholars and physicians who wrote, compiled, and used them or to the scribes who copied them, but also to noblemen who sponsored and collected the texts. It seems that early medical practitioners of the Former Han initially acquired knowledge through oral tradition: teachers would pass on their knowledge to their selected disciples by word of mouth. But committing medical knowledge to writing was a respected and well-established practice during the Han period, encouraged by the imperial court, which collected technical writing.

These texts attracted a deep reverence as a kind of scripture: their purported antiquity and lack of reference to actual authorship conferred an unchallenged authority on the knowledge contained therein. The texts themselves, in the form of scrolls made of silk or bamboo strips, were valuable objects with special powers themselves. Practitioners in possession of these texts acquired great prestige, something all the more important in a world where most physicians were itinerant and needed ways to establish their reputations quickly to their changing clientele. They could reinforce their claim to authority by handing down their knowledge, and eventually the texts themselves, to their pupils in a process shrouded in esoteric ritual. This marked the texts as precious and the transmission as exclusive, and underscored the bond between teacher and pupil.

Although it recounts an episode between figures we know to be mythical, the Yellow Emperor and Lord Thunder, an extract from *The Numinous Pivot* (probably compiled between the first century B.C.E. and the first century C.E.) gives an insight into the kind of ritual that may have accompanied the transmission of high-prestige texts from master to disciple during the Former Han:

> The Yellow Emperor then entered the purification chamber with him. They cut their forearms and smeared the blood on their mouths. The Yellow Emperor chanted this incantation: "Today is True Yang. Smearing the blood I transmit the remedies. May he who dares to turn his back on these words himself bear calamities." Lord Thunder bowed twice and said: "As a young child, I receive them." The Yellow Emperor then with the left hand gripped his hand and with his right gave him the texts, saying: "Pay heed! Pay heed!" (*Huangdi neijing lingshu* 1995, 8 [48 "Jinfu"], 1a–b; translation modified from Harper 1998, 63)

Such was the status of medical manuscripts that editions were also placed in tombs as part of the all-important provisions and conspicuous display that served to enhance the status of the family and sustain the deceased in the afterlife. This has meant that a large number of medical manuscripts have survived in tombs belonging to elite families, as revealed in several major archaeological finds of recent years. Among the most significant are Mawangdui tomb 3 (Changsha Guo, present-day Hunan; closed 168 B.C.E., excavated 1973), Zhangjiashan tomb 247 (Nanjun, present-day Hubei; closed 186 B.C.E., excavated 1983–1984), Shuihudi (Yunmeng, Hubei, closed ca. 217 B.C.E., excavated 1975), and Wuwei (Gansu, closed first century C.E., excavated 1959).

Medical manuscripts tend to tell very different stories from the medical canons preserved in print, and to reveal more diverse forms of healing, ones that are distinctively local or religious. Other manuscripts found in the tombs relate to philosophy, astronomy, divination, government affairs, and military strategy—which underlines the relative importance given to the healing arts in the context of knowledge overall. Indeed, out of the thirty or so manuscripts buried in Mawangdui tomb 3, seven are devoted to the healing arts—an astonishing number.

The wealth of information provided by these texts has helped to fill in great gaps in the history of innovations during Han times. They contain, for example, the earliest extant set of Yin-Yang correspondences, recorded in a philosophic treatise excavated from the Mawangdui tomb. Set out as two lists, the qualities concerned with Yin and Yang provide a simple opportunity to explore what is and what is not universal about core divisions in our human tendency to think in opposites: down/up, outer/inner, night/day, warm/cold, female/male, autumn/spring, winter/summer, younger/older, inaction/action, earth/heaven, host/guest, silence/speech, receiving/giving, mourning/having a child, common

TABLE 1

Mawangdui: Earliest Yin-Yang correlations

Yang	Yin
Heaven	Earth
Spring	Autumn
Summer	Winter
Day	Night
Big States	Small States
Important State	Unimportant state
Action	Inaction
Stretching	Contracting
Ruler	Minister
Above	Below
Man	Woman
Father	Child
Elder Brother	Younger Brother
Older	Younger
Noble	Base
Getting on in the world	Being stuck where one is
Taking a wife/begetting a child	Mourning
Controlling others	Being controlled by others
Guest	Host
Soldiers	Laborers
Speech	Silence
Giving	Receiving

or base/noble (*Mawangdui hanmu boshu* 1984). (See Table 1.) While the initial pairs might seem to be more "natural," there is an increasing cultural specificity as the list progresses until the oppositions of "host/guest" or "mourning/having a child" become arresting enough to make the modern reader question the kind of social and cultural environment that produced them.

The Mawangdui manuscripts, for instance, contain treatises on exercise, breathing control, sexual techniques, herbs, superficial surgery, and magical procedures. They speak of spirit healing, the persistence of the belief that the body served as a dwelling place for spirits, and the notion that good health involved avoiding the wrath of ancestors and the malevolence of demons. They include household manuals presenting remedies for a variety of illnesses ranging from hemorrhoids to convulsions, the latter described as having the characteristics of horses, sheep, and snakes, perhaps by analogy with the noises emitted during episodes or with the quality of the involuntary movements. Charms, exorcism, many kinds of heat treatments, and basic surgery appear among the proposed cures. The tomb also contained the earliest specimens of Chinese medical herbs yet found, including magnolia, Chinese prickly ash, cassia bark, and wild ginger—all of which are used by Chinese herbalists today.

The tomb texts paint a picture of the realities of early Chinese medicine that is considerably more diverse than was previously deduced from the received canons alone. They reveal, rather, the complexity of the medical landscape from which the medical theory of the received canons emerged, and this evidence helps to support the hypothesis that the years marking the end of the Warring States period and the beginning of imperial rule were critical for the writing that was later gathered and compiled in the *Inner Canon of the Yellow Emperor* and formed classical medical theory.

Canonization

The classic texts were known as *jing*, a term normally translated, not unproblematically, as "canon," and meaning something akin to "standard" or "main" text (as opposed to commentary on it). As we have seen, they contain selected writings about the fundamental principles of Chinese medical theory.

The *History of the Former Han*, introduced above, includes the first recorded mention of the *Inner* and *Outer Canon of the Yellow Emperor*, which through the acceptance of the imperial bibliographers provides some of that sense of official authentication involved in the creation of a canon. However, none of the books associated with these titles has come down to us in its original state; what have survived are versions that have been edited, amended, and altered over subsequent centuries, and were eventually printed in the twelfth century. Thus, we can only hope for a partial reconstruction of their content in Former Han times by comparing the received literature with passages in ancient manuscripts and with quotations in works that are more certainly dated to the early dynasties.

Teachers and students in the various medical traditions built up collections of texts and passed them on in manuscripts that had prestige and ritual significance. The content of the texts was often obscure and contradictory, even to readers at the time. Annotations and commentaries, easily differentiated at the time of writing, were designed to elucidate difficulties in interpretation. In successive compilations the scholarly apparatus became embedded into the main text, serving to add confusion and further confound the modern scholar.

By accident or design, and particularly when printing was developed more than a thousand years later, these texts would cease to change, and at this point they became the revered canons or classics that we know today. How our received canons of medicine relate to those standard texts (also named *jing*) as they were recorded in the ancient bibliographies and prefaces is a tricky subject still undergoing philological analysis.

It was only toward the end of the Han period that ancient canonical works began to move from under the cover of secret transmission (or, at least, the ideal of secret transmission) into the public domain. This period was marked by an increasing tendency toward the systematization of knowledge by individual writers and the rise of the preface, which served to make authorial intent explicit. These factors point to a wider audience and greater literacy. Produced during the early second century C.E., the *Canon of Difficult Issues (Nanjing)* set out to appraise, analyze, and explain many of the assumptions of the Yellow Emperor corpus. Still using the question-and-answer format, it represents both the apogee and the concluding chapter of that ancient form.

By now, learned physicians were beginning to express and take credit for their own individual opinions, outside the framework of canonical literature. Rather than ascribing their work to legendary figures, they attached their own names to treatises, effectively mounting a public challenge to the tradition of secret and ritual transmission of medical texts. Zhang Ji (fl. 196–205), for instance, wrote two works on febrile disease in the wake of an epidemic in his town. In these, he charts the progress of the disease in terms of which of the Yin and Yang systems was under external attack, and he suggests remedies for each phase. The treatises were later amalgamated to form the *Treatise on Cold Damage Disorders (Shanghan lun)*. Given that there were many references to it in the received and manuscript traditions, the text clearly circulated widely in the medieval period. It underwent a further renaissance in the eleventh century, when it was heralded in imperial circles as the basis for great theoretical and practical innovations associated with the treatment of epidemic disorders. (See Chapters 4 and 6.)

By this time increasing numbers of physicians were no longer itinerant but instead belonged to family practices in fixed locations. Reputation thus increasingly attached to identifiable medical lineages, rather than to the prestige of claimed provenance. Alongside this change, remedy books now began to multiply. These collections also garnered authority through reference to a received corpus of ancient texts, rather than simply to the legendary bringers of culture, further breaking from the heritage of ritual and secrecy. Families and individuals could build up substantial collections of texts by copying them for themselves, and also through the emerging book trade.

Moving Qi: Acupuncture?

Three of the tomb texts from Mawangdui echo—in both style and content—treatises contained in the received canons of acupuncture and moxibustion cautery. But the way they differ from the received canon is also significant. The Mawangdui texts place the emphasis squarely on moxibustion, not needle or stone therapy. The channels described do not follow the linked pathways of the received tradition, nor do they connect to the internal organs or describe any loci for needling, but instead run as separate lines on the surface of the body and the limbs. Also absent from the texts is any reference to a circulation of *qi* or a system of correspondences like the Five Phases theory, even though by the second century B.C.E. this was well developed in a ritual context.

With the addition of *Writings on the Mo (Channels) (Moshu)* from Zhangjiashan, four early Han tomb texts map some eleven *mo* on the body, a contrast with the received traditions based on late Han writings. Oddly, the tomb texts make little mention of *qi,* except in the context of breathing disorders or Wind trapped in the belly. But there is one important exception, a passage from *Moshu* in which the text speaks of piercing the *mo* to influence the movement of *qi*:

> As for *qi,* it benefits the lower body yet harms the upper; follows heat and keeps a distance from cold. So, the sages cool the head and warm the feet. Those who treat illness take the surplus and supplement the insufficiency. So if *qi* goes up, not down, then when you see the *mo* that has overreached itself, apply one cauterization where it meets the articulation. When the illness is intense, then apply another cauterization at a place two *cun* [Chinese inches; 4.6 cm] above the articulation. When the *qi* rises at one moment and falls in the next, pierce it with a stone lancet at the back of the knee and the elbow. (*Zhangjiashan hanmu zhujian [Moshu],* nos. 57–58)

If we consider that the treatment proposed here is acupuncture because it involves piercing the body to regularize the flow of *qi,* this is the earliest extant reference to it. By contrast, the widespread use of moxibustion to "draw the *qi*" in Han times is clearly attested to in the tomb texts (*Mawangdui hanmu boshu,* vol. 4), and is, significantly, the only form of treatment explicitly cited in the three Mawangdui texts describing the routes taken by the *mo.*

Mawangdui and Zhangjiashan tomb texts always show eleven *mo* channels in the charts. By the late second and early third centuries C.E., the medical canons had settled on twelve circulation Channels associated with the organs, bowels, and functions of the body, with two more associated with extremes of

Yin and Yang, respectively. These, along with a number of subsidiary Channels, were to become the basis of classical acupuncture. But it seems that for centuries there was no consensus on this central aspect of the new medicine. For example, the names given to the eleven *mo*, as well as their descriptions, vary somewhat. It is possible that the number eleven was derived from the numerical system that associated the number six with heaven and five with earth, as recorded in the *Discourses of the States (Guoyu)* and *Zuo's Commentary*; eleven is also the number of the lunar phases of Yin and Yang, according to the early ritual calendars called Monthly Ordinances (Kong 1965, 708 "Zhao Gong" 1], 26b; *Guoyu* 1983, 3 ["Zhouyu"]). In later medical canons, eleven appears as the five internal organ systems and six bowels, but none of the excavated texts make this connection, nor do they show the *mo* linking with the inner body.

Moving Qi: The Arts of the Bedchamber

It is interesting to note that the Mianyang figurine (see Figures 2.5–2.6) has no genitalia. In their general approach to body systems, Han physicians did not tend to distinguish between male and female: rather, the physical differences were seen as equivalents. For instance, men and women both have Essence (*jing*), manifesting in their reproductive fluids: semen for men, menses, fetus-nourishing blood, and breast milk for women. In the twenty-five case histories recorded in the *Historical Records* biography of the physician Chunyu Yi (active from about 170 to 150 B.C.E.) neither gender differences nor even their essential Yin and Yang nature are given any particular emphasis, either in the description of ailments or in their treatment (Furth 1999; Raphals 1998a) (see "The Treatment of Women").

THE TREATMENT OF WOMEN

Lisa Raphals

The most important historical source for the treatment of women in early Chinese medicine is the physician Chunyu Yi's collection of twenty-five medical cases (Sima 1959, 105.2794–2820, translated in Bridgman 1955). It describes the diagnosis and treatment of eighteen males and seven females of all ages, ranging in social status from rulers to slaves (Loewe 1997; Raphals 1998b). From these cases we learn that, unlike physicians in later periods, Chunyu was able to examine women directly. It is also immediately striking that while Yin and

Yang correlate to gender in other writings, in the physiological theory of these case studies they do not (see Raphals 1998a). Although gender affected the handling of highly gendered sociobiological functions such as the treatment of male potency and the care of women through childbirth, with few exceptions it was not a salient category in diagnosis and treatment. For example, there were two cases of women and one of a man who suffered from difficulty in urination. Chunyu Yi assigned different names to their ailments and used different pulses in their diagnosis but cured all three with the same drug.

In another case, both a man and a woman suffered from a fatal spleen disorder. The woman was a slave who used remedy master *(fangshi)* techniques to maintain the appearance of normality in her pulse and color (Sima 1959, 105.2805). The other was a male physician who had unsuccessfully attempted to treat himself. Chunyu presented the male physician's theories and methods in detail and used Yin-Yang theory to argue that he had misdiagnosed himself (Sima 1959, 105.2810–2811). In contrast, he gave only a tantalizingly cursory description of the young female slave as "skilled in secret formulae *(fang)*, capable in several arts, and knowing how to use the newest methods" (Sima 1959, 105.2805). We do not know, though, what formulas she knew or how she learned them (Raphals 1998b). Women may have mastered and used such skills at home, as was the common pattern in more complete later accounts; at least one other rare Han account of a woman remedy master tells us that she learned her skills from her father and used them in a domestic context (*Hou Hanshu* 82A.2717, translated in Ngo 1976, 94–95).

Excavated texts from the period do sometimes state that a treatment may be used by women, or provide variants for men and women. For example, in *Recipes for Fifty-two Ailments (Wushier bing fang)*, a collection of 282 magico-medical recipes excavated at Mawangdui, only seven recipes refer to gender (translated in Harper 1998, 221–304). Two state that the recipe may be used by both men and women, two (on female urine retention) refer specifically to women, and three prescribe different numbers of repetitions of ritual procedures (seven for men, fourteen for women). The same gender-specific numbers of repetitions appear in another recipe collection from Zhoujiatai (Guanju, Hubei). Pregnancy, on the other hand, is treated as a distinct issue. Another Mawangdui text, *Book of the Generation of the Fetus (Taichan shu)*, prescribes diet, ritual behavior, and methods of fetal instruction at each stage of pregnancy, as well as medical recipes specific to pregnant women (translated in Harper 1998, 372–384).

In summary, none of these texts suggests essential differences or ascribes Yang or Yin natures to men and women. For the most part, men and women appear to be medically identical, with a few specific exceptions involving sexuality and childbirth.

Yet when it comes to the important health issue of sexual cultivation, gender difference becomes a salient issue. The tomb texts show that the function and stimulation of the sexual organs were the subject of considerable scrutiny. A Mawangdui tomb text, given the modern title *Remedies for Nurturing Life (Yangsheng fang)*, includes a depiction of the female genitals, including the "red pearl" (clitoris) and the "wheat teeth" (pubic hair), and offers instruction on how to enhance female sexual pleasure.

Yin and Yang and *qi* are all brought to bear on the subject of a woman's sexual satisfaction and male potency. The Mawangdui text given the modern title *Harmonizing Yin and Yang (He Yin Yang)* describes how for the male partner, bringing the woman to orgasm was an opportunity to absorb life-balancing Yin, as its availability increased with the pleasure experienced by the woman as *qi* flooded through her body, bringing a brightness of the spirit (see *Mawangdui hanmu boshu* 1984, 4 *[Tianxia zhi dao tan]* nos. 12–67, esp. 39; Li L. 2006, 315, plate 7; *Huangdi neijing lingshu* 1995, 2 [9 "Zhongshi"], 10b). According to the same source, both successful breath cultivation and sexual cultivation produce the following effects: "The *qi* arrives, blood and *qi* flow freely, the ears and eyes are keen and bright, the skin gleams, the voice is clear, and the back, thighs, and buttocks are sturdy, so that one 'attains a brilliance of the spirits' *[tong shenming]*" (*Mawangdui hanmu boshu* 1984, 4 *[He Yin Yang]*, no. 133; *[Shi wen]*, nos. 15–41).

In these writings we find some of the earliest ideas about influencing the balance and movement of Yin and Yang in the inner body. The texts are often written in beautiful but rather obscure language, with techniques described by euphemisms that are now hard to interpret. Fortunately, lest we imagine that sexual cultivation was an entirely esoteric matter, practical remedies survive telling us that achieving "brilliance of the spirits" was inseparable from technologies of pleasure. Aphrodisiacs, for example, play a large part in recipe literature. A second-century B.C.E. text recovered from the Mawangdui grave site offered these suggestions for arousing passion in a woman (although some words were illegible on the excavated manuscript, indicated here by ellipses, the general sense is clear):

> *Increasing Craving*
> . . . *fuling* (pine truffle) and discard the dregs. Use the liquid to fatten a suckling pig. Feed it to the woman. It makes her increase in sweetness and makes her inside become fine. Incinerate and smith the inner part of cow horn . . . dried *jiang* (ginger) and *jungui* (curled cinnamon). Combine them . . . put in a sack. Soak it in gruel vinegar and insert into the inside.

Another. Blend . . . liquid with choice beef or venison. Have the woman insert it herself deep inside her prohibited part. (Harper 1998, 336; see also Harper 2005a; Lo 2005, 165–170)

Assisting the Flow

These remedy texts concerned with sexual stimulation are kept in close proximity to others that describe the techniques for harmonizing Yin and Yang and the proper control of *qi*. This involved both careful observation of the external signs of arousal and micromanagement of the inner sensory world through bodily discipline. Variations that occur in the medical concepts of *qi* are partially explained by the different practices through which the ideas developed. In some contexts this essence was thought to flow downward through the body like floodwaters, or to rotate on the breath (Kuriyama 1999, 102–104, 223). Daily physical and breathing exercises, much like those depicted in a silk painting found at Mawangdui, were prescribed to assist this flow, for fear that otherwise it would stagnate around the internal organs and cause disease. (See Figures 2.2–2.4.) The joints were considered natural points on the body where this flow might be interrupted, and so treatment often focused on these areas, such as the elbows and the back of the knees. The Zhangjiashan *Writings on Pulling (Yinshu)* describes techniques to make *qi* move downward and into the limbs. One offers treatment for a hangover:

> The prescription for ailing from *liao* [too much liquor]: Grasp a staff in the right hand, face a wall, and do not breathe; with the left foot tread on the wall, resting when tired. Then do likewise with the left hand and the right foot, again resting when tired. When the *qi* of the head flows downward the foot will no longer be immobile and numb, the head will not swell, and the nose will not be stuffed up. Whenever there is free time, practice this often. (*Zhangjiashan hanmu zhujian* [*Moshu*], nos. 36–37)

Thus the imagery of flowing water structured the imagination of early technologies of *qi*, as knowledge of the natural courses of rivers and other waterways began to be applied to the understanding of *qi* physiology, and measures for preventing flood and drought were adapted to conserving all the essences that were the target of bodily cultivation (Allan 1997). By the end of the Han period, acupuncture theory and the names of acupuncture points are replete with references to water, from the "Sea of *Qi*" to the "Crooked Spring" and the

Figure 2.2. Illustration from the silk "Daoyin tu" (chart for leading and pulling), excavated from the Mawangdui tomb [tomb closed 168 B.C.E]. Courtesy of the Wellcome Library, London.

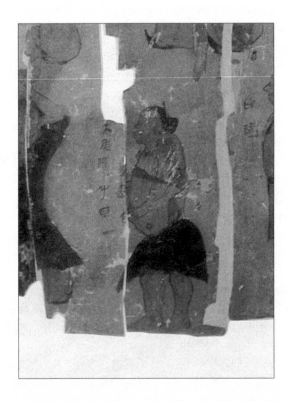

Figure 2.3. "Tree monkey bawling to pull internal heat," from the "Daoyin tu." Courtesy of the Wellcome Library, London.

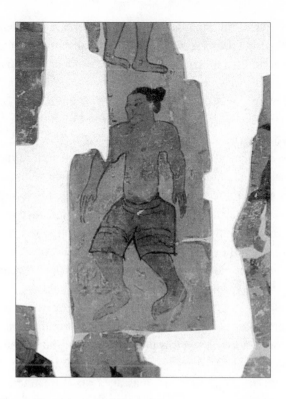

Figure 2.4. "Bear walking," from the "Daoyin tu." Courtesy of the Wellcome Library, London.

"Celestial Well." Treatises on sexual cultivation, in particular, also provide early examples of the propensity to give lyrical, poetic names to points on the body where practitioners could assist the flow of physiological essences (Lo 2001b; *Mawangdui hanmu boshu* 4 [*He Yin Yang*], nos. 102–105). Elaborate concepts of bodily *qi* and of Yin and Yang are found in the medical canons that date from the second and third century C.E. But it is clear from the tomb texts that they were already being aired during the early Former Han, and applied in particular to the fields of breath, exercise, and sexual practice. There was also precedent in the self-cultivation literature for emphasis on Yin in longevity practices aimed at enhancing and sustaining the body, as will be discussed later in this chapter.

Needles, Stones, and Artemisia

Acupuncture emerged out of this complex of diverse healing arts during the Han period, a product of *qi* and Yin/Yang practices, divination, numerology, minor surgery, and bloodletting, plus elements of spirit healing. Its material origins, stones (*bian*, "medicinal stones") for healing the body, may date to

Neolithic times. Treasured stones and pottery tiles excavated from tombs of the Warring States period show signs of heating and stains left by liquid, suggesting that they were tools used for treatment by hot pressing or cauterizing *(yunju)*, a practice that is affirmed in manuscripts predating the Yellow Emperor canon. Alternatively, some stones (also found in tombs in similar contexts) were evidently used for apotropaic purposes (i.e., to ward off evil) (Lo 2002a).

It is clear that by the early second century B.C.E., such techniques already were being used specifically to influence the flow of *qi* around the body along the *mo* channels to free up the blockages that were deemed to be causing ailments, in particular at the places where the channels crossed and around the joints, the sites of frequent pain and discomfort. The intended outcome of the most subtle form of needling was consistent with the aims of sexual and breath cultivation: adjusting the *qi*, Yin, and Yang would make the senses astute, ensure proper flow of the blood, and make the voice and appearance radiant and bright (*Huangdi neijing lingshu* 1995, 4 [9 "Zhongshi"], 2b).

Popular histories of Chinese medicine tend to overstate the importance of acupuncture and the use of needles at named acupuncture locations to move *qi*, especially for Han times, when available archaeological evidence testifies to emerging ideas about body channels but offers hardly anything about this innovative practice. At the gentler end, massage or heat treatment could be applied to the points of blockage, but if a more subtle effect on the flow of *qi* was called for, needles might be used. This is affirmed by the "Nine Needles" (*jiuzhen*) chapter in *The Numinous Pivot*, in which the Yellow Emperor complains about the crude use of stone lancets in *qi* work. But it should be noted that similar procedures cited in this text refer mainly to small-scale surgery, bloodletting, and the treatment of abscesses, not to *qi* therapy. Those needles designated for moving *qi* were of very high quality and likened to "fine hair."

Technically, Chinese smiths were capable of producing fine metal needles at this time, but none have been found. The earliest extant references to piercing the body at named acupuncture points on the body date to the first century C.E. There was nonetheless always a residual concern about the use of needles. A first-century C.E. manuscript recovered from an archaeological site in Wuwei warns against harming the seasonal movement of the spirits and souls within the body and proscribes needling in specific locations at given times of the year.

Compared to needling, heat treatment tended to offer a more accessible and cheaper alternative, and the most popular and widespread technique was *jiu*, translated as "moxibustion" and referring to a variety of heating and cauterization procedures using different materials. Taking the smoldering tip of a plug of herbal plant matter, the practitioner moved it into close proximity to the skin to apply heat to specific points on the body. Moxibustion is sometimes referred to as "cauterization" or "cautery" in the more general sense of applying searing heat, but only occasionally was it used as a means of cauterizing wounds.

It is likely that moxibustion derived from the practice of manipulating spirits around the body. In ancient times, sweet-smelling mugwort (ai; Artemisia vulgaris)—the main herb used by acupuncturists for moxibustion today—was believed to be efficacious in both driving out malevolent spirits and attracting benign ones, and it was burned on or over the body for this purpose. By early Han times, its more refined and targeted application to relieve weakness and treat pain through manipulating qi probably provided a model for later acupuncture formulations.

Cultivating the Jade Body

In different early Han contexts the supreme goal of the healing arts could be not only curing illness but immortality of the physical body or transcendent states of the living body; for the last two, jade was a potent symbol. It combined hardness and durability with an appearance of glossiness—a shining quality that also conveyed the illusion of moistness. Jade lying beneath a mountain was a source of clouds and rain and might stimulate luxuriant growth. It is the resonance of these qualities of strength, radiance, and secretion with youthful sexuality that definitively linked jade with the ability to sustain sexual competence into old age and with the perception of invulnerability to deterioration. Regardless of their function, jade objects always signified a sacred space, impervious to decay (Lo 2002b).

For this reason jade was widely used in ritual and medical writings. The ultimate expression of good health was in the "jade body," yuti (mentioned in Mawangdui hanmu boshu). While in the Warring States period the encasement of the corpse in a funerary suit of jade pieces sewn together with fine gold thread testifies to a very real hope of preserving the mortal body, in Han times one medical text makes reference to the jade body as the result of successfully cultivating Yin and Yang through assisting the movement and flow of the body so as to prevent stagnation in the viscera (Zhangjiashan hanmu zhujian [Moshu], no. 53).

Another contemporary tomb body from along the Yangzi Valley, which has been taken to corroborate the Han tendency to structure the body in lineal tracts as expressed in the early writings on mo, actually tells us more about how to sustain the sensual nature of the body beyond death. Buried next to the corpse of a high-ranking military commander excavated at Shuangbao Shan (Guanghan commandery; in present-day Mianyang, Sichuan, ca. 118 B.C.E.) was a black lacquer figurine with ten red lines painted on its torso and vertically the length of the limbs. (See Figures 2.5–2.6.)

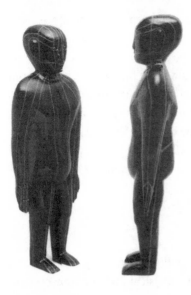

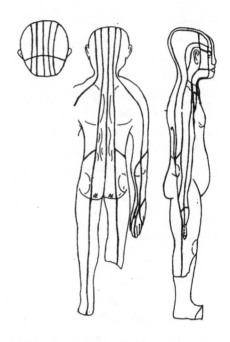

Figure 2.5. Black lacquer figurine from a tomb at Shuangbao shan (Guanghan commandery; in present-day Mianyang, Sichuan, c. 118 B.C.E.). Facsimile. Anterior and side views. Courtesy of Vivienne Lo. Photography by Peter Barker.

Figure 2.6. Drawings of the lines illustrated on the Mianyang tomb figurine. Courtesy of Vivienne Lo.

The conventional analysis is that the figurine illustrates the medical theories found in the manuscripts, with which it shares some similarities, notably an absence of acupuncture loci. It is 28.1 cm high and was wrapped in red fabric and placed in the "outer chamber" tomb *(guo)* (Lo and He 1996, 96, line D.10; Tang 1999; *Mianyang Shuangbao Shan hanmu* 2006, 125, Plate 191). These lines may have served as a map of the *mo* channels, to be used as a medical teaching device or visual guide, in the manner of much later acupuncture models. However, given its ritual position, the figurine is more likely to have been designed as an effigy that could assist the deceased in channeling vitality in the afterlife (Lo and He 1996; detailed discussion in He 1995). With the lines clustering around the sense organs, it also seems to provide new eyes and ears for the corpse.

Cultivating the jade body in life was the preserve of the wealthy, those who had the leisure to indulge themselves in therapeutic exercise and breathing away their excesses. The *Writings on Pulling* from Zhangjiashan suggests that the very lifestyle of nobles gave them a propensity to an excess of emotion that made it necessary to adjust their Yin and Yang *Qi*:

If they (the nobles) are joyful *(xi)* then the Yang *Qi* is in excess. If they are angry then the Yin *Qi* is in excess. Therefore, if adherents of the Way are joyful then they quickly exhale (warm breath), and if they become angry they increasingly *(ju)* puff out (moist breath), in order to harmonize it. (*Zhangjiashan hanmu zhujian [Yinshu]*, nos. 107–108)

In this way the tomb texts offer clear observations about how social status plays a role in health and how people suffer illness. The same text tells us that a common person is subject to elements beyond his or her control, including the vicissitudes of labor and the weather.

As China's healing arts documented the aesthetic internal experience of how it felt to be well and strong, and experiences of pain, passion, and pleasure, it began to medicalize the sensory world. And it is in the language and theories generated by this culture of animating the inner body that we find a core innovation in early Chinese healing arts—one that survives to confound simple articulations of difference between mind, emotion, and body. The semantic circuits invoked by *qi* unite precisely these changing states of the inner sensory world (Ots 1994). They echo the sensibilities of an ancient time in which the boundaries between these experiences were less distinct (Jütte 2005).

The Healers

Given the wide definition of the body and practices concerned with healing and self-improvement, a plurality of different practitioners were called on to service different needs. The pursuit of longevity sometimes meant simply warding off illness and keeping the body supple; at other times it aimed at states of divine transcendence *(xian)*. Yet there is also plenty of evidence that people in Han times entertained the notion of, indeed strived for, physical immortality—a quest that had obsessed the first emperor, Qin Shi Huangdi, who reportedly sent thousands of virgins to sea in search of herbs of immortality (they never returned) and the Han emperor Wudi, who sponsored shamans purveying techniques for long life, including one shaman who also persuaded the emperor he could revive his late consort.

The bibliographic section of the official *History of the Former Han*, compiled by Ban Gu (32–92 C.E.) around 82 C.E., lists twenty-nine medical titles (*Hanshu, Yiwenzhi* 10, 1701–1780). These show the range of strategies associated with the healing arts, including the pursuits of longevity and immortality or transcendence. Under the broader heading of remedies and techniques *(fangji)* we find: (1) Medical Canons *(yijing)*, 7 items; (2) Standard Remedies *(jingfang)*, 11 items;

(3) Arts of the Bedchamber *(fangzhong)*, 8 items; and (4) Arts of Transcendence *(shenxian)*, 10 items, the last group containing titles on massage and therapeutic movement.

Learned physicians *(yi)* were guardians of the most respected texts and practitioners of their contents, which show a marked abstraction of those kinds of ideas developed in ritual and spirit healing. Yet we should be cautious in reading this as evidence of a hard and fast boundary between healers and their practices. A distinction is sometimes drawn between the physicians and specialists in making and prescribing remedies, divination, and more esoteric arts. In fact, these categories are broad and overlapping, the former sometimes subsumed in the latter. We know that noted physicians, including the very few named ones such as the legendary Bian Que and Chunyu Yi (see "The Treatment of Women"), are also likely to have been classified as remedy masters on account of the kind of techniques they used. The remedy masters fulfilled a wide variety of functions, including divination, self-cultivation, early forms of acupuncture, and minor surgery. Distinctions, therefore, can be overstated since they were no doubt established to delineate boundaries of expertise in a competitive environment. Both groups are likely to have consulted a variety of authoritative texts and were certainly collectors of remedy books. Yet as a broader category, the remedy masters were sometimes criticized, and physicians sought to distinguish themselves by possession of theoretically more ambitious texts and by the quality of their learning.

Further blurring any attempt to draw sharp distinctions between healers are contemporary accounts that associate remedy masters and physicians with spirit teachers and supernatural skills. China's most celebrated historian, Sima Qian (ca. 145–90 B.C.E.), included a biography of the physician Bian Que in the *Historical Records* (Sima 1959, 105.2785–2794). Sima tells us that Bian Que gained his healing powers not through study but from taking drugs received from a mysterious stranger he served at an inn. These gave him great diagnostic skills, including the ability to "see through walls" and presumably into people's bodies (Sima 1959, 105.2785). One can see parallels to this story, including the magical acquisition of healing skills, in the *History of the Later Han* biography of Fei Changfang. (*Hou Hanshu* 1965 82B.2743–2745) (See "A Late Han Adept.")

A Late Han Adept

TJ Hinrichs

Many legends grew up around famous adepts, attributing to them superhuman abilities, often gained from divine teachers. These masters, though in human form, tended to ignore common social conventions, and appeared to society merely as eccentrics. Prospective adepts often demonstrated their potential simply by recognizing the teacher's exceptional qualities, which were imperceptible to ordinary people. Such perspicacity was the basic qualification for receiving occult teachings. Before transmitting their most esoteric secrets, however, teachers often tested students by ordeal. The mundane contexts of these encounters with the occult show us a world that is both capricious and numinous. The interactions of mortals and divinities, and the similarities of their day-to-day concerns, reveal great permeability and interpenetration of the two levels of existence.

The following account of the adept Fei Changfang appears in the biographies of technicians (*fangshu*) section of the official dynastic *History of the Later Han*.

> Fei Changfang was from Runan [in modern Henan]. At one time he was a marketplace superintendent. In the marketplace there was a codger who sold medicinal drugs, and had a gourd hanging over his stall. When the market closed he would jump right into the gourd. None of the market people saw him except for Changfang, who observed it from his [guard] tower's upper floor. Finding this uncanny, he went over and repeatedly bowed, offering him ale and dried meat.
>
> The codger, realizing that Changfang had perceived his divinity, said to him, "You can come back tomorrow." Changfang visited the codger again in the morning, and the old man then took him into the gourd. [Changfang] saw only majestic jade halls with a great abundance of delicious liquors and savory meat dishes spread out inside. When they had drunk their fill they went back out. The codger swore him to secrecy.
>
> Later the codger went to the guard tower seeking Changfang and said to him, "I am a divine transcendent. I was stuck here as punishment for my transgression, but as of today I have served my time and shall depart. Would you like to come with me? Downstairs there is some wine for you by way of parting." Changfang sent someone to fetch it, but they were

unable to budge it. He then dispatched ten men to tote it, but they could not [even] pick it up. When the codger heard about it, he laughed, went downstairs, and with one finger carried it up. The vessel appeared to hold about a pitcherful, yet even with both men drinking from it, in a whole day it was not emptied.

Changfang desired to pursue [the codger's] Way, but was worried that he would be missed by his family. The codger therefore broke a green bamboo measured to match Changfang's height, and had him hang it behind his house. When his family saw it, it seemed to them to be Changfang, and they thought he had committed suicide by hanging. Old and young shouted in alarm, and then encoffined and interred him. Changfang stood [watching] by their side, but none could see him.

Thereupon Chanfang followed [the codger] deep into the mountains, where they trod on brambles and thorns and went amongst tigers. The codger left him all alone there, but Changfang was unafraid. The codger furthermore laid him in an empty room, and over his chest, by a rotten rope, hung a 10,000-catty rock. A multitude of snakes swarmed in and gnawed the rope to the breaking point. Changfang again remained unmoved. The codger reappeared, patted him, and said, "You I can teach." Next, [the codger] set [Changfang] to eat worm-infested excrement. Its extreme stench and vileness repulsed Changfang, and the codger said, "You nearly attained my Way, but with your disgust have fallen short. How can this be!"

When Changfang took his leave, the codger gave him a bamboo staff, saying, "Mount this; it will bear you thither. When you arrive, toss the staff into Ge Lake." He also made a talisman for him, saying, "With this you can control the demons and spirits of the earth." Changfang got onto the staff, and in a moment was returned home. He thought he had left his family ten days before, but it had been over ten years. He took the staff and threw it into the lake, and when he turned back to look, it had become a dragon. His family thought he was long dead and did not believe it was him. Changfang said, "What you buried back then was just a bamboo staff; that is all." So they opened the tomb and broke open the coffin, and there was the staff.

After this [Changfang] was able to cure all sorts of diseases, to beat demons, and to coerce the compliance of the [local] Lords of the Earth [gods]. Sometimes he would be sitting somewhere, and become inexplicably enraged. People would ask why, and he would say, "I was chastising demons for breaking the law."

. . .

Later on, the Lord of the Eastern Ocean visited the Lord of Ge Lake and had improper intercourse with the latter's wife. Thereupon Changfang judged him and imprisoned him for three years, and the Eastern Ocean suffered a great drought. [Note: Dragons, like the one the staff became when Chanfang threw it into the lake, ruled bodies of water and produced rain.] Changfang went to the seaside, and seeing the people praying for rain, he addressed them, saying, "The Lord of the Eastern Ocean committed a crime, and I have immured him at Ge Lake. Today I will release him and make him give you rain." And immediately the rains came.

. . .

Sometime later Changfang lost his talisman, and was killed by a horde of demons. (*Hou Hanshu* 82B.2743–2745; DeWoskin 77–81; also see Campany and Ge 166–167)

Skill in prognosis was an important aspect of medical practice and an extension of the practice of remedy masters inasmuch as their work involved divination (based on different types of calculation according to a variety of calendrical systems) and their association with, for example, spirit or stellar beings.

Such powers could also be useful against demonic entities that caused illness on certain days and in certain places. In these cases, specialists usually appeased or banished the demons through ritual and sacrifice. Besides remedy masters, people commonly called on male and female shamans or spirit mediums *(wu)* for this purpose. *Wu* claimed to have special links to the many deities, nature spirits, and ancestors, whom they could contact and summon by invoking the supernatural beings' secret honorific titles. Shamans used effigies of the gods and demons that had caused the illness to influence the course of the disease, and performed dances, prayers, and songs in healing rituals, sometimes alongside priests and physicians. Some remedy masters and physicians were said to have great powers of divination, in their case through their ability to see the nature and course of a person's illness from the expressiveness of the person's body or to communicate with the spirits. The terms "spirits" *(shen)* and "brilliance of the spirits" *(shenming)* had appeared in Warring States literature referring to divine entities, the gods of Heaven and Earth, or the ancestors; such entities were usually believed to dwell outside the human body, but some sources claim that they also dwelled in the human heart, producing a distinctive kind of radiance and enhanced sensory perception (also referred to as *shenming*) (Kong 1965, 562; *Guanzi* 16 [49 "Neiye"], 3a; see also Knoblock 1988, 145–146 and 252–254).

In Han medical writings *shenming* is used more clearly as a type of perspicacity, although the spirits are still rather freely lodging in the body, able to come and go through its various gates and passes as well as circulate regularly around the interior (*Huangdi neijing lingshu* 1995, 1 [1 "Jiuzhen shi'er yuan"], 1a–1b, and [3 "Xiaozhen jie"], 1a). However much shamans and physicians shared healing ideas and techniques, patrons, and client bases, shamans were distinguished, both among themselves and by others, by their relative emphasis on ritual and distinctive regional religious traditions.

Han period terminology used for healers clearly referred to overlapping categories of practitioners, where shamans were sometimes also known as physicians *(wuyi)*, and physicians certainly had resort to the spirits and ritual practice. Nonetheless, by the end of the Han period scholarly medical treatises had come to deride shamans for their lack of knowledge about the new medicine, the ignorance of their clientele, and, presumably, their failure to own appropriate texts.

Imperial Process

In grappling with the perplexing behavior of illness, Han physicians and medical writers were guided by a new belief in the essential unity of the human body with the state and cosmos and in the resident spirits that provided their potency. The unifying quality of *qi*, linking the smallest phenomena, whether object or experience, with the movement of the stars, the intention of the gods, and the spirits of dead ancestors, mirrors rulers' aspirations for the extension of imperial sway. (See Chapter 1 for the earlier etymology of *qi*.) As administration became more centralized, it fell to the emperor to play a pivotal role in mediating between Heaven and Earth, a task performed mainly through a succession of elaborate rituals. The pursuit of virtue, proper reverence for the ancestors, and correctly performed ritual would ensure the approval of Heaven, conceived as the harmony of the celestial bodies and their deities. Disorder, on the other hand—civil strife, natural disasters, sickness—was a manifestation of Heaven's displeasure. Good government was therefore the expression of a synchrony of contiguous worlds that placed humanity in direct relation to pantheons of local and national gods but which was simultaneously as impersonal and calculated as the divisions of the calendar.

One core way in which *qi* was to be categorized during the course of the Han period was into "Oblique" or "Deviating" *(xie)* and "Physically Upright" or "Proper" *(zheng) Qi*, an opposition frequently invoked in Chinese discourses on morality and ritual in relation to governing the people. Here we see the ways in which Han political theory imagined governance to profoundly integrate individual people into the imperial order. For example, the ancient kings, taken to be paragons of virtuous and effective governance, were said to have used proper music to reinforce political control; harmonious ritual music moderated physical desire, thereby mitigating deviant social behavior and political disorder. Common translations of *xie* in a medical context include "evil," "heteropathy," or "perversity," and there it refers to invading agents, both demonic and manifestations of naturalistic phenomena such as unseasonal wind or damp that caused varying degrees of devastation upon entering the body. In this sense we find what might previously have seemed like ontological causes of disease invading the body conceived of in terms of the new medicine of *qi*, *mo*, and descriptions of the functions of the organs.

In the same way that deviant or proper music could incite or calm the passions, so the nurturing of Upright *Qi* would protect against harmful influences such as pathological Wind or other environmental or climatic irregularities, attacking the body, or indeed moral depravity inducing sickness through demonic possession.

Just as good government and the judicious management of highways and waterways mirrored the divine order of heaven, so too did the healthy body. This was more than just an analogy: all formed part of an interconnected continuum. The power and prevalence of this belief go some way toward explaining why Chinese medical theoreticians showed little interest in following up investigations of the internal physical structures of the body known to them through dissections: their vision of the functioning of the human body rested almost entirely on relationships and correspondences perceived in the external world, with which it formed an indivisible bond. This approach to medicine has been called the "medicine of systematic correspondence" (Unschuld 1985, 51–92).

The homologies between empire and person extended to the internal organs and bowels, taken by medical theorists to interrelate in a manner similar to the bureaucratic offices. *The Basic Questions (Suwen)* of the *Inner Canon of the Yellow Emperor* relates:

> The Heart is the office of the lord and ruler whence the brilliance of the spirits emerge; the Lung is the office of the minister whence regulation and economies emerge; the Liver is the office of the generals of the army, whence strategies emerge; the Gall Bladder is the office of the rectifier, whence judgments and decisions emerge; the Chest is the office of minister and envoy, whence joy and happiness emerge; the Spleen and Stomach are the bureau of storehouses, whence the five flavors emerge. (*Huangdi neijing suwen* 1995, 3.8, 1–1b)

The organs are thus described in terms of official functions and bureaucratic interdependence. In another example, from the political treatise *Discourses on Salt and Iron* (*Yantie lun*, composed ca. 60 B.C.E., concerning court debates over fiscal and frontier policies), the way that the legendary physician Bian Que used the "needling stone" *(zhenshi)* to redistribute and balance *qi* in the body is taken as a model for discussions about government distribution— likely a reflection of the new disparities between the wealthy and the poor.

> Now the crude physician does not know the patterns on the skin formed by the arrangement of the *mo*, the division of blood and *qi;* he blindly stabs yet does not benefit the illness, only damaging the skin and flesh. Now you wish to *cut down on the surplus to replenish the insufficiency,* but the rich grow increasingly rich and the poor grow increasingly poor. By deploying the punishments of severe laws you wish to stop villainy with prohibition and violence, yet villainous plots do not stop. Your intention is not that of Bian Que's use of the needling stone [which carefully adjust the flows of *qi* as prudent policies redistribute wealth], so the multitude have not yet received direction. (*Yantie lun* 1936?, 3)

The flow of *qi* in the body came to be imagined as in need of regulation, as were the highways, waterways, and canals that allowed the smooth passage of traffic essential for the well-being of the empire; disruption to the flow of *qi* had consequences parallel to those associated with the disruption of transportation and called for analogous remedies. By the time of the Former Han, in the second and first centuries B.C.E., similar analogies were widely applied to the fourteen Channels of the acupuncture body. Correlating the circulation Channels of acupuncture with natural waterways, the Yellow Emperor asks Qi Bo:

> On the outside the twelve standard Channels *(jingmo)* are in harmony with the twelve rivers, yet on the inside they correspond to the Five Yin Organs and the Six Yang Organs (bowels). Now, each of the twelve main waterways *(jingshui)* is not the same in size, depth, breadth, and proximity. The volume and quantity of grain that the Five Yin Organs and the Six Yang Organs can receive is unequal. How do they correspond? Now, the main waterways are moved by the water that they receive, and the Five Yin Organs become storehouses as they join with spirit, the soul, and the corporeal soul; the Six Yang Organs are moved by the grain they receive and flourish with the *qi* that they receive. The standard Channels are constructed with the reception of blood and one treats where they conjoin. And may I ask, how does one know how deep to pierce or the

number of moxa-cauteries to apply? (*Huangdi neijing lingshu* 1995, 3 [12 "Jing shui"], 11a–13a)

Han preoccupation with facilitating the movement of goods and people (troops and tax collectors) throughout the empire and with establishing regularities in the calendar for ritual and tax collection purposes found reflection in an unprecedented concern with enumerating and calculating the body and its inner organs and bowels, as well as the physiology of its inner fluids.

The Reckoning Arts

The concepts of Yin and Yang, which had been established during the Warring States period, mostly in the descriptions of changes in the external environment (see Chapter 1), were brought into medical knowledge and practice through the course of the Han period. At heart, this binary divides both space and time; it is the harmonious balance of two complementary opposites (or "complementary opposition") that together makes a whole. Implicit in this conception is the idea that all things have some relationship to one another that can be perceived in terms of degrees of Yin and Yang and their dynamic interactions.

Although, like the Five Phases, the Yin/Yang opposition originally appeared in the context of ritual, by the imperial period it was being systematically applied to all activities, including law, government, and military tactics. Inevitably, it also applied to medicine and health, as evidenced in the tomb texts and treatises of the *Inner Canon of the Yellow Emperor*. Yin/Yang correlations appear not only in physiology but also in etiology (study of the causes of disease). Yin, as noted above, was associated with the inside of the body and the internal organs, and the spatial progression of disease this far into the body was taken to make for serious illness. Hence, reinforcing Yin was an important feature of the health care proposed by learned physicians.

As the binary system demonstrates, there was a strong belief in the power of numbers. Numerology (*shushu*, literally "numbers techniques") applied to the human body, just as it did to celestial patterns. Although no doubt of ancient origins, such concepts had come to the fore during the Warring States period. The external world was regulated by the passing seasons, which in turn were in harmony with the sun and the changing patterns of the night sky. Because of the need to perform vital rituals at precisely the right time, analyzing the rhythms of the cosmos was a core activity in the reckoning arts. This applied to understanding the human body as well as to charting the passing seasons and the movement of stars and planets around the heavens; if it was possible to master the structure of the body and identify its rhythms and patterns, physicians would be able to diagnose problems when illness struck, predict the course of the disease, and determine auspicious times for treatment.

The complex calculation of things considered equivalent and resonant is first evident just before the beginning of the Han period in *Mr. Lü's Spring and Autumn (Lüshi chunqiu)*, an encyclopedia of ritual and statecraft compiled around 239 B.C.E.:

> During the third month of Spring, the sun is in Stomach [Astral Lodge]. At dusk the Seven Luminaries are high in the sky and at dawn the constellation Herdboy culminates.
>
> The correlates of this month are the days *jia* and *yi,* the [stellar spirits] Sovereign Taihao, his assisting spirit Goumang, creatures that are scaly, the musical note *jue,* the pitch standard named Maid Purity, the number eight, tastes that are sour, smells that are rank, and the offering at the door. At sacrifice, the spleen is given the preeminent position.
>
> The paulownia trees begin to bloom, the mole is transformed into a quail, rainbows begin to appear, and the duckweed starts to grow.
>
> The Son of Heaven resides in the right apartment of the Green Yang Bright side of the Illuminated Hall *(mingtang).* He rides in a chariot with *luan* phoenix bells, pulled by gray-green dragon horses and bearing green streamers. He is clothed in green robes and wears green jade ornaments. He eats millet accompanied by mutton. His vessels are carved with openwork and are thus porous. (Lü 1936?, 13 [2 "Ying tong"], 677; Liu 1936?, 11.18a; translation adapted from Knoblock and Riegel 2000, 95)

Later such observations were subjected to a more systematic analysis under the Five Phases theories (Lloyd and Sivin 2002; Needham 1956; Loewe 2004). The number five came to dominate ritual, divination, calendrical analysis, and medicine by the third century B.C.E. The universe could be broken down into sets of five assigned to one of the Five Phases (Wood, Fire, Earth, Metal, and Water); there were five seasons of the year (spring, summer, autumn, and winter, with the extra season of "late summer" added to the traditional four to complete the number); and there were equivalent correspondences with the five directions or locations, the five flavors, five planets, five affects, five primary colors, five body textures, and so on. All phenomena could be attributed to an appropriate phase. In medicine, therefore, there were five main internal organs (liver, heart, spleen, lungs, kidney) and five sense organs (eyes, tongue, mouth, nose, ears). As each season flowed into the next, so each phase was thought to propagate the next, Wood generating Fire, Fire generating Earth, and so on.

The ritual calendar provided a link between the positions of the stars and planets and the kind of human activity that would align the workings of Heaven and Earth harmoniously, with the ruler in a pivotal role. Where the hydraulic and water homologies in medicine, described earlier, imagined *qi* as flowing, the most powerful model for circulation and the idea of an entity moving from and returning to a source location lay in the calculation of the circuits of the heavenly bodies. Correlations and numbers were applied to the Chinese body in many ways. As we have already seen, the *Inner Canon of the Yellow Emperor* records the concept of *qi* circulating around the body, and it does so in a pattern that mirrors the movement of the stars and planets across the sky (*Huangdi neijing lingshu* 1995, 15).

This pervasive culture of calculation during the Han period formed the basis through which physicians, diviners, and spirit mediums made diagnoses and predictions about health. Whether the intent was to identify an illness as the interference of a malevolent spirit associated with a particular day, to ascertain the place of the human spirit or *qi* in the body in order to avoid damaging it with an acupuncture needle or stone, or to discipline sexual activity and pick herbs according to the phases of the moon, knowledge of the calendar and phases of time structured medical activity in the household as well as under the physician's care.

The prohibitions concerned with preserving, improving, and predicting the health of the body were based on a number of different systems for dividing time. The twelve Earthly Branches and ten Heavenly Stems that formed the core of the calendar were the temporal organization for a large body of Han technical literature. In medical literature, the terrestrial branches provided a rubric for a variety of predictions, prescriptions, and proscriptions. (See Figure 2.7.) So too the Five Phases and Yin and Yang systems provided important methods for divinatory and hemerological (the science of determining lucky days) calculations, a key to choosing auspicious times for everyday technical and ritual activities including medical interventions (Kalinowski 2005). By the first century C.E. there were so many traditions for determining prohibitions and for selecting lucky days that Wang Chong (27–ca. 100 C.E.), the voice of Han skepticism, railed against the restrictions placed on ordinary people by adherence to Day Books, almanacs that served as guides to everyday activities. Wang Chong was committed to the proper deployment of the Five Phases as a principle of governance, and his prejudice was directed against their popular application.

Equally these systems were at the foundation of the all-important skill of predicting on what day a patient was to get better, worsen, or die. How to treat a patient, and indeed whether to do so at all, was critical to the professional

Ten Stems

甲	乙	丙	丁	戊	己	庚	辛	壬	癸
jia	yi	bing	ding	wu	ji	geng	xin	ren	gui

Twelve Branches

子	丑	寅	卯	辰	巳	午	未	申	酉	戌	亥
zi	chou	yin	mao	chen	si	wu	wei	shen	you	xu	hai

The Sexagenary Cycle

1	2	3	4	5	6	7	8	9	10	11	12
甲子	乙丑	丙寅	丁卯	戊辰	己巳	庚午	辛未	壬申	癸酉	甲戌	乙亥
jia	yi	bing	ding	wu	ji	geng	xin	ren	gui	jia	yi
zi	chou	yin	mao	chen	si	wu	wei	shen	you	xu	hai

13	14	15	16	17	18	19	20	21	22	23	24
丙子	丁丑	戊寅	己卯	庚辰	辛巳	壬午	癸未	甲申	乙酉	丙戌	丁亥
bing	ding	wu	ji	geng	xin	ren	gui	jia	yi	bing	ding
zi	chou	yin	mao	chen	si	wu	wei	shen	you	xu	hai

25	26	27	28	29	30	31	32	33	34	35	36
戊子	己丑	庚寅	辛卯	壬辰	癸巳	甲午	乙未	丙申	丁酉	戊戌	己亥
wu	ji	geng	xin	ren	gui	jia	yi	bing	ding	wu	ji
zi	chou	yin	mao	chen	si	wu	wei	shen	you	xu	hai

37	38	39	40	41	42	43	44	45	46	47	48
庚子	辛丑	壬寅	癸卯	甲辰	乙巳	丙午	丁未	戊申	己酉	庚戌	辛亥
geng	xin	ren	gui	jia	yi	bing	ding	wu	yi	geng	xin
zi	chou	yin	mao	chen	si	wu	wei	shen	you	xu	hai

49	50	51	53	53	54	55	56	57	58	59	60
壬子	癸丑	甲寅	乙卯	丙辰	丁巳	戊午	己未	庚申	辛酉	壬戌	癸亥
ren	gui	jia	yi	bing	ding	wu	ji	geng	xin	ren	gui
zi	chou	yin	mao	chen	si	wu	wei	shen	you	xu	hai

Figure 2.7. Stems and branches and the sexagenary cycle. Courtesy of Vivienne Lo.

and personal survival of physicians, who were vulnerable to reprisals when, for example, wealthy and powerful clients came to misfortune under their care.

The demonological and spiritual dimensions of Han numerology and medicine have been obscured by successive editors in the received histories. The early and medieval hemerological and medical manuscripts discovered in more recent archaeological finds, however, exhibit rich descriptions of spirit and demonological interventions, showing this to have been an enduring part of the culture of calculations. Scholars and practitioners interpreting the received classical tradition in modern times have mostly chosen to ignore its surviving demonological aspects, much of which have been read as if they were abstract rather than referring directly to the spirit world.

Dynastic Decline and the Rise of New Religious Organizations

Social disruption marked the close of the Han era, and with it came the loss of a centralized government, a hierarchy of nobles, and the ranks of scholarly officials. New, often millenarian religious organizations developed fresh understandings of how spiritual matters caused ill health and new approaches to treatment. Retrospectively labeled as "Daoist" (*daojiao*, also transliterated "Taoist") in the Six Dynasties, these movements had been growing in momentum since the first century C.E. By the mid-second century, Daoist cults of healing such as the Celestial Masters *(tianshi)* blossomed, focusing on the confession of sins, spirit possession, and worship of the deity Most High Lord Lao *(taishang laojun)*, understood to be the divine form of Laozi, the putative author of Daoism's sacred text, *Scripture of the Way and Its Power (Daode jing)*, a book also widely read as a guide to self-cultivation, philosophy, and statecraft. Their techniques built on the practices of shamans—for example, by treating illness with incantation and remedies made with infusions of the ashes of talismans.

The Yellow Turbans, or "Way of Supreme Peace" *(Taiping dao)*, formed one such group, and healing was at the center of their popular appeal. Led by Zhang Jue (d. 184 C.E.), in 184 C.E. they rebelled against prevailing social inequalities. Although the Han dynasty succeeded in suppressing the revolt, the government never recovered and finally disintegrated in 220 as power reverted to competing local governors and warlords. Its final years also witnessed the rise to prominence of another Daoist cult that had been founded by Zhang Daoling in the second century C.E. The cult was led by the Celestial Masters, the healers who claimed that the cause of illness was sin and that the cure lay in confession and acts of charity and public works. Some of our evidence for the healing methods of these movements comes from a text adopted by a number of them, the *Canon of Heavenly Peace (Taiping jing)*, parts of which probably date to the first century C.E. It is an early collection of healing techniques and prescriptions for longevity, including meditation, moral self-cultivation, dietary control, *qi* and breath cultivation, medicinal substances from plants and animals, and talismanic medicine, none of which is associated with any specific author.

This eclectic work stands in contrast to slightly later medical works that attempt to systematize treatments in the acupuncture tradition, structuring them around the acupuncture loci and the channels. The late Han trend of distinguishing religious healing (and its transformations of the self-cultivation traditions in the arts of the bedchamber and exercise/meditation traditions) from a more scholarly medicine based on Yin, Yang, and the physiologies of *qi* was to become increasingly prominent in the work of the bibliographers and in the efforts of physicians seeking to distinguish themselves from spirit mediums, religious masters, and common people. These other groups sometimes likewise distanced themselves from physicians, as is evident in the proscriptions laid out by religious organizations, such as the Celestial Masters, who went as far as banning medicines altogether. Yet despite the visible textual boundaries and social distinctions, the wide range of healing modalities and techniques for cultivating the body available in Han times allows us to begin to imagine a rich and plural medical environment.

NOTES

1. The variety of translations of *xing* provides clues to the range of meanings referred to by the term. "Elements" is a rather materialistic European rendering of the powers of each *xing* (Wood, Fire, Earth, Metal, and Water); "phase" refers to their status as divisions of temporal cycles within a calendrical and seasonal context, and "agency" to their potency in dynamic interaction as an explanatory model for change in the phenomenal world.

THREE

The Period of Division and the Tang Period

Fan Ka-wai

Introduction

The Period of Division, also known as the Six Dynasties for the series of Han Chinese regimes that ruled in the south, refers to the time between the fall of the Han Empire in 220 and unification by the Sui (581–618). After the Han finally disintegrated, the territories it had controlled divided into what became known as the Three Kingdoms (220–280). The Jin Dynasty (265–420) regained hegemony for a short time (280–316), but the subsequent 265 years, the Northern and Southern Dynasties period, were marked again by division between north and south. Most of the Sixteen Kingdoms (316–387) and succeeding dynasties in the north were governed by non–Han Chinese rulers, and it was ethnically mixed northern clans who founded the Sui and Tang (618–906) Empires. The Tang achieved unprecedented heights of power and prestige and maintained contacts not only throughout East Asia but across South and Central Asia. Traders, diplomats, and Buddhist monks traversed these vast regions, exchanging knowledge and goods, including important methods of healing, approaches to medical relief, and pharmaceutical drugs.

Except for the rare work that might be inscribed on wood or stone, books were still duplicated by laborious hand copying. Many books of the Warring States and Former Han periods, known from bibliographies such as that of the *History of the Former Han*, dropped from circulation. Literate physicians and learned aristocrats, though, many of whom practiced healing and life-nurturing arts, edited and annotated Han classics, preserving for posterity those books

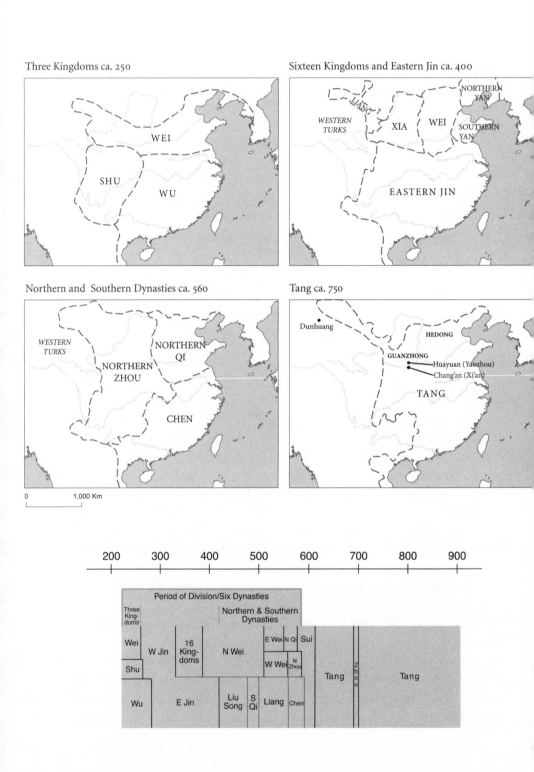

Three Kingdoms ca. 250

WEI

SHU

WU

Sixteen Kingdoms and Eastern Jin ca. 400

NORTHERN YAN

LIANG

WESTERN TURKS

XIA

WEI

SOUTHERN YAN

EASTERN JIN

Northern and Southern Dynasties ca. 560

WESTERN TURKS

NORTHERN QI

NORTHERN ZHOU

CHEN

0   1,000 Km

Tang ca. 750

Dunhuang

HEDONG

GUANZHONG

Huayuan (Yaozhou)

Chang'an (Xi'an)

TANG

200   300   400   500   600   700   800   900

Period of Division/Six Dynasties

Three Kingdoms

Northern & Southern Dynasties

Wei

W Jin

16 Kingdoms

N Wei

E Wei | N Qi | Sui

W Wei | N Zhou

Shu

Tang

Zhou

Tang

Wu

E Jin

Liu Song

S Qi

Liang | Chen

they chose to study and transmit. They also continued developing those traditions, and authored new works in which we can see their innovations.

The chaos toward the end of the Han encouraged the expansion of religious movements and gave Buddhists opportunities to spread their teachings. Healing played a significant role in the rise and expansion of religious groups, which possessed distinctive therapeutic systems and explanations for the causes of disease. Buddhist monks imported South and Central Asian healing modalities. Adepts ("remedy masters," *fangshi*) and members of movements such as the Celestial Masters continued to practice varied transcendence-seeking, life-nurturing, and related healing traditions, and during the Northern and Southern Dynasties period came to be collectively labeled as "Daoist,"

Those Buddhist monks and Daoist priests who sought to convert commoners often pitted themselves against indigenous religious officiants/healers, in the common language labeled "shamans" (or "mediums," *wu*). Thus, the strategy by which physicians sought to distinguish themselves from shamans and marginalize the latter received reinforcement from the missionaries of expanding organized religions. (See "Shamans.") The tendency to demarcate one type of practice or practitioner from others, though, did not inhibit a widespread tendency toward eclecticism: the incorporation and adaptation of ideas and techniques across traditions.

Shamans

Lin Fu-shih

Over the course of the Han period, as we saw in Chapter 2, even though shamans and physicians shared overlapping approaches to healing and elite clients continued to rely on both services, the term "shaman" increasingly came to stand for humble, poor, and illiterate ritual and healing specialists. In contrast to physicians, distinguished by their mastery of universal medical knowledge, shamans were associated with particular indigenous and therefore limited traditions. In their divergence from "high" cultural norms, shamans could be considered deviant; because of their local power, they could be threatening to central control. Thus, shamans occasionally became the objects not only of scholars' and physicians' denigration but also of persecution by local government administrators.

In the medieval period, the proliferating number of Buddhist and Daoist figures—who, like scholars, physicians, and officials, grounded their authority in texts—joined in reviling shamans, criticizing them especially for their "impure" animal sacrifices and for their worship of "demonic" local spirits. Nevertheless, like physicians, Buddhist and Daoist healers held in common with shamans the idea that spirits could cause diseases, as well as responses employing talismans and invocations. All groups' healing rituals could be dramatic, colorful, and even raucous, with such feats as self-mortification, resistance to sword and fire, and the manifestation and killing of bestial demons.

Sources of the period tended to portray shamanic women in "double standard" stereotypes familiar to many cultures: as exotically seductive and corrupting to young men's morals, or, as in the following atypically sympathetic dynastic history account, as vulnerable and virtuous.

> Miss Tu (*fl.* 481) was a native of Dongwuli in Zhuji District [modern Zhejiang]. [Because] her father was blind and her mother suffered from chronic disease, she and her parents were neglected by relatives and not allowed by the villagers to live in their community. She and her parents then moved to live on Mount Zhule far from their homeland. To support her parents, [Miss Tu] gathered firewood and mulberry leaves by day and spun cotton and hemp every night. When her parents died, she personally managed the funerary affairs and carried soil to build her parents' tombs. Out of the blue, a voice in the air announced, "Your extreme virtue is admirable. [I], the deity of the mountain, intend to select you to serve me. [If you assent], you will be able to cure illness for people and, as a result, you will acquire great wealth." Thinking the deity was a bewitching goblin, she did not comply, and so became sick. Over a certain period she cured a next-door neighbor who suffered from brook sprite *(xiyu)* poisoning. After this she too recovered from her illness. Henceforth she used the Way of Shamans *(wudao)* to treat people's ailments, and all of them recovered. Her wealth increased, and many villagers of her hometown wanted to marry her. (*Nan Qishu* 55.960; Lin 1994, 45–46)

Although shamans did not leave their own records, and even though written sources take the perspective of outsiders and are usually hostile, sometimes we see hints of the ways in which shamans such as Miss Tu might have lived and worked. Like ecstatic healers in other parts of the world whose powers derive in part from spirit travel or possession, medieval shamans were often reported to acquire powers not by learning specific skills but by being called by a deity whom they served only reluctantly, often after an ordeal of sickness (Lewis

1971, 59–89; Taussig 1986, 261). Many were marginal figures, and their shamanic abilities helped them find productive, integral, and sometimes even powerful roles in their communities.

Social and Institutional Contexts

The Period of Division, Sui, and Tang were marked by the dominance of aristocratic clans, the rise of organized Buddhist and Daoist religions, and the establishment of medical governance. These social and institutional changes produced new forms for the transmission of medical knowledge, new forms of healing, and new types of healers, all of which left important legacies.

Aristocratic Clans and Civil Officials

From the late Han through the Tang, through the dissolution, fragmentation, and re-formation of so many regimes, governments were largely staffed by a stable group of aristocratic clans. These families maintained their power through the possession of large estates worked by serf-like dependents, by intermarrying with each other, and by inculcating in each generation traditions of learning that gave them the cultural capital and skills to hold high official positions. Period of Division governments recruited them by systems of nomination, reinforcing the class's near-exclusive hold on power. The Sui, Tang, and Tang-interregnum Zhou Dynasty (690–700, with rule by the much reviled empress Wu Zetian) developed civil service examination systems that in some ways reinforced the authority of aristocratic elites but also brought increasing numbers of men from new families into provincial administrations and into the lower tiers of government.

Aristocrats played a central role in transmitting and creating medical knowledge. Why were they so concerned with medicine? As in earlier periods, they were deeply imbued with the sacredness of filial devotion, which entailed caring for one's parents and ancestors, caring for the body they bequeathed, and ensuring the continuation of the family line into the future through progeny. (On medical responses to concerns over reproduction, see "Prerequisites for Treating Childlessness," "Nurturing the Fetus," and "Childbirth.") This multifaceted commitment elevated day-to-day health practices, healing, longevity, and reproduction to paramount concerns, as we can see in their writings. For example, Cui Hao (381–450), a member of the most powerful aristocratic family in the Northern Dynasties, produced the *Dietary Classic (Shi jing)*. Yan Zhitui (531–591), a member of a prominent southern family, devoted a whole chapter of his *Family Instructions of the Yan Clan (Yanshi jiaxun)* to nourishing life. He advised his sons to be vigilant in preventing disease and for cases of urgent need to cultivate basic medical knowledge, specifying study of medical works such as those on acupuncture by Huangfu Mi (215–282) (Yan 1968).

PREREQUISITES FOR TREATING CHILDLESSNESS

Jessey J. C. Choo

Sun Simiao opened his monumental work *Priceless and Essential Formulae for Emergencies* with remarks on the training of physicians in medieval China. He stressed that the mastery of theories of Five Phases, Yin and Yang, Fortune *(lu)*, and Destiny *(ming)*, as well as various divinatory methods, were of equal importance to the command of the medical classics. Sun contended that a physician without such occult knowledge was a man who "sightlessly wandered in the night stumbling each step of the way." (Sun 1992, 1.1) Unsurprisingly, the first advice he gave to couples who desired children was to know their Original Destiny *(benming)*—the various kinds of fortune that Heaven and Earth endowed upon each individual at the time of birth. Sun insisted that medicine could do very little for those fated to have no progeny, and that the efficacy of any treatment hinged on the individual's Heaven-allotted Original Destiny. In other words, medicine could only restore a person to the condition that she or he was born with.

Knowing the Original Destiny was hence central to the prevention and treatment of childbirth-related illnesses and to a child's future well-being. Sun states:

> Those who desire children should first learn the Original Destinies of the husband and wife. Only a couple whose Five Phases are mutually generated *(xiansheng)* and Heavenly Stems auspiciously matched, as well as whose Original Destinies do not have Heaven-Suspending ([*tian*]*xiu*), Heaven-Discarding ([*tian*]*fei*), Death *(si)*, and Grave *(mu)* stars in the Northern *(zi)* [lunar] Palace will be successful in conceiving a child.... Without such due diligence, even if they succeed in having [a child], they will later suffer complications. (Sun 1992, 2.16)

Sun urged those couples whose Original Destinies were favorably matched to follow a series of avoidances and prohibitions so that the child born to them would be "perfect beyond description." He advised couples to avoid copulating on *bing* or *ding* days of the sexagenary cycle (see Figure 2.7); on the first, third, seventh, eighth, fifteenth, twenty-second, and thirtieth days of the month; and during adverse weather, earthquakes, and solar and lunar eclipses. Children conceived at those times, he warned, would be mute, deaf, insane, lame, blind, otherwise infirm, short-lived, unfilial, or cruel. Besides temporal prohibitions, Sun offered spatial ones: sexual activity in certain places—outdoors under the Three Radiances (Sun, Moon, and Stars), inside temples and shrines, and in the vicinity of graves and corpses—could offend important spirits or provoke dangerous ones. Sun concluded that while adherence would result in having smart and healthy children, noncompliance would bring wicked and foolish children and lead to misfortune for the whole family. (Sun 1992, 27.490)

Sun's treatment of childlessness epitomizes the importance of cosmological considerations not only in medical training but in everyday life as well.

Nurturing the Fetus

Sabine Wilms

Pregnancy is a time of great hope, but it also brings concern for the well-being of the mother and child. Prenatal care was not only an arena of oral household traditions or illiterate midwife specialists. Literate physicians developed models of the physiology of pregnancy and fetal development that informed their methods for "nurturing the fetus" *(yangtai)*. The earliest known work of this genre, the *Book of the Generation of the Fetus (Taichan shu)*, was lost, but later was found among the Mawangdui manuscripts from the second century B.C.E. (see Chapter 1; book translated in Harper 1998, 372–384). Another important work, with even more elaborate illustrations, is the *Classic of Childbirth (Chanjing,* fifth-sixth century C.E.). The *Classic of Childbirth* similarly disappeared from the textual tradition in China, but its text and illustrations come down to us as quoted in a tenth-century Japanese compendium of Chinese medical texts, *Formulae from the Heart of Medicine (Ishinpō)*.

The illustrations depict the progression of pregnancy from month to month, showing a naked female body drawn in fine lines. The figures depict overall changes in the woman's form, from the increasing size of her thighs to the

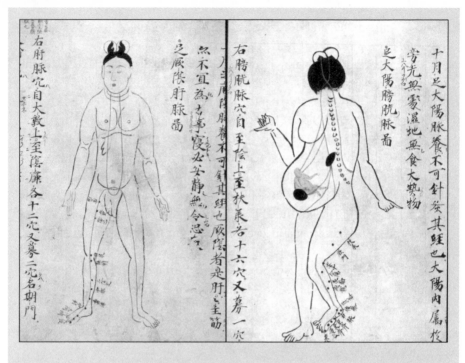

Figure 3.1. *Classic of Childbirth*, months one and ten. Mayanagi Makoto has convincingly argued that these two drawings were copied from the *Classic of Childbirth* by the compiler of the *Formulae from the Heart of Medicine*. While the illustrations include red lines that could have been added by the Japanese compiler, the black line drawings as such appear to be Chinese in origin. Seikaido Library scroll, 1145 C.E. Courtesy of Li Jianmin.

curvature of her back and her painfully protruding belly, emphasized by the sideways perspective in the drawing of the last month. The body is transparent, revealing the normally hidden interior. Inside, we see a fetus (which gradually evolves from a dot into a monkey-like and then human figure) and anatomical features that appear to depict the internal organ responsible for nurturing the fetus in the given month. Symmetrical pairs of red lines link the fetus in the womb to a number of points marked on the body's surface in the extremities, as well as to the head or neck.

The supplementary text offers month-by-month information on the development of the fetus, on behavioral and dietary recommendations and prohibitions, and on the Channels that nurture the fetus. It identifies the points marked on the body's surface as precluded for acupuncture or moxibustion during the given month of pregnancy because of danger to the fetus. The text's description of the course of the Channels is incongruent with the position of the red lines in the drawings, so scholars still debate whether those lines were meant to correspond to the Channels mentioned in the text and therefore to acumoxa

Channels. Some argue that the lines could even be additions by the Japanese editor of the original Chinese source, therefore reflecting a Japanese tradition of acumoxa or gynecology. Because the Chinese source text is lost and no other depiction of pregnancy exists from this early period, the controversy has yet to be settled.

Medieval formularies such as Sun Simiao's *Priceless and Essential Formulae for Emergencies* supplemented this information with correlations between the months of pregnancy, the Five Phases, and the internal organs according to the theory of systematic correspondences; detailed descriptions of fetal development; and complex medicinal formulas for the prevention and treatment of pregnancy-related disorders.

In "nurturing the fetus," early and medieval physicians' classical medical training made them attentive to physiological transformations through time; to methods of preserving and nurturing health, not only curing disease; and to matters of daily hygiene, especially diet. They gave great priority to prenatal care and childbirth, as we can see in the ways in which they systematized their knowledge and devoted entire books to it.

CHILDBIRTH

Jen-der Lee

Childbirth may have been the most important experience of women in traditional society. The behaviors prescribed for women before, during, and after delivery tell us much about the medicine of the period and about women's roles in this patrilineal society.

While earlier recommendations varied, by the eighth century medical texts came to focus on the last month of pregnancy and the first month after delivery as especially critical. These texts advised the expecting mother to take herbal medicines of a "slippery nature" only in the last month of pregnancy to ensure a quick and safe delivery, and instructed her family to prepare a place for the childbirth according to "delivery diagrams." These showed, for example, the proper locations and directional orientation of a tent specially set up for delivery, squatting positions for labor, and burial of the placenta, with different configurations depending on the month of the year. People believed that powerful spirits circulated through various places in and around the house, making it essential to avoid those locations (and those spirits) during the

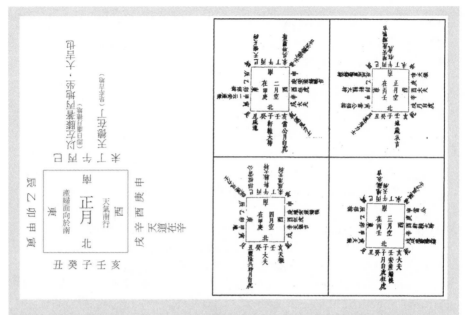

Figure 3.2. *Left:* Childbirth diagram for squatting positions in labor (the first month). Reconstructed by Chen Shiau-yun based on *Chanjing* of the sixth century C.E. Lee, *Nüren de Zhongguo yiliaoshi*, 2008, p. 82. *Right:* Integrated diagram for childbirth in the seventh-century *Cuishi chantu* (for the first four months of the year). Wang, *Waitai miyao*, 1964, pp. 927–928.

stages of childbirth. Although medical texts sometimes emphasized certain marvelous midwifery techniques, most also warned that indiscretions toward the spirits could bring harm to mother and child.

Male-authored medical texts after the sixth century sometimes accused female attendants of hasty and unnecessary interventions. However, most deliveries were handled successfully through the cooperation of women, including the pregnant mother, her female relatives, and midwives. Women usually assumed squatting positions during delivery, either clinging to fastened ropes or supported under the arms by midwives.

Responses to complications such as breech presentation included both manual manipulations and ritual techniques, and they brought attention to the father's importance in delivery and the resonant relations between him, his wife, and their baby. Doctors employed methods such as scratching with fingernails or poking with needles to make the child turn back around by itself. They wrote the father's name on the fetus's sole to cause the child to emerge smoothly. On the basis that the fetus would recognize its own father, they had mothers swallow a pill made of cinnabar paste combined with the husband's pubic hair, maintaining that the child would then correct its movements and emerge holding the pill in its hand.

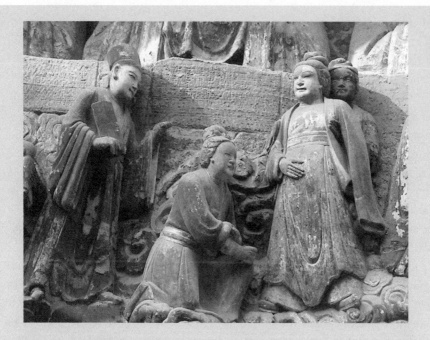

Figure 3.3. Sculpture showing vertical position in delivery. Dazu, Sichuan, twelfth century. Courtesy of Jen-der Lee.

During the month right after the delivery, the new mother would be kept from social contact. This seclusion was due both to her need for time to recover and to fears that she was polluting, either because she had shed blood in the delivery or because she had changed roles from wife to mother. Still, the confinement did give her a chance to rest. Friends and relatives would bring over precious and nutritious food to "nourish her body," medical texts reported, "not just to celebrate the child."

Most aristocratic clans were followers of Daoism and aspired to transcendence or at least to extending their life span. To do so, they needed to acquire a thorough understanding of treatments for different diseases. But they did not feel a need to draw clear distinctions between these different parts of their lives. Ge Hong (281–341) and Tao Hongjing (456–536) were members of important clans who became famous for their Daoist learning—Tao was a prominent priest— and also compiled collections of medical remedies that included discussions of medical topics. In his work *Medical Remedies (Yaofang)*, the renowned Southern Dynasties aristocratic physician Yang Xin included the quintessential Daoist therapy of ingesting the ashes of burned paper talismans dissolved in drinking water. Some major aristocratic medical writers also studied with Buddhist monks. Cui Yu (Northern Wei), a member of the Cui clan of Qinghe, began his career after a chance encounter with a monk. He took in many students who also went on to win fame, and his descendants practiced medicine as well.

During the Six Dynasties period, medical knowledge and skills were transmitted mainly through familial and, less commonly, extrafamilial apprenticeships; officials in the nascent medical bureaucracy sometimes spread their knowledge more widely. We find all three modes of transmission exemplified in the Xus of Donghai. Xu Xi of the Eastern Jin dynasty (317–420) learned medicine from a Daoist priest and went on to found a family tradition. While many of his descendants joined the government as regular officials, in the Song and Qi dynasties they also served emperors, aristocrats, and government officials as physicians. They produced Xu Zhicai's (505–572) *Tested Formulae Transmitted by the Xu Family for Eight Generations (Xuwang bashi jiachuan xiaoyan fang)* and *Secret Formulae Transmitted by the Xu Family (Xushi jiachuan mifang)*. Such texts were usually transmitted only within families. Outsiders might have heard of the titles but rarely had occasion to read the works in their entirety. The Xus' works nevertheless appeared in the *Sui History (Suishu)* bibliographical monograph and were quoted in major Sui and Tang medical works. The Xus were especially known for their skills with Cold Damage epidemic disorders, a new southern disease known as foot *qi (jiaoqi)* (see below), the treatment of children and women, and the production of pharmaceuticals including "immortality pills." They were famous for a remedy popular among elites during the Period of Division called Five Minerals Powder or Cold Food Powder *(hanshi san),* referring to the need for patients to consume cold food after taking it because it led to an increase in body temperature.

In the Tang a number of civil officials took an active interest in medicine because of the danger of demotion, which often entailed being sent to southern jurisdictions. Tang officials came mainly from northern families and were vulnerable to the diseases they encountered in the south; many died at their new posts or even on the way to them. Wang Tao (ca. 690–756), for example, wrote that on his way to a southern posting, he found that many of his fellow travelers fell ill but were able to recover thanks to medical books they consulted. This convinced Wang to write a book of his own geared to easy reference during times of urgent need: *Secret and Essential Formulae from an Outer Censor (Waitai miyao fang).*

Tonics, many of which were mineral-based and potentially toxic, were widely used and studied by Tang bureaucrats. Wang Tao, citing the works of several fellow officials, wrote on the dangers of brews made from pulverized stalactites, and on treatments for the poisoning that sometimes resulted from their use. Other officials explained how to distinguish poor-quality stalactites from high-quality ones. Some, while acknowledging the harmful effects of the former, also reported that the latter could produce smooth internal flows of *qi* and relaxation.

Traders, Students, and Envoys

We know that many traders, envoys, students, and Buddhist monks traveled to and from China during the Period of Division and Tang. Travelers brought drugs and books, and often took the same back with them. For example, in 803, the kingdom of Silla (located on the Korean peninsula) sent envoys to Chang'an specifically to copy a collection of medical recipes. Heian Japanese physician Tanba Yasuyori's 984 *Formulae from the Heart of Medicine (Ishinpō)* included quotations from numerous Period of Division and Tang texts.

Materia medica (compilations of information on medicinal drug ingredients) of the period include many South and Central Asian drugs. We know that the Tang produced at least two works devoted to pharmaceutical resources from abroad: *Overseas Materia Medica (Haiyao bencao)* by Li Xun, who was of Persian origin, and Zheng Qian's *Materia Medica of Northwestern Barbarians (Hu bencao)*. The Tang court's *Newly Compiled Materia Medica (Xinxiu bencao)* included such imports as *ferula communis, terminalia chebula retz*, theriac *(diyejia)*, and various aromatics (Schafer 1985). Theriac was introduced into China by Nestorian missionaries and presented as tribute from Byzantium (Schafer 1985, 184). The major transportation routes were along the so-called "Silk Roads" of Central Asia. Dunhuang was a major stop for these travelers, and in the early twentieth century modern scholars found sealed in its cave complexes a great cache of manuscripts that included many medical works (Lo and Cullen 2005). (See Figure 3.4.)

Buddhism

Three types of medical texts reflecting South Asian influence stand out in the *Sui History* bibliographic monograph: those identified with Hinduism, such as *Remedies of Brāhman Deities (Poluomen zhuxian fang)* and *Brāhman Pharmaceutical Remedies (Poluomen yaofang)*; those that refer explicitly to Buddhist origins, such as *Pharmaceutical Remedies of Bodhisattva Nāgārjuna (Longshu pusa yaofang)* and *Bodhisattva Nāgārjuna's Methods for Nurturing Nature (Longshu pusa yangxing fa)*; and those written by Buddhist monks, which included works on acupuncture, tested prescriptions, and diseases treated with Cold Food Powder.

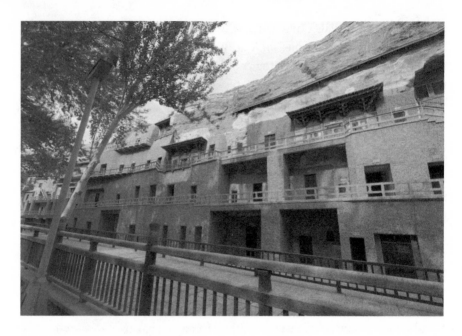

Figure 3.4. Mogao Caves at Dunhuang. Courtesy of Fan Ka-wai.

As a result of Buddhism's expansion, medical concepts embedded in Buddhist texts such as the Four Elements (Earth, Water, Fire, and Wind) and theories explaining disease according to karma and retribution assumed profound importance. In Buddhist writings, the human body was made up of the Four Elements, with illnesses and diseases attributed to discord among them. Each element could trigger 101 diseases, adding up to a total of 404. This idea appeared not only in Buddhist works but also in three key medical texts that attempted to reconcile Four Elements with Han Five Phases theory: Chao Yuan-fang's (550–630) *Comprehensive Treatise on the Origins and Symptoms of Diseases* (*Zhubing yuanhou zonglun,* 610), Sun Simiao's (d. 682) *Priceless and Essential Formulae for Emergencies (Beiji qianjin yaofang),* and Wang Tao's *Secret and Essential Formulae from an Outer Censor.* Sun Simiao also recorded Buddhist curative incantations and the prescriptions of the renowned South Asian physician Jivaka in his own book.

Central values of Buddhism such as benevolence and compassion exercised a noticeable influence on medicine, with notable physicians including Sun Simiao among those who emphasized their importance in medical ethics. Sun advocated, for example, that "when the sick come and ask for help, a physician should not concern himself with whether they are of high or low social position, rich or poor, old or young, pretty or ugly, enemies or friends, Chinese or foreigners, stupid or wise. They should be treated equally, as if they were the physician's close relatives." He also advised that if it was necessary to use animal-derived substances as medicine, physicians should wait until the animals died naturally before buying the carcasses on the market (Sun 1997).

Many hagiographies of eminent monks described their successes in treating patients. During the Eastern Jin Dynasty, for example, the monk Yu Fakai from Khotan in Central Asia proved proficient in applying South Asian medicine, and stated that medicine served two purposes: first, to help oneself, and second, to help others. Chinese Buddhist monks also developed life-nourishing practices derived from South Asian medicine and from indigenous traditions. Tang emperors such as Taizong (r. 626–649) and Xianzong (r. 805–820) recruited monks from South Asia to make longevity pills. Ironically, although some of these monks possessed great medical skills, others were criticized for treating people in an unskillful manner, leading Emperor Guozong (r. 649–683) to ban Buddhist monks and Daoist priests from practicing medicine.

Buddhist temples provided philanthropic medical services and dispensed medicines for the poor. In his list of what should be stored in a temple, Tang monk Dao Xuan (596–667) logged supplies such as needles and knives, and medical books, including works on acupuncture, prescription texts, pulse canons, rhyming guides to drugs, and *materia medica*. Temples that stored large quantities of drugs sometimes functioned as hospitals, taking in the indigent sick. They also looked after people who suffered from serious skin problems such as *lai* (a disease of skin ulcers with pustulent discharge).

During the Tang period, Buddhism became increasingly popular. Temples owned large tracts of land, which allowed them to set up and maintain "Compassionate Field Homes" (*beitian yuan* or *beitian fang*) to treat and feed poor patients. Between 701 and 704, Empress Wu Zetian, a devout Buddhist, sponsored many such homes. Tax exempt, Buddhist institutions eventually became so powerful that they undermined the state's revenue base, and Emperor Wuzong (r. 840–846) broke up the great temples, returning their monks to the laity, restoring their lands and tenants to the tax rolls, and removing Compassionate Field Homes from their management, converting them into "convalescent homes" (*yangbing fang*).

Buddhist philanthropists also had medical recipes, or formulas, inscribed on stone and displayed in order to give more people access to medical knowledge; even illiterate travelers could make rubbings from these inscriptions. An extant example from between the late Northern Dynasties and early Tang, known as the *Longmen Formulary (Longmen yaofang)*, was engraved on a stele

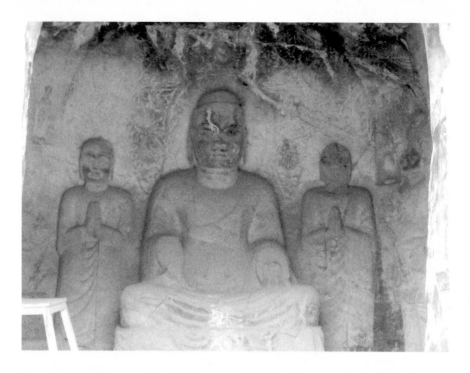

Figure 3.5. Buddhist statues from the Longmen medical formulary grotto. Courtesy of Fan Ka-wai.

that was erected in one of the Buddhist grottos at Longmen. It included about 140 entries and covered subjects such as internal medicine, surgery, treatments for women and children, and madness. It described the preparation of pills, powders, plasters, potions, and salves, all made with ingredients easily collected by common people.

Buddhism also influenced personal hygiene by encouraging practices such as bathing and tooth brushing. Buddhists scriptures mentioned instances of diseases being cured through bathing, and Buddhists taught that baths could dispel malefic Wind from the body, harmonize the Four Elements, prolong life, and cure diseases. Under these influences, hot springs became popular. In his *Annotated Classic of Water (Shui jingzhu)*, Li Daoyuan (Northern Wei, d. 527) listed thirty-eight hot springs and pointed out that most of them could heal diseases. During the Tang, government funds paid for the maintenance of public hot springs. Emperor Xuanzong (r. 712–756) was notorious for bathing in the Huaqing Palace springs with his concubine Yang Guifei (719–756), a woman infamous in legend as the femme fatale blamed for the devastating An Lushan Rebellion (755–763). (See Figure 3.6.)

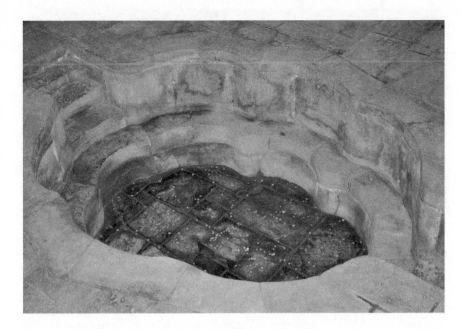

Figure 3.6. Springs at Tang Huaqing Palace, Chang'an. Courtesy of Fan Ka-wai.

Daoism

During the Period of Division, the practices of various adepts, religious lineages, and movements began to be treated as belonging to a more coherent set of traditions that came to be known as Daoist teachings *(daojiao)*. Intensifying competition for followers and patronage provoked contrasts with Buddhists, making the common ground of diverse indigenous groups more obvious. Systematizers and scholars such as the Liu Song Dynasty's Lu Xiujing (406–477) and the Liang Dynasty's Ruan Xiaoxu (479–536) assisted the process by combining the works of these scattered groups together into single collections and categories: Lu in his edited compilation of Lingbao sect scriptures, Ruan in his catalog classification "Records of Transcendents and Daoists," under which he grouped "scriptures," "dietetics," "arts of the bedchamber," and "talismanic diagrams." Daoist texts could be devoted to strictly religious topics such as liturgies or codes of priestly and lay behavior, but they also included *materia medica,* collections of medical remedies, instructions for talismanic cures and exorcisms, and methods for circulating *qi* such as breathing meditation, guiding and pulling exercises, and massage. (See "Ingestion of the Five Sprouts.")

INGESTION OF THE FIVE SPROUTS

Gil Raz

The Daoist lineages that appeared beginning in the late second century tended to eschew medical practices such as acupuncture and the ingestion of medicines, viewing these techniques as merely treating secondary symptoms. Both physicians and Daoists subscribed to correlative cosmology and viewed the human body as homologous to the cosmos, but medieval Daoists developed more esoteric notions to explain and manage the intricate patterns that linked humans and the Way (Dao). For Daoists health was not the final objective but an important basis of the higher soteriological goal of transcendence. They thus sought direct communication with the Way, the fundamental unity that, through the emanation of *qi,* the most ethereal and elemental material aspect of the world, generated the myriad manifestations, processes, and patterns that constituted the cosmos. It was by interacting with the subtle and refined potencies of the Dao that the bodily microcosm could be harmonized with the macrocosm, thereby leading to transcendence. Daoist techniques for cultivating *qi* included dietary regimens of minerals and herbs, sexual practices, and alchemy.

The most basic forms of Daoist cultivation, however, involved methods for absorbing and circulating the *qi* (vital pneumas) of the macrocosmic celestial matrix, with its regular patterns of transformation, through the microcosm of the human body. Among the most popular of these practices was ingestion of the Five Sprouts *(wuya).* The Sprouts were the celestial effluvia of the five directions at their nascent and most potent moment of emergence, correlated with the temporal, spatial, and mythical scheme of the Five Phases. Ingesting the Sprouts would lead the adept to literally embody the primordial essences of the cosmos. The practitioner would thus refine the body, quit regular foods, and gain access to the deities' powers and abilities.

Several versions of this method are preserved in medieval Daoist texts. One of the earliest examples is found in the *Central Scripture of Laozi (Laozi zhongjing).* The text provides the names of the five directional effluvia, along with the sources from which they are imbibed (see Table 2). These mysterious fonts are in fact saliva glands activated by complex and precise movements of the tongue. Daoists viewed the body as inhabited by a variety of ethereal entities, and the final attainment of Five Sprouts practice involved their control and activation. Practitioners eradicated the "Three Worms," harmful beings that resided within the body but sought to destroy it, and refined their beneficial body spirits. The adept would thereby "become a spirit transcendent and not die; [his name] inscribed with jade characters on gold, he would ascend riding clouds" (*Laozi zhongjing* 18.22a–b).

TABLE 2

The Five Sprouts (in the *Central Scripture of Laozi*)

Direction	East	South	Center	West	North
Sprout	Green Sprouts	Ruby-Cinnabar	Yellow Pneuma	Bright Stone	Dark Shoots
Liquid	Dawn Blossoms	Cinnabar Pool	Liquor Font	Metallic Fluid	Jade Syrup

The *Scripture of Initial Vitality of the Green Sprouts of the Most High from the Cavern of Perfection (Dongzhen taishang qingya shisheng jing)* preserves an intriguing variant. Practiced together by a pair of initiates between the ages of twelve and fifteen, ingestion of the Sprouts caused them to "unify with the spirits." Ultimately, the adepts would "roam with the Five Thearchs," the celestial rulers of the five directions, and "ramble freely among the Three Purities," the even higher primordial emanations of the Dao that were the highest Daoist deities.

Between the late Han and the Six Dynasties periods, one of the great attractions of movements such as the Celestial Masters and the Way of Supreme Peace lay in their claims to protect devotees from the epidemics that ravaged many populations at the time. They attributed sickness to divine punishment for human wrongdoing, and offered disease prevention and cure through confession, repentance, chanting scriptures, prayer, and protective or curative incantations and talismans (Lin 2002). Some groups prohibited medical treatment, insisting that followers rely solely on moral rectification, but many also offered acupuncture and herbal treatments.

The Celestial Brigand and Illness

Donald Harper

The Bureau of the Grand Diviner at the Tang imperial court included specialists in the "occurrence of illness," and in the Imperial Medical Office there was an Erudite of Exorcism. While the Tang elite did not hold the same view of human illness as their kinsmen of the first and second millennia B.C.E., the connection between illness and the spirit world remained ever-present to the medieval mind. Certain forms of illness bore the mark of spirit world interference, which might also manifest itself in other human calamities. The goal of iatromancy—the use of divination and related methods to diagnose and treat illness—was to identify spirits responsible for illness and to eliminate the calamity with sacrifices, exorcistic acts, and talismans.

In 1900 roughly a dozen iatromantic writings were discovered in a cache of medieval manuscripts found near Dunhuang, Gansu Province, in a cave that had been sealed for nearly a millennium. Specialists in iatromancy were responsible for creating these writings, which were intended for everyday use by nonspecialists. They provide invaluable evidence of popular ideas about illness and medicine and must be included among the textual sources for medieval medicine. The longest, with 309 columns of text arranged in twelve sections, has a colophon with the title *Book on the Occurrence of Illness (Fabing shu)* and a copy date of 862 C.E. The manuscript, a paper scroll, was acquired by Paul Pelliot at Dunhuang and is now in the Bibliothèque nationale de France (numbered P2856).

One example of iatromantic diagnosis and treatment from the *Book* illustrates perfectly the nature of medieval Chinese iatromancy. The fifth section explains illness as a function of spirit interference, based on the set of twelve Earthly Branches used in the compound cycle signs assigned to calendar days. (See Figure 2.7.) The section introduction instructs the reader to determine the sign for the day the illness began, to make the image of the spirit identified with the day, and to write in red cinnabar ink the talisman that controls the spirit. The first spirit, identified with the day *zi,* is the Celestial Brigand *(tianzei):*

> If a person becomes ill on a *zi* day, the spirit's name is Celestial Brigand. It
> has four heads and walks on one foot with its tongue sticking out. It causes
> a person to be unable to raise the four limbs; the five organs do not main-

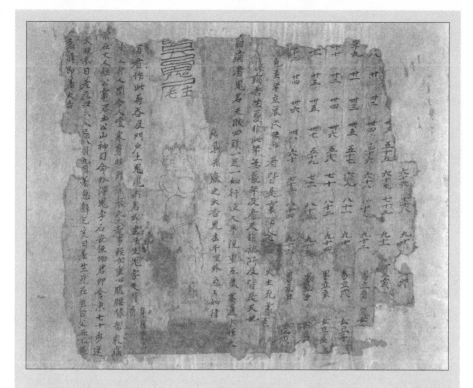

Figure 3.7. An image and talisman for the Celestial Brigand, preserved in another medieval manuscript acquired by Aurel Stein at Dunhuang, and now in the British Library. Courtesy of the British Library.

tain a proper flow; there is edema and the abdomen is enlarged; half of the body is immobilized. It causes a person to suffer violent death. Using the spirit's image to suppress it is auspicious. Write the talisman in red. The ill person may swallow it or attach it over the doorway. Quickly, quickly—in accordance with the statutes and regulations.

Whoever copied the manuscript left blank space for drawings of the twelve spirits, but the drawings were never made. Fortunately, the image and talisman for Celestial Brigand are preserved in another medieval manuscript acquired by Aurel Stein at Dunhuang, now in the British Library (numbered S6216). (See Figure 3.7.)

Images of spirits and talismans are often associated with medieval Daoist religion. Yet iatromancy, as documented in the Dunhuang manuscript copy of the *Book,* has roots in common religious practices that preceded Daoist religion. The Celestial Brigand, the image, and the talisman derive from this ancient religious core. The *Book on the Occurrence of Illness* and other Dunhuang iatromantic manuscripts reveal an important aspect of medieval medical knowledge at the same time as they show us religious healing in everyday practice.

In the quest for the god-like state of transcendence, which became irrevocably associated with Daoism, some adherents tried the alchemical concoction of elixirs using such expensive and often toxic ingredients as gold, mercury, cinnabar *(dan)*, sulfur, and arsenical compounds. Blood-red cinnabar, a mercury ore that had a long association with vitality, came to stand metonymically for elixirs and for alchemy in general. The highly complex and ritualized processes by which these alchemical mixtures were created were generally understood to reverse cosmogonic processes so as to return to a more primordial and perfect state (Ware 1966; Campany and Ge 2002; Pregadio 2006). Many of those who imbibed these elixirs, including a number of emperors, died, something that could be interpreted as successful metamorphosis and release from the world. During the Tang, "external" alchemical methods became fully internalized, so that adepts visualized, for example, the crucible and production of elixir in their bodies but did not actually create the elixir in the outer world. (See "Legendary Daoist Women" in Chapter 4 and "Female Alchemy" in Chapter 6.)

Daoist salvation, whether aiming to lengthen life and ensure a good afterlife or focused on the achievement of divine transcendence, built on a foundation of physical wellness, and physicians and Daoists borrowed extensively from each other. Daoists produced two of the best-known *materia medica* of the time, Tao Hongjing's *Annotated Collection of Classics of Materia Medica (Bencao jingji zhu)* and Li Hanguang's (Tang) *Guide to the Meaning of Materia Medica with Pronunciations (Bencao yinyi)*. The Sui and Tang Imperial Medical Offices included a Department of Incantations and Talismans that used and taught Buddhist and Daoist rituals. Sun Simiao saw no difference between the beneficial effects of medical decoctions, acupuncture, talismans, and incantations, and included a substantial section on apotropaic measures in his *Priceless Supplemental Formulae (Qianjin yifang)*.

Sun Simiao

Victor Xiong

Historical records show the physician, herbalist, and Daoist Sun Simiao to have been active mainly in the Guanzhong area, with close ties to the Tang court early in the dynasty. He was said, though, to have repeatedly declined official appointments. Sun's approach to medicine was eclectic. He merged longevity techniques—including dietary regimens, breathing exercises, and alchemy—with traditional herbal, acupuncture, and moxibustion treatments. Like the *Inner Canon,* though, Sun emphasized the primary importance of maintaining good health and preventing disease through proper diet, exercise, and hygiene.

Among Sun's many works, the best-known is the *Priceless (One Thousand in Gold) and Essential Formulae for Emergencies,* so named because "human life is so precious that it is worth a thousand pieces of gold." This book holds a unique place in the history of Chinese medicine as the first encyclopedic work on therapeutics. Completed in 652 C.E., it comprises thirty chapters covering 232 categories and more than 5,300 remedies. In its introductory chapter Sun lays out general principles of medical practice, including ethics, treatment, diagnostics, prescriptions, and the application of medicine. In the main body of the work he pays particular attention to gynecological and pediatric medicine and deals with themes as varied as external medicine, epidemics, and treatments for poisoning and other emergencies.

About thirty years later, probably shortly before his death, Sun completed a sequel to the *Priceless Formulae.* Entitled the *Priceless Supplemental Formulae (Qianjin yifang),* the work gathers more than 2,000 additional prescriptions in thirty chapters. Of particular value is its extensive coverage of 853 largely herbal pharmaceuticals. Proceeding along the lines of a *materia medica,* it deals with these herbs' attributes, areas of distribution, harvesting, and application.

Sun's search for cures for illness and perfect health show the influence of Daoism. He sojourned on Mount Emei in Sichuan to alchemize the "Great Monad elixir of the divine essence" *(taiyi shenjing dan).* Taiyi is an ancient astral god, often identified with the Polestar or Heaven. In Daoism, it also refers to the original primordial state of the cosmos, and is identified with the Dao itself. This elixir is reminiscent of the Daoist longevity drugs so popular among Tang royals. In a chapter entitled "Interdiction Classic" ("Jinjing") in his *Priceless Supplemental Formulae,* Sun also described exorcistic rituals and demonic medicines, some of which are likely of Daoist origin.

In medieval China, medicine was strongly influenced by South Asian ideas and methods, including occult practices. Sun's writings show knowledge of South Asian massage techniques and describe treatments borrowed from Buddhist works. Some of his exorcistic formulas were originally in Sanskrit, which was believed to give them efficacy against demons. At the same time, Sun's approaches were rooted in correlative cosmological traditions that drew parallels and connections, for example, between the four seasons and the four extremities of man, and between the Five Phases and the Five Viscera. In a similar macro-/microcosmological vein, in Sun's work we see the idea that just as areas stricken by disasters can be succored, so can diseases in human bodies be cured.

Sun Simiao achieved fame in his own time for his remarkable abilities and erudition. He left subsequent generations the invaluable resource of his medical works and eventually achieved legendary and even divine status as the "King of Medicine."

Daoist practices included the activation through visualization of the many spirits understood to be part of the body, such as spirits that reside in and maintain the proper functioning of each of the viscera. Daoists believed the body was born not only with beneficent spirits but also with antagonistic ones: the Three Corpse Worms (sanshi[chong]), which resided in each of the body's three Cinnabar/Elixir Fields (dantian), one in the head, one in the middle of the chest, and one in the abdomen below the navel. In contrast to the other body spirits, which contributed to the health of the body unless weakened, the Corpse Worms actively sought the death of their host so that they could be freed to feed on others' ancestral offerings. To bring about an early death, the upper Corpse Worm tried to incite such unhealthy and immoral urges as ambition, the middle one attempted to promote gluttony, and the lower one provoked lust. The Corpse Worms were understood to emerge on the gengshen night, the fifty-seventh of the sexagenary cycle, during sleep, when the boundaries that separate the person's internal spirit world from the external spirit world become more permeable. (See Figure 2.7.) The Corpse Worms would ascend to the Jade Emperor's court, report on the person's misdeeds, and ensure that the requisite days be deducted from his or her life. People gathered to hold vigils on gengshen nights to help each other stay awake, and to hold rituals and drink medicines intended to kill the Corpse Worms. These gengshen observances were less common in China after the Tang, but became popular at the Heian court and persisted in Japan into the twentieth century (Kubo 1956, 1961; Kohn 1995).

Medical Governance

The Southern Dynasties had medical offices, but they were short-lived and poorly defined. The Northern Dynasties established better-organized and functionally distinct medical bureaucracies. The Sui and Tang inherited and built on those northern institutional structures, establishing a Palace Medical Service (shangyaoju), a Pharmacy in the Secretariat of the Heir Apparent (taizi yaozangju), and an Imperial Medical Office (taiyi shu). The Palace Medical Service, working under the command of the Palace Administration (dianzhong sheng), provided medical care only to the emperor and the imperial family. The highest officials in the service were the two chief stewards of palace medication (shangyao fengyu). Their staff included four chiefs, four imperial physicians-in-attendance, twelve pharmacists, thirty apprentice pharmacists, four palace physicians, eight medical assistants, four erudites of massage (anmo shi), four erudites of incantations and talismans (zhoujin shi), and two preparers of drugs. The Pharmacy in the Secretariat of the Heir Apparent, a subdivision of the Chancellery, was responsible for treating the crown prince. In the Tang, the Pharmacy had a director, a pharmacist's aide, an apprentice pharmacist, and a manager of medicines.

Imperial Medical Office duties ranged from training students to producing remedies for the Palace Medical Service and Pharmacy. It was under the Court of Imperial Sacrifices (taichang si) and was administered by imperial physicians and aides, including erudites of general medicine (yishi boshi), erudites of acupuncture (zhenshi), erudites of massage, and erudites of incantation and talismans. The office also administered the herbal garden and managed medicinal tribute from the prefectures (zhou) (Needham 2000). Erudites and their aides taught medical students, who regularly sat for examinations and attended clinical practice. Every practitioner and medical student was tested on a range of works, including *The Illuminated Hall Canon (Mingtang jing), The Basic Questions, Yellow Emperor's Canon on Acupuncture (Huangdi zhenjing), A and B Canon of Acupuncture and Moxibustion (Zhenjiu jiayi jing), Canon of the Pulse (Mojing),* and *materia medica*. Erudites of acupuncture taught such topics as Channels, acupoints, and the "nine needling methods for supplementation and drainage."

Sui and Tang medical institutions drew practitioners from aristocratic families into public medical teaching service, creating new avenues for the transmission of medical knowledge. The Sui and Tang courts were able to collect more medical texts in one place, making it possible for their medical officials to produce more ambitiously comprehensive and synthetic works. Notable Sui works include Chao Yuanfang's *Comprehensive Treatise on the Origins and Symptoms of Diseases* and *A Collection of Classified Formularies of the Four*

Seas (Sihai leiju fang); the Tang court produced *The Illuminated Hall Illustrated (Mingtang tu), Newly Compiled Materia Medica*.

Appropriating Buddhist strategies for making medical care more widely available, Tang emperors Xuanzong and Dezong (r. 779–805) also commissioned *Formulae for Widespread Benefaction (Guangji fang)* and *Formulae for Widespread Benefit (Guangli fang)*, shorter collections of simpler remedies, to ensure that "medicine is easily acquired" by "removing what is superfluous and assembling what is precise and proven." For even greater dissemination, in 746 Xuanzong decreed that important entries from *Formulae for Widespread Benefaction* be inscribed on wooden blocks and posted on thoroughfares.

The establishment of official medicine in the Sui and Tang provided new avenues for the development and dissemination of learned medicine. It brought together erudite physicians, gave them access to imperial libraries, and encouraged them to produce texts geared toward the formal education of groups of students. Knowledge transmitted from father to son and from master to disciple, even when it employed texts, tended to leave much room for oral or even tacit communication. Institutional instruction required medical teachers to formalize knowledge: to organize it into distinct curricular categories, to systematize it for clear explication, and to state information explicitly. In order to reach wider audiences, as Xuanzong and Dezong sought to do through their formularies, medical officials had to produce more simplified and standardized forms of knowledge.

Medical Texts

As medical writers gave more thought to reaching wider audiences and to teaching larger groups, they produced works that have revealed to historians much more information about healing practices and about daily life. At the same time, new textual forms also produced and transmitted new types of knowledge and practice.

Formularies

This period saw the growing production of practical books of therapeutic recipes, or formularies *(fangshu)*. Ge Hong, also famous for his writings on alchemy, in place of the haphazard organization of earlier formularies, introduced a rational structure to his *Formulae to Have on Hand for Emergencies (Zhouhou beiji fang)*, making it more useful as a reference for laypeople. As we have seen, some devout Buddhists and emperors produced, inscribed, and posted collections of simpler, more accessible formulas for laypeople. Some formularies targeted specific diseases, especially southern ones, such as miasma *(zhang)* and foot *qi (jiaoqi)*. Some focused on the care of children and women, such as *Yu's Formulae for Treating Children (Yushi liao xiao'er fang), The Classic of Children's Medicine (Xiao'er jing), Xu Wenbo's Treatments for Conglomerations in Women (Xu Wenbo liao furen jia),* and *Fan's Formulae for Treating Women (Fanshi liao furen fang).*

Perhaps with the development of larger, less personally connected audiences for medical knowledge, writers sometimes made a point of noting that a remedy had been proven in practice *(yan fang),* and many medical books came to use the phrase "collection of tested formulas" *(jiyan fang)* in their titles. On being told that a remedy that used the ashes of burnt beards had been tried and proven, Emperor Taizong trusted it enough to shave off his own beard to prepare medicine for Li Ji (571–649), a beloved official.

In addition to shorter formularies designed for laypeople's practical reference, the period saw the production of works that aimed to comprehensively collect and organize therapeutic knowledge, something more useful to the learned physician, serious medical scholar, or official educator. In this category we find the Sui government's massive *Collection of Classified Formulae of the Four Seas (Sihai leiju fang,* twenty-six hundred scrolls), Sun Simiao's *Priceless and Essential Formulae for Emergencies,* and Wang Tao's *Secret and Essential Formulae from an Outer Censor.* Although the Sui work was lost, Sun's and Wang's were printed by the Song government in the eleventh century (see Chapter 4) and became great classics of the genre. Together, these works assembled thousands of remedies, from which we can learn much not only of Tang medicine but also of daily life. Wang's collection quoted extensively from no longer extant Six Dynasties works, preserving much that otherwise would have been lost.

Consolidation and Annotation of Medical Canons

Books of formularies mainly recorded practical information on how to combine medical ingredients to treat the ill; they seldom discussed medical theory or pathology. For that, I learned physicians of this period relied on the medical classics bequeathed by the Han. In the Six Dynasties classical texts circulated in multiple versions, but during the Sui and Tang dynasties, medical scholars compiled, reorganized, and annotated many of these classics, producing standardized authoritative versions and interpretations.

The *Sui History* listed many versions of the same classical medical texts. *The Yellow Emperor's Basic Questions (Huangdi suwen)* appeared in eight-scroll and nine-scroll versions; *A and B Canon of the Yellow Emperor* appeared in ten-scroll and twelve-scroll versions; *The Yellow Emperor's Acupuncture and Moxibustion*

Classic (Huangdi zhenjiu jing) in nine-scroll and twelve-scroll versions. Early authors had no standardized way of dividing books into volumes, and later generations freely rearranged the books according to their own preferences. Often, different master-disciple lineages also transmitted different versions of a given text. For instance, in the Southern Dynasties, Quan Yuanqi compiled and annotated *Basic Questions*. Quan's version was in turn revised by Yang Shangshan (ca. 575–670) and then Wang Bing (eighth century). Wang Bing claimed he had received a secret version of *The Basic Questions* from Guo Zizhai, which allowed him to add to his version seven chapters *(zhang)* said to be missing since Quan's time. He also added annotations by Xuanzhuzi (a Daoist priest and Wang's teacher), known as *Secret Words of Xuanzhuzi (Xuanzhu miyu)*.

Materia Medica

Tao Hongjing stated that successful medical practitioners all began from a strong foundation in *materia medica*. Generally speaking, books of *materia medica* recorded essential information about medicinal plants, animals, and minerals, including their names, natures (Cold, Heat, Warmth, and Coolness), flavors (Acridity, Sourness, Sweetness, Bitterness, and Saltiness), appearance, the best time and place to pick herbs, how to prepare them for treatment, and what conditions they alleviated.

The *Materia Medica of the Divine Husbandman,* compiled in the Former Han, is widely regarded as authoritative, but there were other sources of knowledge, and not all of them were in accord. In the Three Kingdoms period, Wu Pu's *Materia Medica* listed alternative and even contradictory descriptions, citing legendary sources ranging from the Divine Husbandman to the Yellow Emperor, Qibo, Bian Que, Tong Jun, Yi He, Li Shi, and Lord Thunder (Fan 2004a). A number of books on *materia medica* were written by single authors, and each physician might write his own version in keeping with both the teaching he received from his masters and his practical experience. Tao Hongjing reported there were "four classics and three schools" *(sijing sanjia)* related to the *Materia Medica of the Divine Husbandman*. Noting that the place names used in the book were those current in the Later Han, sometime after the book was ostensibly composed, Tao inferred that Zhang Ji and Hua Tuo had revised and augmented it. Other scholars, including Wu Pu (an apprentice of Hua Tuo) and Li Dangzhi, are known to have revised the book.

Tao Hongjing himself produced a pioneering and influential revision of *Materia Medica of the Divine Husbandman* entitled *Annotated Collection of the Classic of Materia Medica,* adding 365 drugs to the 365 found in the original. He categorized drugs into seven groups: "jade and stones," "herbs and trees," "insects and animals," "grains," "fruits," "vegetables," and "miscellaneous," and many later medical practitioners followed his classification system.

Tao Hongjing's *Annotated Collection* served as an important reference for *A Newly Compiled Materia Medica,* produced by a group of imperial physicians led by Su Jing at the behest of Tang emperor Gaozong (650–683). *A Newly Compiled Materia Medica* became an official textbook and standard manual. According to Tang law, if a physician failed to follow the formula presented in this book and his patient died as a result, he would be subject to two and a half years of imprisonment (although given how few physicians likely had access to the book, it is doubtful that the law was rigorously enforced). This book had special significance, not only because it was the first officially compiled *materia medica* in China but also because it standardized the knowledge of *materia medica* developed since the Eastern Han Dynasty.

Acupuncture

Like *materia medica,* acupuncture practice had a long history marked by competing approaches. By the Six Dynasties, there were already several versions of the seminal acupuncture treatise *Illuminated Hall Classic.* In the Western Jin, Huangfu Mi wrote *A and B Canon of Acupuncture and Moxibustion,* claiming in the preface to have combined the finest parts of *Basic Questions, Numinous Pivot,* and *Essentials of the Illuminated Hall's Acupuncture and Moxibustion Healing (Mingtang zhenjiu zhiyao).* This book became the standard work on acupuncture and an important reference for later generations.

From the *Sui History* bibliography we learn three things about acupuncture knowledge in the Period of Division: first, many works were written in the name of the Yellow Emperor and—what comes down to the same thing—the Illuminated Hall (The *Inner Canon of the Yellow Emperor* places the Yellow Emperor and Qibo in the Illuminated Hall when they discussed the Channels). Second, many books from the Six Dynasties focused on moxibustion, sometimes preferred as a less dangerous alternative to acupuncture. Third, it soon became standard for works on acupuncture to be complemented by illustrations. Zhang Ji, Ge Hong, and Chen Yanzhi all mentioned the importance of combining text and illustrations. Wang Tao said that texts "speak of the essentials of the illness," while illustrations "exhibit the positions of the named acupoints," as one would expect.

By the Tang, as the number of acupuncture textbooks and illustrations in circulation increased and as physicians increasingly shared their knowledge, the contradictions in acupuncture knowledge became obvious. Physicians

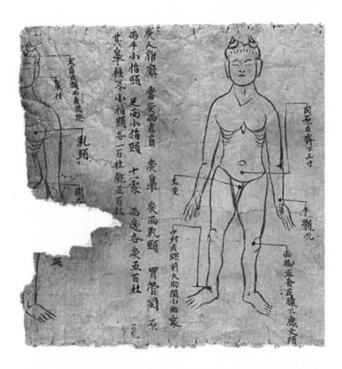

Figure 3.8. Chart of moxibustion methods *(Jiufa tu)*, Dunhuang. Courtesy of the British Library.

assigned different names to the same position and the same name to different positions, and there were different understandings of many points' physiological effects. They often located acupoints in different positions.

Zhen Quan (ca. 541–643) was renowned in the Sui and Tang as an acupuncture systematizer and produced such works as *Acupunctural Remedies (Zhenfang)*, *The Manuscript Classic of Acupuncture* (Zhenjing chao), and *Illuminated Hall Figurines Illustrated (Mingtang renxing tu)*. His compiled version of *The Illuminated Hall Illustrated* was Sun Simiao's principal reference in his own comparisons of pre-Tang acupuncture works.

Sun developed tools to resolve the acupuncture perplexities faced by physicians of his day. His first step was to redraw the figures for *Illuminated Hall Figurines Illustrated*, showing them lying on their back, their stomach, and their side. His second step was to advocate a consistent system of functional names for acupoints, making it unnecessary to separately memorize names and functions. Next, he insisted on matching acupoints and corresponding symptoms ("needling corresponding to acupoints"), listing corresponding symptoms under the names of the acupoints. He also developed the concept of an *"a-shi* point" or what we might call a "touch point," meaning treatment would be applied directly on the spot of pain rather than at a distant but functionally related acupoint along the Channel. Sun made it easier for even untrained laypeople to locate the points of treatment. Sun also advocated the "same-body-inch" *(tongshencun),* using the patient's finger as the standard unit of measurement, immediately eliminating inaccuracies that arose due to discrepancies between measuring systems and bodies of different shapes and sizes. Sun was less an innovator than a shrewd systematizer and popularizer who assembled a coherent program that became a conventional reference for later generations.

New Disease Issues

From the end of the Han to the Southern and Northern Dynasties, China experienced a cooler period, often referred to as a "little ice age," which appears to have contributed to an increase in floods, droughts, and virulent respiratory epidemics, driving mortality rates far beyond their normal levels (Ishida 1992). In earlier times, epidemics had been referred to generically as *jiyi,* or simply *yi,* but late Han and Period of Division physicians gave the subject more attention and made finer distinctions. Ge Hong classified epidemics into three categories: Cold Damage *(shanghan),* Seasonally Spread *(shixing),* and Warmth *(wenyi).* His classification was adopted by physicians of later generations such as Sun Simiao and Wang Tao. The advent of the Tang brought not only greater sociopolitical stability but also a warmer and moister climate. Unification and an established medical bureaucracy, though, allowed the government to record epidemics more regularly, and from those documents we know that outbreaks struck the Guanzhong (modern Shaanxi and Henan) and Hedong (modern Shanxi) regions in the north between 636 and 658. In the century between 790 and 891 the south coast was continually afflicted by epidemics (Twitchett 1979).

At the end of the Western Jin, many fled the chaotic north, heading to Jiangdong (present-day Jiangsu and Zhejiang) and Lingnan in the south. Moving from a dry environment to the damp south exposed these migrants to new diseases, such as foot *qi,* characterized by swelling beginning in the lower extremities and sometimes attributed to bad diet (Smith 2008); miasma, characterized mainly by fever and associated with noxious southern landscapes; and *gu* poisoning, an abdominal ailment that came to be often attributed in this period to a type of witchcraft practiced on visitors by indigenous southerners (Feng and Shryock 1935).

Perhaps due to the increasing importance of scholarship, a trend related to the growth of the civil service examination system, medical works pay more attention to eye problems. Both Bo Juyi (772–846) and Liu Yuxi, prominent Tang poets, had severe eye problems. Sun Simiao listed sixteen causes contributing to the decline of eyesight: three of them were "reading small print in the dark," "reading by dim moonlight," and "copying for many years." South Asian works such as *The Indian Classic That Discusses Eyes (Tianzhu jing lun yan)* and *Bodhisattva Nāgārjuna's Discussion on Eyes (Longshu yanlun)* enjoyed a vogue. Some techniques were fully absorbed into Chinese medicine, although the process inevitably involved reinterpretation and adaptation. A good example is the "golden comb technique" *(jinbishu)* imported from South Asia, which is also known as couching for cataracts *(jinzhen bozhang fa)*. Physicians inserted a sharp needle into the limbus or clear cornea, aiming at the opaque white cataract. Then, with a downward movement, the lens was dislodged away from the pupil. After continuous modification, the technique is still practiced by physicians today (Fan 2005; Deshpande 2000; Unschuld 1985)

Conclusion

The third through the ninth centuries were notable for the increasing circulation of medical knowledge, both throughout the lands governed by the Han and unified again under the Sui and Tang, and between China and other parts of Eurasia. The period also saw the emergence of new groups actively engaged in the development and transmission of medical knowledge: aristocratic elites, Buddhist and Daoist priests, and medical officials. In their teaching and health practices and in their textual productions, these new groups produced new forms of medical knowledge, recorded and embodied in edited and annotated Han period medical classics, and compilations of medical formulas and *materia medica,* leaving important resources for later physicians and scholars. The Sui and Tang medical bureaucracies, medical relief policies, and textual productions also laid important foundations for those of the Song state (960–1279).

FOUR

The Song and Jin Periods

TJ Hinrichs

THE SONG EMPIRE WAS SMALLER and less cosmopolitan, and faced greater external threats than the Tang had. For a few decades after Tang's collapse, no single state rose to recentralize power across the territories that it had controlled. In the northeast, the Khitan Yelü clan unified Manchuria and parts of Mongolia and went on to conquer sixteen of Tang's provinces, founding the Liao Empire (907–1125). Descendants of the Tuoba clan of the Tangut (Xianbei) peoples, who had ruled several of the Northern Dynasties (386–581), established the Western Xia (1038–1227) in the northwest. For several decades various leaders struggled to hold a succession of Ten Kingdoms in the south and Five Dynasties in the northern plains. The last of the Five Dynasties, the Later Zhou, reconquered most of the south and inaugurated the Song Dynasty in 960. In the 1120s, the Jurchen people toppled the Liao and then captured the Song's northern territories, establishing the Jin Dynasty (1115–1234). The Song moved its court from Dongjing (Kaifeng) in the north to Hangzhou (renamed Lin'an) in the south, and maintained control there until they were conquered by the Mongol founders of the Yuan (1206–1368). Historians refer to the period preceding the Jin conquest as the Northern Song (960–1126 C.E.) and the period following as the Southern Song (1127–1279).

With these regime changes came the violence of warfare, famines caused by disruptions to agriculture, and epidemics most likely spread by the movement of refugees and armies. Despite this turmoil, the tenth through the thirteenth centuries saw a doubling of population over Tang levels, perhaps in good part due to relative stability within Song territories and growth in agriculture and commerce, including specialized production of and trade in medicinal drugs. The Song state also expanded programs of poor relief, including medical care,

Ten Kingdoms and Five Dynasties ca. 950

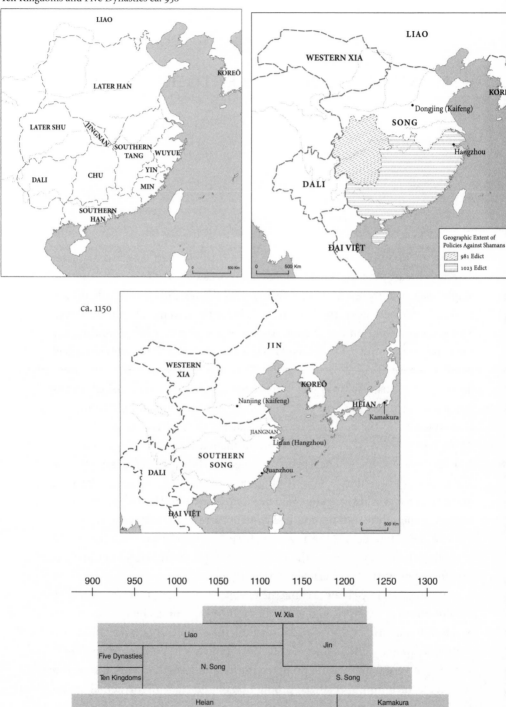

although those policies' demographic impact may have been small compared to those of adequate nutrition and secure livelihoods. Printing and literacy spread, fostering an explosion in medical publishing. Barriers to social mobility were eroded, contributing to the emergence of new types of healers, such as elite scholar-physicians *(ruyi)* and Daoist Thunder Rites exorcists.

Medical Governance

Prior to their displacement from the north by the Jin regime, Song courts and local officials, more than had their predecessors, tended to seek social transformation through centralized state policies, including medical relief and education. Some of these expansions of medical governance occurred as part of such famous institution-building episodes as the Qingli Reforms of 1043–1044, the New Policies of 1069–1085, and the restoration to power of New Policies proponents under Emperor Huizong (r. 1101–1125). These well-known movements, however, merely punctuated a continual growth of state involvement in medicine, already apparent in the first years of the dynasty. While state-centered solutions to social problems generally lost favor under the Southern Song, the 1150s saw another round of expansion of state medical institutions.

Inseparable from social reform, and the underlying rationale for the role of medicine, was the government's responsibility for the material welfare of the people. In its earliest Confucian formulations, this usually comprised proposals for low taxation and for tax remissions after natural disasters. Governments had since at least the Han period distributed medicines to the populace during epidemics on an ad hoc basis, but not until the Song did this become an established policy. In fact, the need for relief was seen as a profound failure: cosmologically, natural disasters were taken to be Heaven's response to misrule; morally, epidemics were punishment for misdeeds; and pragmatically, epidemics were consequences of imperial improvidence. A Tang official thus opposed state medical relief as detracting from the fundamentals of Confucian governance. But, as we saw in Chapter 3, Buddhist establishments strongly reinforced the idea of charity as a basis of morality, and introduced institutions like Compassionate Field Homes for administering medical care to the poor. In many ways, late Tang and early Song policies for distributing medical texts and medicines, and particularly Song charity clinics, drew on Buddhist models (Scogin 1978).

The primary areas of innovation in medical governance were the extension of medical policies and institutions (medical schools, regularization of medical relief) from the center to the prefectural level, and the creation of new institutions for the delivery of medical services (pharmacies and hospitals) and for the production and distribution of medical texts (Bureau for Editing Medical Treatises *[jiaozheng yishu ju]*). The Song state also used medical texts and relief for the novel purpose of reforming popular healing customs in the south.

Institution Building

Some of the most enduring medical departments in government were those dedicated to treating the imperial family. The Song retained the Tang's Imperial Medical Office *(taiyi shu)*, and by 992 had renamed it Hanlin Physician Service *(Hanlin yiguan yuan)* and broadened its functions to include, for example, producing medical texts. The court made it subordinate to the Hanlin Artisans Institute *(Hanlin jishu yuan)*, which also oversaw departments for astrology, divination, and artistic painting. Until 1044, recruitment to the Physician Service appears to have been carried out on an ad hoc basis. As part of the Qingli Reforms, Hanlin Physicians came to be drawn from a bureaucratically endorsed pool (Liang 1995, 99–100; Miyashita 1967, 139; Fu 1990, 220).

The Song also continued the Tang's Imperial Medical Service *(taiyi ju)*, responsible for instruction in medical subjects and clinical practice and certifying physicians for government service. Medical students were tasked with treating their fellow students, soldiers of the garrisons, and residents of the capital, and were graded on their success rates. The Qingli Reforms mandated the creation of Medical Schools *(yixue)* at the prefectural level, and in 1083 medical training was extended from the prefectural to the district level.[1] In contrast to places for forty medical students in the Tang, the Song Imperial Medical Service began with 80, increasing to 161 in 1060 and 300 in 1076. In 1076 the curriculum was expanded from nine to thirteen subjects, including women's and children's disorders, acupuncture, and moxabustion. State medical education thus encouraged functional specialization, which may have contributed to theoretical development in certain fields. For example, in women's medicine *(fuke,* literally "women's department"), female bodies came to be theorized as dominated by Blood (as Yin Vitality) over Qi (as Yang Vitality), and on that basis remedies were differentiated according to patient gender, even for disorders that were unrelated to traditionally female issues such as pregnancy. While in later centuries this therapeutic distinction fell out of favor, the approach focused attention on menstrual regulation as a basis of women's health (Furth 1999, 59–93). Similarly, in children's medicine *(youke,* "children's department"), Qian Yi (1032–1113), an instructor in the Imperial Medical Service, developed diagnostic approaches that took into account children's limited communication skills and the delicacy of their bodies, emphasizing the reading of signs in the face and eyes over verbal interrogation and pulse-reading.

Qian also argued that physicians needed to take children's physiological differences into account, that their viscera were more "weak and fragile and [could] be weakened or strengthened easily, [and] thus they suffer more easily from cold and fever" (Hsiung 2005, 36).

Among the types of medicine taught by the Song state, the one most employed was probably the diagnosis and treatment of epidemics. Imperial medical students were responsible for distributing aid during epidemics. In 992, Emperor Taizong's (r. 976–997) court regularized medical relief for the capital with an edict allocating monies from the annual budget for the purchase of medicines, and assigning ten physicians from the Imperial Medical Office to make rounds among city residents (*Song dazhaoling ji* 1962, 219.842). In the same year Taizong revived the Tang era prefectural medical post, of Medical Erudite *(yiboshi)* (*Tang huiyao* 1991, 82.1806; Okanishi 1969, 713–720).

Local officials seem to have become more active in epidemic relief in the Song. The official Su Shi (1036–1101), still famous for his genius in composition and calligraphy, was also in his own time known for his energy and innovation in public works and welfare. In 1089, as prefect of Hangzhou, Su distributed medicines for an epidemic, following a formula called Sagely Powder that he said had been transmitted to him by a mysterious traveler (Su 1908–1909, 24.11). He also established a hospital for the indigent, which within three years was tending to more than a thousand patients. Su used a Buddhist monastery as a base for these operations and named the hospital Ward of Tranquility and Joy *(anle fang)* after the Buddhist Western Paradise (Hinrichs 2003, 121; Scogin 1978, 32). In 1098 the court followed Su's lead, mandating that poorhouses, charged with housing and feeding the indigent and with distributing medicine, be set up in all prefectures. In 1103 these were put on a firmer financial footing, expanded to accommodate more people, and maintained throughout the year rather than only seasonally. The state also established charity clinics modeled on Su Shi's hospice and called "Tranquility and Relief Homes" *(anji fang)*, each with a kitchen, dispensary, staff physicians, and four administrators (Scogin 1978, 32–35).

As part of the New Policies, the state entered into the pharmaceutical trade. In 1076, the same year that it expanded the Imperial Medical Service, the court created the Pharmacy Service. The new institution consolidated administration and pharmaceutical processing being conducted under separate offices. The Pharmacy Service acquired medicines, prepared them for sale to the public in the capital at below-market prices, and distributed them gratis during epidemics. In contrast to small commercial shops, which mainly packaged raw ingredients for each customer on the basis of physician prescriptions (see Figure 4.5), the Pharmacy Service mainly sold powders, pills, or pastes made to standardized formulae (Liang 1995, 86; Miyashita 1967, 141; Goldschmidt 2009, 123–128).

In 1085 a change of emperor and shift of imperial favor inaugurated a period of reaction and the dismantling of many New Policies institutions. The thirteen subjects of the 1076 curriculum were recombined back into nine, although acupuncture and moxabustion remained separate (Liang 1995, 99–100; Miyashita 1967, 139; Fu 1990, 220). Under Huizong, in 1103 the court restored the New Policies group, renamed the Imperial Medical Service the Medical School (yixue), and restored the number of students to three hundred (Fu 1990, 220; Miyashita 1967, 139). Huizong's court expanded the Pharmacy Service to seven branches in the capital and opened more branches in the prefectures (Miyashita 1967, 141). It had the preset formulas of the Pharmacy Service published in 1107 as the *Formulary of the Pharmacy Service for Great Peace and for the Benefit of the People (Taiping huimin hejiju fang)*. In 1113, it had Medical Schools set up in the circuits, and increased the number of medical students by 733. The Pharmacies and the medical schools were scaled back in 1120 due to the cost of fighting Jurchen invaders. In 1136, after the Song court had reestablished itself in the south, it set up five pharmacies in the new capital, Lin'an (Hangzhou), where Su Shi had founded his hospital and distributed Sagely Powder. In the following years branches of the Pharmacy Service were opened in the circuits, and by 1151 reached a peak of seventy outlets (Miyashita 1967, 139–141; Fu 1990, 226–227).

An important adjunct to epidemic relief in general and the Pharmacy Service in particular was the publication of formularies to guide prescription. For similar purposes, the Song state produced *materia medica* texts, listing drugs and their properties. Besides supporting the Pharmacy Service, Song state medical publishing also sought to disseminate and shape medical knowledge throughout the realm. This aim could have been achieved without printing, but the technology facilitated and perhaps inspired the wide distribution of these texts, which, like medical relief, reached ever broader sections of the populace.

Production of Medical Texts

In European history, printing is often seen as a radical invention that, by greatly accelerating the circulation of ideas, spawned revolutions in both learned and popular cultures. Print certainly contributed to the historical changes of the Tang-Song period, but its emergence was a more gradual process than in Europe. In China, print was a refinement of the ancient technologies of official seals used to imprint documents; stamps used to make talismans; and texts engraved on stelae, from which rubbings could be made on

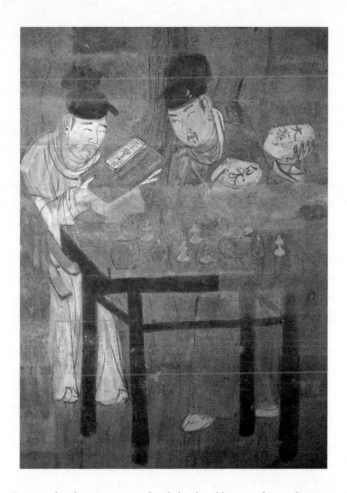

Figure 4.1. Two merchant's assistants, standing behind a table covered in medicine containers, consult a volume of the *Taiping Era Formulary of Sagely Grace*. One holds two packages of herbs, the first labeled "*dahuang*" (rhubarb) and the other "*baizhu*" (white atractylodes rhizome). Portion of a mural showing what appears to be a commercial workshop for packaging medicines for market. From tomb discovered in 2009 near Hancheng, Shaanxi; visited by author in November 2010. Photograph by TJ Hinrichs, with thanks to the Shaanxi Archaeological Institute.

paper. Actual printing, the production of many copies of a text, usually from carved woodblocks, is thought to have first appeared in Tang Buddhist contexts, where the replication of sutras was believed to generate good karma. The Five Dynasties and Song states began using printing in the tenth and eleventh centuries, and commercial printing spread in the eleventh and twelfth centuries (Chia). Printing stimulated the reproduction of existing texts, including works on medicine, and the compilation of new ones for larger markets.

The first known medical text created by and for a court was Chao Yuanfang's nosological work *Comprehensive Treatise on the Origins and Symptoms of*

Diseases of 610 C.E., and the following 350 years saw just four more, two *materia medica* and two formularies. In contrast, in its first two centuries, the Song central government compiled and produced sixteen authoritative editions of medical classics, and produced and printed eighteen new medical texts. Local governments published another twenty-four medical books (Hinrichs 2011).

The first Song court-initiated medical text publishing projects appeared when the Song founders were still completing their territorial conquests and building a new government. As they worked to incorporate and centrally administer territories and peoples, they also moved to centralize medical knowledge and the management of medical relief. The early courts therefore commissioned and printed encyclopedic works, collecting information on drugs and remedies from throughout the empire, and redistributing this knowledge to key offices. Amid ongoing military resistance (the last resisting state fell in 979) and while also printing a new legal code, Emperor Taizu's (r. 960–976) court commissioned the *Kaibao Era New and Detailed Definitive Materia Medica* (*Kaibao xinxiang ding bencao,* 973, revised and republished 974). It contained 983 drug descriptions, contrasted to 850 in the Tang state's 659 C.E. *Newly Compiled Materia Medica* (Unschuld 1986, 47, 55–60). As its title shows, they sought to create an exhaustive, authoritative work.

The court of the second emperor, Taizong (r. 976–997), is perhaps most famous for establishing firm civil control over the military and strengthening the objectivity of the civil service examination system. Taizong himself collected medical formulas, and, putting out a call to gather remedies from throughout the empire, had a team of court-appointed physicians compile them into the mammoth *Taiping Era Formulary of Sagely Grace (Taiping shenghui fang),* a project that took a decade to complete. In contrast to the Tang court-commissioned *Formulae for Widespread Benefaction (Guangji fang)* and *Formulae for Widespread Benefit,* each of five chapters, *Taiping Era Formulary* had one hundred chapters and 16,834 formulas. This work applied the rationalized nosological system of Chao Yuanfang's 610 C.E. *Comprehensive Treatise on the Origins and Symptoms of Disease* and incorporated its essays on the origins of disease. The court had the work printed and two copies distributed to each prefecture. It was at this time that they established the prefectural post of Medical Erudite, given the responsibility of "taking charge of" the text. Presumably these erudites were to use it as a reference for administering medical care to the prefectural office personnel and the populace, but Taizong also ordered them to make it available to functionaries and commoners who might want to copy it (Okanishi 1969, 713–720).

The state also produced texts specifically for use by the imperial medical schools and examinations. The Hanlin Medical Institute *(Hanlin yiguanju)*

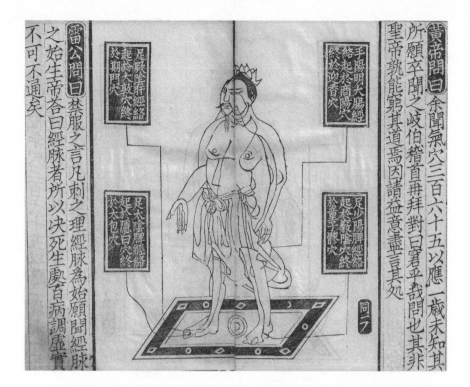

Figure 4.2. Starting points for Channels. Reading labels clockwise from upper right: Hand Yang Brightness Large Intestine Channel, Foot Lesser Yang Spleen Channel, Foot Greater Yin Spleen Channel, Foot Reverting Yin Channel. From reproduction of 1186 C.E. Jin Dynasty republication of Wang Weiyi's 1023 work *Newly Printed and Supplemented Illustrated Canon of Loci for Acupuncture and Moxibustion for Use with the Bronze Instructional Statues (Xinkan buzhu Tongren yuxue zhenjiu tujing)* (Guichi: Liushi Xuantong jiyuan,1909). Image courtesy of the Needham Research Institute.

produced authoritative editions of three Han and Sui period classics, which the Directorate of Education *(guozi jian)* printed in 1027: *Inner Canon of the Yellow Emperor, Basic Questions (Huangdi neijing suwen), Canon of the Yellow Emperor's Eighty-One Difficult Issues (Huangdi bashiyi nanjing),* and *Chao's Comprehensive Treatise on the Origins and Symptoms of Disease (Chaoshi zhubing yuanhou zonglun).* In the same year, they published Hanlin physician Wang Weiyi's (fl. 1023–1031) *Illustrated Canon of Loci for Acupuncture and Moxibustion for Use with the Bronze Instructional Statues (Tongren yuxue zhenjiu tujing,* written between 1023 and 1026). Where different medical lineages had disagreed on the locations of Channels and the acupoints, this work produced a standardized, authoritative map. (See Figure 4.2.) The statues in question were made with front and back halves inscribed on the inside with the internal viscera and on the outside with the Channels, with holes drilled in them cor-

TABLE 3

Books edited and published by the Bureau for Editing Medical Treatises

Bureau publication date	Author, title, length (original date of compilation/authorship)
After 1057	*Inner Canon of the Yellow Emperor, Great Simplicity (Huangdi neijing taisu)*, 30 chapters (1st c. B.C.E.)
After 1057	*Canon of the Numinous Pivot (Lingshu jing)*, 12 chapters (1st c. B.C.E.)
After 1057	Huangfu Mi, *A-B Canon [of Acupuncture] (Jiayi jing)*, 8 chapters (256–282)
1061	*Jiayou Period Supplemented and Annotated Divine Husbandman's Materia Medica* [a revision of the *Kaibao Era Materia Medica* (974 ed.)] *(Jiayou buzhu Shennong bencao)*, 21 chapters (fragments extant as quoted in other works)
1062	*Illustrated Classic of Materia Medica (Bencao tujing)*, 21 chapters (repr. 1096; produced to accompany *Jiayou buzhu Shennong bencao*; fragments extant as quoted in other works)
1064–1067	Sun Simiao, *Priceless Supplemental Formulae (Qianjin yifang)*, 30 chapters (682)
1065	Zhang Ji, *Treatise on Cold Damage Disorders (Shanghan lun)*, 10 chapters (205)
1066	Sun Simiao, *Priceless and Essential Formulae (Qianjin yaofang)*, 30 chapters (652)
1066	Zhang Ji, *Newly Edited Treatise on Essential Formulae from the Golden Chest (Xinbian jinkui yaolüe fanglun)*, 3 chapters (205)
1066	Zhang Ji, *Classic of the Golden Chest and the Jade Box (Jinkui yuhan jing)*, 8 chapters (205)
1067	*Revised and Expanded, Supplemented and Annotated Inner Canon of the Yellow Emperor, Basic Questions (Chongguang buzhu Huangdi neijing suwen)*, 24 chapters (1st c. B.C.E.)
1069	Wang Tao, *Secret and Essential Formulae from an Outer Censor (Waitai miyao fang)*, 40 chapters (752)
1069	Wang Shuhe (201–280), *Classic of the Pulse (Mojing)*, 10 chapters (ca. 280)
1069	Huangfu Mi, *The Yellow Emperor's Three Ministries A-B Canon of Acumoxa (Huangdi sanbu zhenjiu jiayi jing)*, 12 chapters (256–282)

(Compiled from Okanishi 1969)

responding to the acupuncture points, which were also labeled. For tests, they were covered in wax and reportedly filled with mercury, or perhaps water. Students would insert needles, and accurate placement would be confirmed by leakage (Goldschmidt 2009, 31–37, 208 n. 67). Toward the end of the twelfth century, the Imperial Medical Service produced and printed even more specialized texts for the schools, *Comprehensive and Subtle Treatises and Formulae for Guarding the Lives of Children (Xiao'er weisheng zongwei lunfang)* and *Model Essays for the Examinations of the Imperial Medical Service (Taiyi ju zhuke chengwen)* (Okanishi 1969, 1053–1059, 1351–1354).

State publishing of medical texts peaked between 1057 and 1069 under the Bureau for Editing Medical Treatises. The bureau's projects included the largest work on *materia medica* produced to that point, containing discussions of 1,084 drug, and accompanied by a volume of illustrations (Unschuld 1986, 60–68). The bulk of the bureau's work, however, was the collection, collation, and production of authoritative editions of medical classics dating from between the Han and Tang periods (see Table 3). Prior to the Song, these had been rare works, and spread slowly, often in divergent versions, through laborious hand copying. Song state-printed editions spread widely beyond hereditary physician lineages and state Medical School libraries. The recensions that we have today date to those Song imprints (Sivin 1993, 196–215). By lending certain works official approval, the Song state established a medical canon, a set of texts taken to be authoritative foundations of the tradition. It also made previously obscure ideas more widely available, sparking great theoretical innovation.

As we have seen, the Song state increasingly regularized medical relief under the Imperial Medical Service, the Pharmacy Service, and Medical Erudites. The encyclopedic *materia medica* and formularies, while useful for gathering and organizing knowledge for this purpose, could be unwieldy for daily use. The medical canons revived by the Bureau for Editing Medical Treatises tended toward theoretical discussion, useful for training but not handy. The bureau did republish smaller medieval formularies, but many of their remedies were deemed unsuited for "modern diseases." In response to these needs, *Formulae of the Imperial Medical Service (Taiyi ju fang)* was published in a streamlined ten chapters in 1080. These publications show different approaches to the production of medical knowledge: *materia medica* texts and encyclopedic formularies were *inclusive* projects, aspiring to collect all available knowledge; the bureau's medical canons were *exclusive* projects, establishing orthodox knowledge and to an unprecedented extent distinguishing medical from nonmedical healing; while the *Formulae of the Imperial Medical Service* was a *pragmatic* project, simplifying and rationalizing medical knowledge for practical application.

Emperor Huizong's court, famous for producing grandiose visions of imperial power through a range of cultural, religious, and institutional works (including, as discussed above, an expansion of medical services), inaugurated another ambitious round of publication, producing texts in all three of these modes. In the pragmatic mode, in 1107, not long after expanding the Pharmacy Service, they commissioned *Formulae of the Pharmacy Service for Great Peace and for the Benefit of the People (Taiping huimin hejiju fang)* in ten chapters. The book became popular and continued to circulate commercially long after the fall of the Song. In the inclusive mode, the regime produced two books. The 1116 *Zhenghe Period Revised Classified Practical Materia Medica from the Classics and Histories (Zhenghe xinxiu jingshi zhenglei beiyong bencao)* expanded on a privately compiled work from sometime after 1080, annotated and published in 1108. The *Zhenghe Period Materia Medica* included an unprecedented 1,748 drug descriptions in thirty chapters (Unschuld 1986, 70–77). The 1118 *Comprehensive Record of Sagely Beneficence (Shengji zonglu)*, like Taizong's 992 *Taiping Era Formulae for Sagely Grace* an encyclopedic formulary, doubled the number of chapters over the previous work, added treatises and charts, and increased the number of remedies by about one-quarter. Huizong's preface boasted, "There is nothing that it does not entirely provide for." Finally, in the exclusive mode, Huizong did not just canonize a classical text but produced the putatively self-authored canonical work the *Canon of Sagely Beneficence (Shengji jing)*, discoursing on theoretical principles (Okanishi 1969, 794–816, 794–811).

Campaigns to Transform Southern Healing Customs

Beginning in the early decades of the Song we find a fourth approach in the state's medical governance: producing and distributing medical knowledge for the purpose of rectifying commoner customs and mores. While this goal was generally encompassed in the inclusive, exclusive, and pragmatic modes of medical publishing and governance, officials serving in southern locales focused on reforming customs and produced texts geared specifically toward that. To understand these policies, we should consider the wider historical contexts and particular dynamics that produced this new attention to southern customs.

In the Late Imperial Period, Jiangnan, the region south of the lower reaches of the Yangzi River, was a wealthy center of high culture. Today in most of China's southern provinces, although people might speak, for example, Min, Wu, or Yue dialects, they also identify themselves as Chinese (Han or Hua). While in modern times people often think of difference in terms of racial or ethnic identities, in the imperial (Han through Qing) period literate elites, at least, tended to make such distinctions in terms of cultural practices. Rather than locating people in one or another category into which they were born, they tended to view people as being along a continuum of literary and ritual/moral transformation. Literate elites, having greater access to education, had greater capacity and responsibility for moral development. Commoners might not be literate but were still capable in their behavior of following elite example and instruction. Song elites generally viewed northern villagers, having lived much longer close to the beneficial influences of traditional centers of culture and power, as embodying authentic traditional norms. Those more distant in habitation and in lifestyle, including southern commoners, were seen as barbaric, usually in a degree increasing with their distance from the northern center. Their deities were labeled "demons," their religious officiants were labeled "shamans" (*wu*, conveying the exotic and derogatory sense of "witch doctors"), and their customs, including healing practices, were described as "noxious" and "polluted" (Hinrichs 2003; on shamans as healers, also see "Shamans," in Chapter 3).

Prior to the Song, officials had occasionally made some effort to reform southerners' customs. A common approach was to introduce the worship of orthodox gods such as deified generals famous for their conquest of the south. Some officials also exhorted people not to consult local shamans, or even destroyed their shrines. As with medical relief, in the Song, campaigns to reform southern customs not only became higher-profile, more regular, and more creative but took on a new focus in the handling of illness and in medical knowledge. Song officials' concerns focused not only on southerners' "demonic" worship but also on (1) their preference for local shamans over physicians, which was often seen as the root of (2) their ignorance of medicine and refusal to accept medical care, and of (3) their avoidance of the sick for fear of contagion.

Scattered prefecture- and district-level cases appear across the south from the 960s and into the twelfth century. Court attention to the issue peaked in 1023, when the prefect of Hongzhou (in modern Jiangxi), Xia Song (985–1051), reported that he had taken action against more than 1,900 shamans in his jurisdiction, or one for every eighty-seven registered households. He had destroyed their shrines, and forced them to "change occupation and return to agriculture, as well as apply themselves to the practice of acumoxa, prescription, and pulse-taking" (Hinrichs 2003, 45). Xia called for "harsher codes," and the court responded with an edict imposing severe penalties on

> shamans who make their reputations by means of heterodox deities; keep clothing, food, and medicines from sick people; cut them off from being seen by their relatives; treat them as though with affection; intentionally entrap people into harm; and hope for illnesses, together with people who conspire with them. (Hinrichs 2003, 25–26)

The decree extended the geographic reach of a 981 court ban on shamans throughout the region corresponding to modern Sichuan, thus covering all of the south. (See ca. 1050 map.) Of course, although local healers and the people they served did not leave us their own accounts, surely they did not consider their own deities "heterodox," were glad to have the contaminated clothing of the sick removed, saw reason in keeping food and medicines from them, and saw shamans giving concern and help rather than entrapment and conspiracy.

How did this polarization of viewpoint and conflict emerge? At the local level, some of these cases arose when officials attempted to distribute medicines as relief for epidemics, only to be informed that the local people would not take them because shamans had told them the gods forbade it. Although officials attributed such taboos to ignorance, the practice was not necessarily restricted to illiterate southern commoners. Religious Daoist texts, diagnosing illness as divine punishment, also told the sick that taking food and medicines would interfere with the process of recovery, which must be based on purification and prayer. Local shamans, who are known to have adapted Daoist exorcistic techniques (Davis 2001), may have shared a similar reasoning. While Daoist traditions developed in distinctive directions, they did also draw on popular practices, and fasting during ritual cures may have been one of these.

From the perspective of the officials, though, for the populace to reject medicines (which in some cases had been purchased by the official with his own personal funds) was a great affront to their authority. As Xia Song put it:

> [The people] receive [shamans] with increasing respect, and trust them to increasing depths. They follow their words more closely than the statutes and regulations, and they fear their power more than that of the officials and clerks. (Hinrichs 2003, 44)

By expanding state functions to regularly include epidemic relief, officials provoked resistance, and local shamans became objectionable to them not only in their capacities as officiants for illegitimate gods, but also as ritual healers.

Officials were notably creative in their responses. Soon after the Song conquest of the Later Shu state in modern Sichuan, an official there, combating the local prejudice against medicine, rounded up and flogged the shamans. (See the ca. 950 and ca. 1050 maps.) The populace anticipated divine punishment against the official by the deities served by those shamans, so to reinforce the point that his was the greater power, after a few days the official had the shamans flogged again. A few decades later another magistrate in Sichuan, facing resistance to his dispensation of medical relief, had his functionaries forcibly administer the decoctions. He reported that he achieved seven or eight recoveries out of every ten cases and that the local people thus learned to trust in medicine. Besides exhortation and distributing medical decoctions, by local officials as early as 971 and by imperial decree as early as 974, we find the state making medical texts, especially formularies, available to the populace to encourage medical over shamanic healing. For example, in some cases, texts were carved in wood or stone and posted, for example, outside government office gates. Some officials commissioned, printed, and distributed new formularies directly to the shamans in question (Hinrichs 2011).

Another major provocation of southern customs, avoiding contact with the sick, seems rational to us today, and seemed reasonable not only to "benighted" southern commoners but also to many—perhaps even most—Song literati. We know that at least one Song hospital separated patients in different wards in order to prevent contagion, and methods for avoiding it even appear in Sun Simiao's *Essential Formulae Worth a Thousand in Gold* and in state-published formularies, from *Taiping Era Formulary of Sagely Grace* to *Comprehensive Record of Sagely Beneficence*. The methods attributed to shamans—putting "talismanic seals on the doorways, prohibiting [family members] from returning home, sending close relatives far away, and discarding personal utensils"— are all well attested in both Daoist and medical literature in the Song; "incantations and talismans" was even one of the major divisions of the Song Medical School. (See Figure 4.3.) Furthermore, both Daoist and medical texts labeled, discussed, and treated contagious categories of disease as demonic in origin, again suggesting common ground between southern commoner and literate elite practices (Hinrichs 2003, 130–202).

If ritual healing and avoidance of the sick were not anathema in state-sanctioned medicine or in literati life, what then was the issue for officials

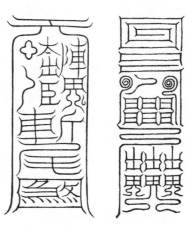

Figure 4.3. Talismans from official medical and Daoist sources. *Left:* Talisman from *Record of Sagely Beneficence*. It came with the instruction "Place over the door to stop Warmth demons." Zhao, *Dade chongjiao shengji zong lu* (1300), 1813, 195.71A. Courtesy of Harvard-Yenching Library. *Right:* "Lord Lao's talisman for quelling [demons] in the house and exorcising Warmth plague": "For over the bed." Lu, *Wushang xuanyuan santian yutang dafa* (1126), *Zhengtong Daozang* (1444–1445), 1926, 24.17.

campaigning against them in the south? As common as such practices were, isolating and avoiding contact with the sick violated ideals of family and community solidarity and mutual care that were important bases of imperial legitimacy and rule. We can find not only negative campaigns against what officials found disruptive but also positive depictions of the world they sought to create. Parallel to the growth of medical relief, education, and publishing, in the eleventh and early twelfth centuries there was an increasing tendency to portray happy commoner life—showing how the types of customs that the court sought to propagate nurtured the populace morally and physically (Cheng 2003; Cheng 2011; Hammers 2002). One such early twelfth-century court painting, attributed to Li Tang (ca. 1050–after 1130), shows an itinerant rural doctor treating a patient. (See Figure 4.4.) In place of quarantined patients and shamanic exorcism, we see family and neighbors sympathetically collaborating to help the afflicted, holding him still while he endures the pain of moxa being burned at points such as those laid out in the state-produced *Illustrated Canon of Loci for Acupuncture and Moxibustion*. The itinerant physician's apprentice cools a healing plaster that will be applied to the resulting blisters. This takes place in an open space near a village wall, not in the dark, enclosed quarters of a sickroom. We can see from the doctor's simple and torn clothes that, virtuously, he serves for little pay.

While attacks on isolating the sick were mainly framed in moral terms, one Southern Song literatus, Cheng Jiong (fl. 1163–1176), did pose the problem in medical terms. He wrote a treatise challenging the idea of contagion, not surprisingly attributing it to southern customs and blaming shamans for it. Cheng Jiong's own starting point was the damage that fear of contagion did to families, and several officials specifically denounced the avoidance of stricken homes by neighbors and the abandonment of sufferers by their relatives. The prominent Neo-Confucian Zhu Xi (1130–1200) wrote in argument against Cheng Jiong that contagion simply did occur, and to tell people otherwise was to undermine their faith in anything officials might say. Rather, he proposed telling people that even though contagion existed, they should put their compassion and integrity before their own interests, thereby teaching them a moral lesson. The issue, then, was often framed more strongly in moral than in medical terms (Hinrichs 2003, 203–226; Hinrichs forthcoming).

On the other hand, by the middle of the eleventh century—as orders to practice "acumoxa, prescription, and pulse-taking" and the distribution of decoctions and formularies opposed medical healing to ritual healing—the choice of particular types of formulas for distribution promoted a way of understanding and treating epidemics that, if it did not entirely dispute contagion, placed it outside the therapeutic framework. A 1065 Bureau for Editing Medical

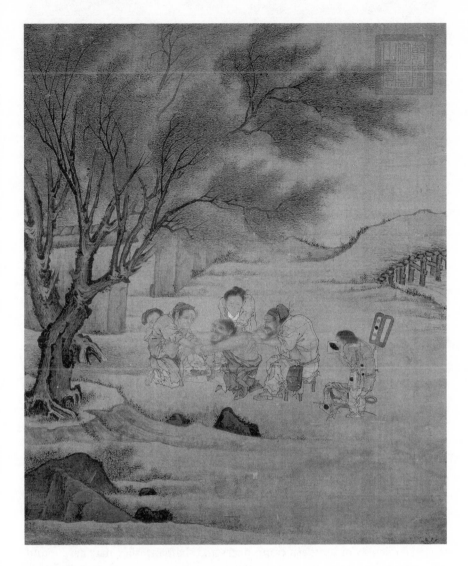

Figure 4.4. Itinerant rural doctor, attributed to Li Tang (ca. 1050–after 1130). Courtesy of National Palace Museum, Taiwan, Republic of China.

Treatises publication, the late Han text devoted to Cold Damage epidemics, Zhang Ji's *Treatise on Cold Damage Disorders (Shanghan lun)*, was helpful in clarifying and putting forward such an approach. Zhang did not look at transmission but rather analyzed the treatment of Cold Damage according to the six Yin and Yang modalities that governed the system of Channels *(jing)* as laid out in the *Basic Questions:* Greater Yin *(taiyin),* Lesser Yin *(shaoyin),* Reverting Yin *(jueyin),* Greater Yang *(taiyang),* Yang Brightness *(yangming),* and Lesser Yang *(shaoyang).* In later times, while some epidemics, especially

Warmth *(wen)* diseases, were treated as contagious (and demonic in etiology), medical authors attributed Cold Damage's spread to external climatic factors rather than person-to-person transmission. The Cold Damage approach also tied disease firmly to *Inner Canon*–style physiology, something that had not always been clear in earlier formularies.

Within a decade of the bureau's publication of Zhang's *Treatise,* two officials commissioned the compilation of Cold Damage formularies in order to combat local customs. To counter influence of shamans and distrust of medicines, a magistrate serving in Huainan produced *Formulary for Cold Damage to Rescue Customs (Shanghan jiusu fang),* clearly stating its purpose—to reform customs—in its title, and had this engraved in stone. Liu Yi (1015–1091), a prefect serving in southern Jiangxi, similarly stated his goal in *Formulae to Correct Customs (Zhengsu fang),* a text again solely devoted to Cold Damage disorders. Rather than simply displaying the text to the populace, however,

> he registered all of the shamans under his jurisdiction, netting over 3,700 people [one shaman for every 26.5 households]. He restrained them, and gave each of them a copy of his *Formulae* so they would make medicine their occupation. (Hinrichs 2003, 37–39)

What these shamans, almost surely illiterate, did with Liu Yi's *Formulae,* the sources do not tell us. For his fellow officials and for local elites, however, the symbolic import of this campaign, pitting shamanic healing against a pointedly canonical style of medicine, occasioned a sharpening of the lines between heterodox and orthodox healing.

While widespread illiteracy alone makes it doubtful that campaigns against southern healing customs could have had much direct effect on their purported audiences of southern commoners and shamans, they may have found more purchase among a growing pool of literate observers, including both literati and physicians. After the eleventh century, along with a general retreat from state-centered approaches to social transformation, we see fewer official campaigns against shamans, but local gentry elites could be seen picking up the slack (Sutton 2000). In the field of medicine, thanks to the bureau's revival of Zhang's *Treatise,* Cold Damage became a great focus of theoretical and therapeutic interest. Its approach was the basis for the systematic extension of classical medical theories to drug therapeutics (Goldschmidt 2009). It also came to be integrated with the Five Circulatory Phases and Six Climatic Qi (*wuyun liuqi,* hereafter Five Phases and Six Qi) cosmological system, one that also incorporated the six Yin and Yang modalities and focused on the prediction and treatment of epidemics. Five Phases and Six Qi was given a central place in Huizong's medical publications and in the official medical curriculum (Despeux 2001; Goldschmidt 2009).

The example of state-produced formularies encouraged both physicians and literati (the prolific Su Shi among them) to privately collect and publish formularies, both to contribute to the spread of medical knowledge and, more cynically considered, to enhance their reputations for concern for the public welfare. The prominence of medicine in governance, along with the greater circulation of both hitherto rare and new medical texts, encouraged literati interest. This began with amateur scholarly avocation but increasingly became an alternative to careers in office or in teaching.

Status Structure and Medicine

While some medieval aristocratic elites had used specialized medical knowledge to enter office, for the most part their interest was directed toward the care of their families and themselves, not to medicine as a vocation. We must understand the emergence of greater Song elite interest in medicine in the context of epochal changes in status structure. While eligibility for office remained the prime demarcation of elite versus commoner status, the terms of that qualification changed.

From the end of the Han through the Tang, a stable and endogamous group of aristocratic clans dominated high office. Under the centralized Sui and Tang regimes, their wealth, power, and prestige became increasingly tied to the court, so when the Tang fell, they effectively ceased to exist as corporate entities. At the same time nonaristocratic literate men were gradually drawn into government service, especially in provincial administrations. The Song thus began with a larger and more diverse pool of civil officials. Many had achieved office during the Five Dynasties and Ten Kingdoms era on the basis of their ability to handle troops or documents rather than their family backgrounds. Emperor Taizong in particular is famous for having put the military under civilian rule and for expanding the role of the civil service examinations as a gateway to office. At the same time, the court increased the system's objectivity, for example, having test essays recopied and names coded so that examiners could not identify examinees and thereby favor their own friends or relatives. These measures contributed to making cultured pursuits more central to elite identity, thus making the term "literati" (wenren) increasingly synonymous with elite status. They also helped open access to office to an ever-widening pool of talent, so that by the twelfth century we have examples of physicians investing in examination education for their sons and succeeding in placing them in office. At the same time, as the number of eligible candidates grew, the number of places remained stable, so their chances of actually passing the examinations and attaining office diminished proportionately. We thus see more and more sons of officeholding families turning their attentions from the central state to local community service and to local marriage alliances. For this reason, social historians often refer to elites from the Southern Song and Jin through the Qing as "local gentry." Besides stronger local orientations, local gentry elites also turned to alternative careers, among them that of physician (Hymes 1987). The social distance between physicians and literati thus narrowed, and they more often socialized together, read and referred to each other's work, and wrote prefaces for each other's books (Hinrichs 2003, 109–114, 125–128).

Early in the twelfth century, Huizong produced the first recorded instance of the appellation "scholar-physician" *(ruyi)*, using it to refer to the type of candidates—literati students proficient in medical arts—that he hoped to attract to his newly expanded Medical School (Goldschmidt 2009, 56–57). The word *ru,* translated here as "scholar," is often rendered into English as "Confucian." In the case of *ruyi*, though, it does not necessarily imply a specifically Confucian orientation or background. In the subsequent decades the term was used to describe both physicians of exceptional learning or moral rectitude and literati engaged in medical practice. Under the Southern Song, and more notably under the Jin, where mainstream government and teaching prospects for literati were even scarcer, so-called scholar-physicians, in some cases reacting specifically against the standardized remedies dominant in the Pharmacy Service and its publications, developed approaches to diagnosis and treatment based on canonical physiologies today often called "pattern diagnosis" *(bianzheng)* (Furth 1999, 65–66). These physicians applied Five Phases and Six Qi theory to methods of pharmaceutical prescription, requiring not only sensitivity to subtle shifts in the patient's underlying physiological condition in order to make a diagnosis, but also calculations based on calendrical cycles, climatic changes, and geographic location in order to design complex mixes of drugs combined according to their qualities.

Such erudite physicians tended to relegate hands-on practices such as acupuncture, bone setting, minor surgeries, the treatment of skin diseases, massage, and ritual therapies to less prestigious practitioners denigrated (as in the past doctors in general had been) as technical specialists (Leung 2003c, 383–386). Nevertheless, well-educated hereditary physicians, including some whom the literati acknowledged as having transcended the level of mere craft to become scholar-physicians, persisted in practicing eclectic styles of medicine. The well-connected third-generation physician and medical writer Zhang Gao (fl. 1189), for example, argued for the irreducible mystery of most healing and pointedly resisted dominant trends toward either simple pragmatic treatment (prominent in most state and private formularies) or the theoretical reductionism of some Five Phases and Six *Qi* theories (Hinrichs 2009).

Although most healing skills continued to be transmitted within families, increasing numbers of aspiring doctors studied from purchased books and traveled to study with renowned physicians. For the most part, they often freely studied with multiple teachers. In the Jin, however, on the model of contemporary Neo-Confucian practice, some physicians began apprenticing exclusively with a single teacher and formed medical lineages (Leung 2003c, 386–396).

Popular Handling of Disease

These ferments in the field of medicine were fed not only by shifts in status structure and approach to governance, but also by accompanying changes in patterns of trade and demographic growth and movement. The wars of the ninth and tenth centuries devastated the northern plains, resulting in population loss through death and southward migration, and a consequent demographic shift to the south. Migrants gradually (and not without conflict) integrated with southern populations and opened up lands to agriculture. Another wave of migration came with the twelfth-century Jin conquest. The establishment of the capital in Hangzhou with its palaces, government offices, and supporting services, attracted more people and accelerated development in the surrounding region (Shiba 1988). By the twelfth century, then, both the demographic and economic center had shifted from the traditional northern heartland to Jiangnan. Overseas trade, notably through the port of Quanzhou in Fujian, continued to grow, contributing to the growth of infrastructure such as roads and bridges and of specialized agricultural and crafts production—including medicinal drugs—for market (Clark 1991).

The growth in commerce led to a proliferation of marketing centers, towns, and cities. While smaller markets met only periodically, larger urban centers developed both wholesale and retail districts. Pharmacies sprouted up with attending physicians. Chengdu in Sichuan, a source of much drug production and trade, held semiannual drug fairs, with merchants trading imported as well as locally grown medicines (Shiba 1970, 49). Itinerant herb sellers and healers traveled the urban and periodic market circuits selling their wares and services.

Like Li Tang's idyllic image of orthodox healing in rural life, vibrant urban life entered the imperial imagination of a prosperous realm. *Qingming on the River* (*Qingming shanghe tu*, late eleventh or early twelfth century), a long scroll depicting daily life from the peaceful countryside to the exuberant and exciting city market, is another such court painting. It includes two commercial pharmacies, one with a full front view. (See Figure 4.5.) One of the latter pharmacy's signs advertises remedies for hangovers, echoing the theme of drink, visible elsewhere in the painting. A smaller but forward-facing sign advertises remedies for the "Five Overexertions and Seven Injuries" *(wulao qishang)*, ailments of overindulgence and overwork. Another sign refers to disorders of the stomach and intestine, also perhaps meant to evoke overindulgence in food and wine. In contrast both to the themes of these signs and to the agony represented in Li Tang's painting, the human scene in the pharmacy itself is a serene one—an island of tranquility, in fact, on a busy street. A doctor quietly examines a small child held on his mother's lap, while a female servant stands next to them. Two of the signs hint at official connections, and hence link the prosperity directly to the trickle-down effects of state medical policies. The sign that ends with "stomach and intestine disorders" begins with "Pills issued by the Imperial Medical Service." Over the main entryway hangs a sign identifying the shop as that of the "Shop of the Imperial [Medical Service] Director" (Zhao 1997, 88, 95–104).

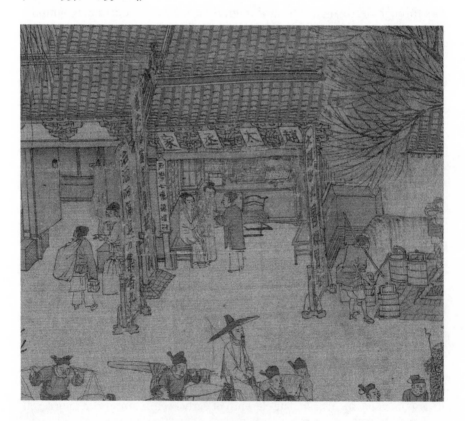

Figure 4.5. Urban commercial pharmacy. "Qingming on the River," attributed to Zhang Zeduan (1085–1145). Courtesy of Palace Museum, Beijing.

Although the vagueness and inconsistency of sources make it difficult to confirm epidemiological changes in this period, the above-described shifts in demographic and socioeconomic patterns have led many scholars to hypothesize an increase in epidemic disease during the Song. The increased circulation of goods and people and their concentration in urban centers may have spread diseases further and more quickly. The migration of northerners to the south may have exposed them to diseases for which neither their immune systems nor their repertoires of remedies left them well prepared. Whether or not epidemics themselves increased in incidence or intensity, innovative responses to epidemics did. We have already noted the attention devoted in state and literate medicine to Cold Damage and Five Phases and Six Qi theories, both primarily concerned with the treatment of epidemics.

In the south, popular ritual handling of disease, including epidemics, continued to flourish despite so many Northern Song officials' opposition. In fact, new Daoist therapeutic and exorcistic movements emerged and spread across the south, especially from the twelfth century on (Davis 2001). The same period saw the spread of cults devoted to plague spirits, the most popular being the Five Commissioners of Epidemics *(wuwen shizhe)* and the Twelve Year-Controlling Kings of Epidemics *(shi'er zhinian wenwang)*. The Five Commissioners were linked to the Five Phases, while the Twelve Kings were worshipped as underlings of the year-controlling deity Taisui (Jupiter). These gods were propitiated during plague offerings *(wenjiao)*, exorcistic rituals that culminated in the floating away or burning of a boat bearing their images. The exact origins of such offerings are unclear, but they appear to derive from boat expulsion rites performed during the Dragon Boat Festival, held annually on the fifth day of the fifth lunar month—the birthday of the Five Commissioners—to prevent outbreaks of epidemics during the summer months (Katz 1995, 49–57). (See "Plague God Cults.") In many ways, despite some officials' efforts to replace shamans' ritual healing with medicine, we find a burgeoning of popular exorcistic rites and festivals.

Plague God Cults

Paul R. Katz

During the Song, new Daoist liturgical movements in the south absorbed plague deity cults. Such processes reflect an age-old reverberation between Daoism and communal religious traditions, with Daoist religion consistently struggling to co-opt, reform, and even eradicate the numerous cults and ritual traditions it encountered in the regions into which it spread. Although Daoist priests made mighty efforts to eliminate "excessive" *(yinsi)* local cults, we also find numerous cases of Daoists grudgingly accepting the hated heterodox deities they had once attempted to destroy.

One example of this interplay involves the Divine Empyrean (Shenxiao) movement, which arose during the Song and proceeded to make a major impact on Daoist beliefs and practices. The origins of this movement are unclear, but its development reflects the ongoing interaction between Daoism and religious traditions indigenous to south China. Although most histories of Daoism emphasize the importance of leading Divine Empyrean Daoists such as Lin Lingsu (1076–1120) at the court of the Northern Song emperor Huizong (r. 1100–1125), this movement also played a vital role in the interaction between Daoism and local cults throughout south China. One example is the plague-quelling deity Wen Qiong, also known as Marshal Wen (Wen Yuanshuai), whose earliest known hagiography was composed by the Divine Empyrean master Huang Gongjin (fl. 1274). Huang and his peers appear to have played key roles in the construction of some of Wen's oldest temples and helped popularize his cult through rituals featuring the expulsion of plague boats. These Daoists also viewed Wen as a compassionate, self-sacrificing hero who had dedicated himself to the service of the Daoist celestial bureaucracy.

Excerpt from the hagiography of Marshal Wen, Huang Gongjin, 1274:

> General Wen was loyal and upright, serving the Deities of the Peaks in protecting the cult of the Supreme Emperor of the Dark Heavens. . . . One day the Northern Emperor transmitted one thousand plague poison pills to the Emperor of the Eastern Peak, and ordered him to deploy a commissioner to spread the plague. [The Emperor of the Eastern Peak assigned Wen to the task.] . . . Wen thought, "One of these pills can kill thousands of people and harm thousands of households, not to mention that the climatic currents will spread this poison even further, causing additional deaths. . . . It would be better for me to die in place of all those thousands. . . . If such is to be my fate, I would feel no bitterness." Thereupon he lifted his gaze towards heaven, faced north, and swallowed all the pills. His body was instantly overcome by an unbearable burning sensation, and his belly ached. He then took burning incense and presented himself before the Emperor of the Eastern Peak, where he metamorphosed into a huge, ferocious demon. Submitting a memorial reporting his acts, he lay prostrate and awaited his punishment. When the Northern Emperor heard of this

incident, he immediately ordered an investigation, at which point the Emperor of the Eastern Peak could do nothing but clearly report Wen's crime of disobedience in a memorial. . . . [The Northern Emperor] ordered the Right Tribunal to reprimand Wen, but because the Supreme Emperor of the Dark Heavens prized Wen . . . he submitted a plea to pardon Wen for his crimes. The Northern Emperor assented, and ordered that Wen should solely serve the Supreme Emperor of the Dark Heavens in his missions of transforming [the people through Daoist] teachings and of punishing demons. (Adapted from Katz 1995, 87–88)

Daoist and Buddhist priests performed the rituals in many of these popular festivals and were often called upon not only by commoners but also by literati to cure disease. On a personal level, literati continued to turn, for health as well as spiritual reasons, to Daoist inner alchemy *(neidan)*, which emphasized meditative breathing and visualization. By this time the concoction of elixirs, typical of "external alchemy," had declined radically in popularity, but its language permeated inner alchemical practice. Most obviously, the word for alchemy was the same as that for elixir and for a common ingredient in elixirs, cinnabar *(dan)*. Highest Clarity *(shangqing)* Daoist traditions of inner alchemy were especially popular, and under the Jin we find the emergence of a major new branch of Daoism, Complete Perfection *(quanzhen)*. (See "Legendary Daoist Women.")

LEGENDARY DAOIST WOMEN

Catherine Despeux

In the Song period, several female figures in Daoism became known for their virtue and attainment of the Way. A collection of hagiographies compiled around 1294 includes some fifteen biographies of women for this period, of which seven were from the reign of the emperor Huizong, known for his support of Divine Empyrean Daoism (Miao 7.11b–12a). Two women in this group stand out. Cao Daochong (1039–1115) is the only woman known to have produced a commentary on the *Scripture of the Way and Its Power (Daode jing)* and to have received high honorific titles from Huizong. Sun Bu'er (1119–1182) came to be included on the list of the seven founders of the Complete Perfection (Quanzhen) tradition, one of the two great Daoist currents at that time.

Cao Daochong (1039–1115)—better known as Cao Xiyun the Poetess or Cao Wenyi the Daoist—had been ordained in a temple on Gezao Mountain (Jiangxi), site of the Gezao School, founded in 1097 as an outgrowth of the Numinous Treasure (Lingbao) branch of Daoism. The principle temple of the area—the Chongzhen Temple—housed hundreds of Daoists and was frequented at the time by a number of literati, some of whom were known for their poetry and their knowledge of internal alchemy (Qing 1994, 123–128, 194–195). Cao's commentary on the *Scripture of the Way and Its Power* was preserved in a collection of commentaries by prestigious authors of the Song, including Emperor Huizong and the celebrated Neo-Confucian Zhu Xi *(Daode zhenjing jizhu)*. Yet although her highly traditional commentary makes several brief allusions to general practices of internal alchemy, it says nothing specific to women's practices.

Sun Bu'er belonged to the Complete Perfection Daoist movement, which was born in north China under the Jin. This branch taught a method of meditation similar to that of Chan Buddhism, as well as a relatively simple version of internal alchemy *(neidan)*. A number of small local societies, among which some were women's, were attached to the great temples of this school. The founding masters—among them Ma Dayang, the elderly husband of Sun Bu'er—addressed poems to these women, often advising them to increase their purity (Despeux 1990, 127–138).

Cao Daochong's and Sun Bu'er's reputations grew in later periods to legendary status. In the Qing, they came to be identified as the matriarchs of the specifically female currents of Daoism that emerged then, and as the purported authors of works derived for the most part from spirit writing *(fuji)* (Despeux 1990, 83–155; Despeux and Kohn 2003, 129–174). (See "Female Alchemy" in Chapter 6.)

Legacies

With the significant exceptions of the Yuan institutions of local Medical Schools and Medical Households (see "Medical Schools and the Temples of the Three Progenitors" in Chapter 5), post-Song states tended to reduce rather than enlarge the scope of medical governance. However, we can still see many effects of their work today. Throughout East Asia, the word for pharmacy means literally "Bureau of Pharmaceutics" (*yaoju*, J. *yakkyoku*, K. *yakguk*), a legacy of the Song Pharmacy Service. With the exception of works and fragments recovered from archaeological sites and from archives in Japan, the publications of the Bureau for Editing Medical Treatises remain our main sources for pre-Song medicine. The interest in Cold Damage medicine spawned by the bureau's revival of Zhang Ji's *Treatise* remained strong in later centuries, engendering a major stream of the medical tradition (see "The 'Warm Diseases' Current of Learning" in Chapter 6; see also Chapter 7). Both government and private imprints of medical texts circulated widely, and were reprinted, quoted, and adapted to local medical practices all over East Asia. (See "Song Printed Medical Works and Medieval Japanese Medicine and "A Chosŏn Korea Medical Synthesis" in Chapter 5.)

Song Printed Medical Works and Medieval Japanese Medicine

Andrew Edmund Goble

For nearly three centuries after the compilation of *Formulae from the Heart of Medicine (Ishinpō)* in 984, medical writing in Japan was limited. The concern of hereditary aristocratic physicians to guard their cultural capital served to restrict the circulation of information, and familiarity with developments in Chinese medicine was minimal. However, beginning in the thirteenth century—thanks to new routes of intellectual interaction facilitated by Chinese and Japanese Buddhist priests, and to access to the fruits of the Song printing revolution—the situation changed dramatically. By the early fourteenth century, the ready availability of Chinese printed texts enabled more extensive dissemination of medical knowledge, the locus of that knowledge shifted from aristocrats to Buddhist priests, and the tool kit of Japanese medicine was markedly enhanced.

The Buddhist priest Kajiwara Shōzen (1265–1337) was active for several decades at the most comprehensive medical facility constructed in Japan to that time. That facility was located in the city of Kamakura at Gokurakuji temple, a major site for the Shingon Ritsu sect, which was devoted to the teachings of the Healing Mañjuśrī Buddha and known for its charity and hospice activities. The medical facilities at Gokurakuji included the Hall of the Healing Buddha, a clinical treatment building, a lodging for *rai* (leprosy) sufferers, a medicinal bathhouse, a dispensary, lodging for the ill, an equine veterinary clinic, and at least one other medical building whose function is left unspecified but which might have been an outpatient clinic. Thousands of people were treated each year.

Shōzen's writings embody the impact of Song and Yuan medicine in Japan. His *Book of the Simple Physician (Ton'ishō)* of 1302–1304 is some 3,000 leaves in length, is written in Japanese, contains some 1,400 formulas, and refers by name to at least 55 Chinese medical titles. The *Myriad Relief Formulae (Man'anpō)* of 1327 is some 6,800 leaves in length. Written in Chinese, it contains approximately 3,100 formulas, refers by name to some 270 Chinese titles, and is the most substantial medical work produced in Japan prior to the seventeenth century. Many of the titles mentioned are also cited in other works consulted by Shōzen, so it appears that he had actual physical access to about eighty of them. This is still a large number, and all are Song or Yuan titles. By contrast, Shōzen mentions only three Japanese works, one being *Formulae from the Heart of Medicine*, but his degree of access to it is uncertain.

Shōzen had access to a broad range of contemporary Chinese medical sources, and the works that appear in *Man'anpō* and *Ton'ishō* provide a rare window into the full dynamics of Chinese medicine. The most heavily represented sources were works compiled under official auspices, such as the Northern Song *Formulary of the Pharmacy Service for the Benefit of the People*, the Yuan printing of *Comprehensive Record of Sagely Beneficence*, or the Yuan *Prescriptions of the Imperial Pharmacy (Yuyaoyuan fang)*. He had several works devoted to particular medical specialties, such as pediatrics, women's diseases, and tropical medicine, plus an innovative work on etiology and Chen Yan's theoretically innovative *Formulae and Treatises on the Three Types of Causes Bringing Ultimate Unity to Diseases and Their Symptoms (Sanyin jiyi bingzheng fanglun*, 1174). He also included a number of working handbooks from southern China, which was the primary region of interaction. The last group were ephemeral texts and either became lost or did not achieve long-term prestige in China, but their presence among Shōzen's works indicates that he, or his suppliers, selected them on the basis of their reputation at the time and not on the basis of any sense of "the tradition," a concept that was perhaps not fully formed.

Shōzen's broad selection of sources and formulas and his commentary confirm that he was well versed in Chinese medicine, was aware of new fields of specialization, and had tested a larger number of formulas than the thousands he listed. Access to printed Chinese medical works permitted him to address what he saw as shortcomings in Japanese medicine. For example, he asserted that Japanese physicians, lacking access to printed works, prescribed medicines based on guesswork. He sought to rectify what he deemed to be deleterious

以至予掌握子孫可秘之〃〃〃
輕於本朝即導生禪師一流傳來
家秘之不令餘家而傳矣禁防不
亦性全傳受之此方於宋朝只俞
亦兄弟之眠實照相傳之自實照
以法養之好傳受之從一圓禪師
傳之自導生比丘一圓禪師 尾州長母寺長老
及脉道針灸口決并此遇仙丹相
仍黑錫丹養生丹靈砂丹等諸方
在唐九ヶ年只為習傳於醫術也
私云此藥参州實相院導生此丘

Figure 4.6. Song printed medical works and medieval Japanese medicine, translation of *Man'anpō*. Kajiwara Shōzen *Myriad Relief Formulae* (*Man'anpō*, 1327), Tokugawa edition. Courtesy of Andrew Edmund Goble.

Translation (from *Man'anpō* chapter 52, Kagaku Shoin edition, p. 1398, leaves 52–134, 52–135):

My comment: Regarding this medicine [the Yū Family Meeting the Transcendant Pill (*Yūke gūsen tan*)], the Buddhist monk Dōshō of Jisshō-in Temple in Mikawa province resided in Tang [China] for nine years in order to learn and have transmitted to him the medical arts. He received the transmissions for such prescriptions as Black Tin Pill (*kokushaku tan*), Nourishing Life Pill (*yōjō tan*), and Spirit Sand Pill (*reisha tan*); for the oral transmissions for pulse analysis, acupuncture, and moxibustion; and for this Meeting the Transcendant Pill (*gūsen tan*). Monk Dōshō then transmitted it to Zen Master [Mujū] Ichi'en (the elder at Owari Province's Chōboji Temple) since [Ichi'en] had such a great interest in all things associated with Buddhism. Then Zen Master Ichi'en transmitted it to his brother Jisshō, and Jisshō further transmitted it to me, Shōzen. In the Song this prescription had been a secret of the Yū's lineage and had not been transmitted to any other families. It was strictly guarded and had not been known in Japan. Thusly it was transmitted in the lineage of Zen Master Dōshō, and came into my hands. Our descendants must maintain this as secret.

practices in pre- and postnatal care, such as the reluctance to prescribe medicines to pregnant women, and the belief that a woman should not lie down or sleep for seven days after giving birth.

Shōzen also spread new approaches to treatment. For example, he identified an ailment previously treated with prescriptions as infant malnutrition, which required an improved diet. Whereas old medical works treated vomiting with warming medicines, he disseminated approaches recommended in newly arrived medical works that contraindicated this strategy, taking the position that vomiting itself arises from heat. Second, he obtained recent and precise technical information such as standards or variations in the weights and measures used in formulas, or corrections to previously inaccurate identifications of *materia medica*. Third, he substantially changed the form of medicines. The information contained in the close to twenty thousand formulas that he encountered in Chinese works, and the several thousand that he included in *Ton'ishō* and *Man'anpō*, ushered in a general replacement of decoctions prepared from minimally processed ingredients with premade pills, pellets, and powders. Access to a wider variety of crude drugs and to compounding approaches that reflected both the Arabic and the Chinese pharmaceutical regimes introduced greater complexity and sophistication to the Japanese pharmacopeia and the medicines themselves.

In sum, the combined effects of the Song printing revolution, the extensive production of medical writings in China, the access to these materials made possible by new channels of exchange opened by Buddhist priests, and the acquisition of a greater range of crude drugs exercised a transforming influence on medieval Japanese medicine.

While shamans remained active throughout China even until today, literate physicians also became more common. Under later regimes, as it became more difficult for literati to attain office, medicine remained an important alternative vocation. Scholar-physicians continued to develop individualized styles of healing, hereditary physicians' sons sometimes gained office, and the two groups were not always clearly distinguishable. Commerce, literacy, and printing continued to spread ever more widely, steadily disseminating the influence of canonical medical knowledge, as well as popular plague god cults, exorcistic festivals, and other ritual modalities.

1. The Song divided its territorial administration into "circuits" *(lu)*. Each circuit was divided into prefectures, and these in turn were divided into districts (*xian*) with populations of around ten thousand to fifteen thousand people. At its greatest extent in the eleventh century, the Song had twenty-four circuits and approximately three hundred prefectures and fifteen hundred districts. The central government assigned separate military, fiscal, judicial, and supply commissioners to govern the circuits. The governors sent to head the prefecture and district administrations were known as prefects and magistrates, respectively (Hucker 1985, 45–46).

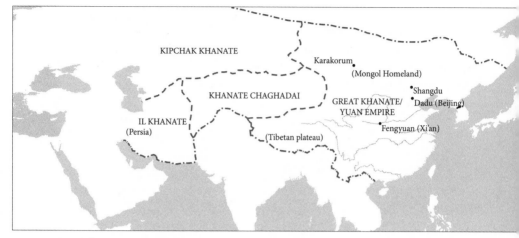

Mongol Empire, ca. 1300

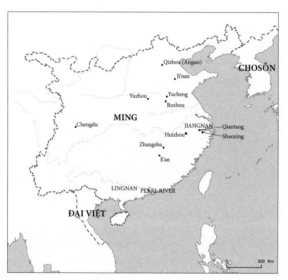

Ming Period

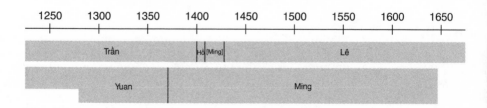

FIVE

The Yuan and Ming Periods

Angela Ki Che Leung

THE MONGOL CONQUESTS of the thirteenth century decimated populations and devastated infrastructures across Eurasia. On the other hand, the Mongol empire, subdivided into four khanates, encouraged trade across the continent (including in medicinal drugs), supported diverse religious and technical specialists (including healers), and promoted cultural exchange (including between Greek-based Arabic medicine and Chinese medicine). (See "Arabic Medicine in China.") The eastern Great Khanate, known in Chinese terms as the Yuan Dynasty (1206–1368), unified long-divided southern and northern territories, enhancing opportunities for exchange, including between medical practitioners.

The Han Chinese–ruled Ming Dynasty (1368–1644) that succeeded the Yuan came to be known as an insular regime, but contact and trade across borders continued. (See "Tuệ Tĩnh—Vietnamese Monk-Physician at the Ming Court" and "A Chosŏn Korea Medical Synthesis.") In the sixteenth century, among literati and at court, Jesuit missionaries found skepticism but also interest in their scientific and technical knowledge and in their religious teachings.

By placing renewed importance on the examination system, the Ming state enhanced scholars' cultural power. At the same time, Jiangnan's already solid agricultural and commercial economy facilitated the growth of its scholar class, whose conceptions of body and health would gradually dominate the medical discourse of the late imperial period. Moreover, the expansion of state power in the Pearl River region during the latter half of the Ming period uncovered for Jiangnan scholar-physicians a different cultural and ecological locus. There, bodies appeared to be different. New contagious diseases seemed to emerge and spread to other parts of the empire. These observations would eventually influence mainstream discourse on the body, diseases, and health.

Practitioner Types and Hierarchies

The consolidation of the civil examination system "Confucianized" medical learning in the Yuan-Ming period. This development produced an increasingly sophisticated scholarly tradition, based on medical classics and emphasizing pattern diagnosis, that was distinguishable from popular, sometimes illiterate traditions that retained local and often hands-on practices.

Learned Traditions

The scholarly medical traditions that had emerged in the Song and Jin continued to flourish, and by the late fourteenth century they came to be represented by the Four Masters: Liu Wansu (1120–1200), Zhang Congzheng (1156–1228), and Li Gao (1180–1251)—all northerners of the Jin Dynasty—and Zhu Zhenheng (1282–1358), a southerner of the Yuan Dynasty (Leung 2003c, 374–375). The three Jin masters, each a revisionist of Song medicine, based their innovations on a return to the classics, especially the *Inner Canon of the Yellow Emperor,* and in their application of Five Phases and Six Qi theory were especially sensitive to environmental elements in explanations of the body, diseases, and therapeutics (Despeux 2001; Leung 2003c, 379–380).

Liu and Zhang favored purgative treatments for the "solid and full" "northern" body. Li, however, responded to a period of wars and famines, when patients were weakened, by stressing replenishing therapeutics. It was Zhu Zhenheng—the southerner living in the unified Mongol Empire, and the synthesizer of the northern masters—who exerted the greatest influence on the learned medical traditions of the Yuan and Ming periods. His motto, "Yang is always in excess; Yin is always deficient," interpreted Fire as a potential source of destructive instability. This perspective "brought the medical body into correspondence with neo-Confucian metaphysics" (Furth 1999, 147). Recognized above all as a Confucian scholar rather than as a physician in his native place, Zhu epitomized the scholar-physician culture that matured in his day (Furth 2006).

Doctors of the learned tradition, rapidly growing in number under the Ming, would follow Zhu's career pattern of learning to become a doctor after repeated failures in the imperial civil examinations. It was certainly not a coincidence that the greatest number of scholar-physicians, fine doctors from med-

TABLE 4

Geographic distribution of known Ming doctors

Province/training	Self-taught doctors	Doctors trained by masters	Doctors trained by family
Jiangsu	27	81	389
Zhejiang	25	41	143
National total	101 (29 in the Yuan)	271 (77 in the Yuan)	769 (282 in the Yuan)

Sources: Li Jingwei 1988; Li Jiren 1990; Gao 1994; Chen and Xue 1985; Zeng 1991; Leung 1995.

ical lineages *(shiyi)* in the Ming, came from the southern provinces of Jiangsu and Zhejiang (the latter being Zhu's native province), which also produced the greatest number of successful candidates for the civil examination (Ho 1962, 227). Using biographies of medical practitioners, we have broken down the numbers of known Ming doctors by province and found that the two provinces produced the greatest numbers of doctors in the empire. The majority of these doctors were known for their healing skills in their locality or for medical texts they authored. Many were summoned by the court to be palace doctors. In other words, the center of medical culture in Ming China was unquestionably the Jiangnan area, more specifically eastern Jiangsu and Zhejiang provinces (Xie 2006, 1207, 1211–1212). (See Table 4.)

As in the Sui-Tang period, when Indian influence was obvious in Chinese medicine, this period was also known for active cultural exchanges between China and other cultures: Arabic, Tibetan, and European Christian medical ideas came to China at different stages and via different channels (Ma, Gao, and Hong 1993; Garrett 2006; Fan 1942). The establishment of the unique Muslim Pharmacy *(Huihui yiwu yuan)* in 1292–1293 at the Yuan capital was a clear indication of Mongol sponsorship of Persian medicine at the height of its development (Song 2001). (See "Arabic Medicine in China.") Three centuries later, the publication of Chinese medical books on anatomy also revealed the introduction of European Christian anatomical knowledge into China by the first Jesuits (Chu 1996).

Arabic Medicine in China

Paul D. Buell

The classic texts of "Arabic medicine" were Arabic translations from the Greek, although Islamic theoreticians and synthesizers made many contributions of their own. Arabic medicine is today the traditional medicine of the Islamic world, but in times past it was also the cosmopolitan medicine of much of Eurasia, reaching its widest geographical extent during the Mongol period. Indeed, it was the preferred medicine of the elite at the time and, in Mongol China, represented serious competition for Chinese medicine.

Arabic medicine first appeared in China during the Tang period. Elements borrowed by Chinese medicine included a modified humoral system, hot-cold classification, many herbs and simples, and medicinal foods. The surviving fragments of the *Iranian Materia Medica (Hu bencao)*, written during the era, and the slightly later *Overseas Materia Medica (Haiyao bencao)* provide early evidence of these exchanges. These texts were two of several specialized herbals devoted to non-Chinese *Materia Medica*. We also may infer foreign medical practice on the part of such men as Li Xun (fl. tenth century), whose family was of Iranian origin and who wrote the *Overseas Materia Medica*.

The Mongol rulers of China actively patronized and promoted the attempt to synthesize Arabic medicine for a Chinese and international court audience. They built on earlier Chinese and non-Chinese roots, including classificatory systems for pharmaceutical substances, materials used, and independent traditions of medicine in the north. One result was a work reedited during Ming times as *Muslim Medicinal Recipes (Huihui yaofang)*. Originally it was a great encyclopedia of 3,500 dense pages, but only 484 now survive, leaving three out of the original thirty-six chapters (12, 30, and 34) and the table of contents for the second part of the encyclopedia. The three content chapters focus, respectively, on various kinds of paralysis and related conditions (chapter 12); general conditions and symptoms of the body (chapter 30); and injuries ranging from arrow and sword wounds to breaks, fractures, burns and bites, and interventions such as cauterization (chapter 34). Some of the procedures for treating skull fracture embrace advanced surgical intervention. Of the sections that have disappeared, as indicated in the table of contents, the most serious loss is the complete list of *materia medica* (chapter 36) and the text's overall conception of the human body and its systems (chapter 29).

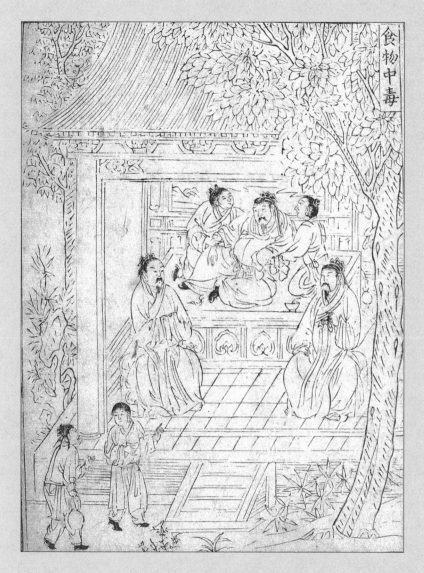

Figure 5.1. scholar-physicians advising food poisoning patient. From Hu Shihui, *Proper and Essential Things for the Emperor's Food and Drink (Yinshan zhengyao).* Courtesy of the Wellcome Library, London.

Muslim Medicinal Recipes is unique in including Arabic script entries for *materia medica* and terms. Despite these primarily Persian forms, the contents in the surviving chapters make clear that more than one medical tradition is at work, including Tibetan. Moreover, the entire work has been assimilated to Chinese views of the body and medicine. For example, it uses Chinese terminology for disease categories such as "Wind," and for physiological systems such as the Viscera *(zangfu)* and the *Qi* and Blood vitalities. The reediting of the work during the Ming shows a continued interest in the contributions of Arabic medicine. The Ming also took over traditions of Arabic medicine found in the Yuan imperial court dietary manual, the *Proper and Essential Things for the Emperor's Food and Drink (Yinshan zhengyao)*, published in 1330. (See Figure 5.1.) Although the long-term influence of Islamic medicine on Chinese medical theory is unclear, Chinese herbals such as the *Systematic Materia Medica* (see "Li Shizhen") draw extensively on items from *Proper and Essential Things for the Emperor's Food and Drink* and other Arabic works.

TUỆ TĨNH—VIETNAMESE MONK-PHYSICIAN AT THE MING COURT

C. Michele Thompson

In 1385 Đại Việt, a state on China's southern border covering the northern third of present-day Vietnam, was ruled by the Trần Dynasty (1225–1400). The Chinese and the Yue/Việt (Yue is the modern Mandarin pronunciation of Việt) had had an uneasy relationship since well before the Common Era. A positive aspect of that relationship was exchange of medical products and medical information. Early evidence of medical contact between Han and Việt comes from manuscripts from the Mawangdui archaeological site that contain a number of Yue medical formulas (Harper 1998, esp. 173–183). During this very early period the ethnic Yue/Việt could be found in a number of polities scattered throughout what is today southeast China and northern Vietnam. Later, during the period of Chinese rule (111 B.C.E.–939 C.E.), local medical products were part of the tribute extracted from the area (Schafer 1967; Li 1979). After gaining independence from China the rulers of Đại Việt continued to acknowledge fealty to China and exchanged presents/tribute with Chinese rulers. This tribute always included *materia medica*, spices, and exotic fruits, plants, and animals. Sometimes it also included people with notable skills in the arts or sciences, and in 1385 the Vietnamese Buddhist monk-physician Tuệ Tĩnh was sent to the Ming Court as a living present.

Tuệ Tĩnh (1330–ca. 1389), meaning "Tranquil Wisdom," is the name Nguyễn Bá Tĩnh took when he became a monk. He was born in Nghĩa Phú village in Hải

Dương province and was orphaned at age six. After this Tuệ Tĩnh was raised and educated by Buddhist monks, who taught him not only Buddhist classics but also Confucian texts for the imperial exams. He passed these exams, but instead of accepting a job as a royal official he became a monk. In Đại Việt, Buddhist institutions were often involved in health care, and Tuệ Tĩnh became a respected doctor and pharmacist. He worked extensively with plants, founded medical gardens at several pagodas, did research into the medicinal properties of local plants, and compiled texts on Vietnamese medicine and pharmacology. His basic medical philosophy was that it is best to maintain good health through a diet of local fruits and vegetables, adequate physical exercise, and moderation in hedonistic activities. He further viewed the plants of Vietnam, if properly used, to be superior to imported Chinese medicines for Vietnamese people and their illnesses (Dương 1947–1950, 73–74; Hoang 1993, 16–17).

Tuệ Tĩnh's renown attracted attention, and when he was fifty-five he was sent to China with the 1385 tribute mission. Tuệ Tĩnh had a successful career in China; indeed, Vietnamese folk beliefs hold that he saved the life of a Chinese empress who suffered postnatal complications. Tuệ Tĩnh's most famous work, the *Nam Dược Thần Hiệu (Miraculous Drugs of the South)*, was written in China. This work, intended to explain Vietnamese medicine to Chinese physicians, consists of eleven volumes covering pharmaceutical ingredients and 184 medical situations that were common in both China and Vietnam. Tuệ Tĩnh sent copies to Vietnam, and copies undoubtedly existed in the Vietnamese royal libraries before the Ming invasion of 1407 (Hoang 1993, 17). During this invasion many Vietnamese texts were destroyed or taken to China (Dương 1947). This important text by Tuệ Tĩnh disappeared from the Vietnamese imperial libraries during this period, but it was reconstructed from partial copies held in private libraries and printed in 1761 (Hoang 1993, 38–39; Nguyen 1986, 49; Thompson 2010, 408).

Tuệ Tĩnh was not allowed to return home, and when he died he was buried in Nanjing. His tomb became a pilgrimage site for Vietnamese visiting the area. In 1676 a scholar from Tuệ Tĩnh's home village recorded the epitaph on the grave stele and had it carved on another for their village (Hoang 1993, 17). Sad to say, the epitaph included a plea for anyone from Vietnam who came to Tuệ Tĩnh's tomb to return his remains to his homeland. (Also see *Southern Medicine for Southern People* 2012.)

Popular Traditions

While classical studies, fine diagnostic methods, and prescriptive art were highlighted in learned, mainstream medicine, other methods and specialties—especially those requiring hands-on technologies or more drastic therapeutics—were gradually marginalized. More to the point, they were increasingly left in the hands of popular, illiterate healers who mostly maintained traditions orally. As learned scholar-physicians skilled in pattern diagnosis applied therapeutic strategies according to their interpretations of medical classics, popular healers often bypassed pulse reading and used manual treatments or administered drugs that produced immediate effects, resulting in quick relief or the disappearance of symptoms.

Such practitioners were mostly skilled in acupuncture, moxibustion, and massage, and in surgical skills that dealt with eye, skin, muscle, or other problems viewed as external medicine *(waike)* disorders. They also applied drugs that induced vomiting and purging effects, which quickly stopped symptoms. Many were, in addition, practitioners of variolation against smallpox. Midwives, who assisted in childbirth and abortion and provided care for newborns, were also trained in this tradition. (See "Variolation.")

Specialists in ritual healing, practicing mostly in temples and shrines, were yet another alternative for those who fell ill. The techniques of ritual healing could sometimes be traced to ancient texts or to late Buddhist and Daoist rituals. Many were characterized by systems of deities and worship in local societies. Ritual healers did not always base their practice on written texts, even though Daoist exorcists relied heavily on the drawing of talismans for healing purposes (Strickmann 2002, 123–193). There was no standard diagnostic procedure for these healers, and the refined art of prescribing was not their main concern. Ritual healers also had to bear the risk of being persecuted by bureaucrats for their "subversive" and dangerous practice, which sometimes attracted alarmingly large followings of believers (Leung 1987, 149; Leung 1999, 121–123). To make matters worse for them, learned physicians criticized these approaches to healing as heterodox.

The separation of the two traditions had already been noted by Yuan doctors such as Ni Weide (1303–77), who deplored scholar-physicians' ignorance of specialties such as treating the eye. He wrote, "On eye-healing, there is no complete work. Although mentioned sporadically in various works, it is treated neither completely nor in depth. Can it be that our ancestors despised it? Or that those who teach it are not authentic, so that those who are taught cannot but learn in futile ways?" (Leung 2003c, 384). The Yuan acupuncturist Hua

Shou (1304–1386) lamented, "The way *(dao)* of acupuncture declines, the channels system has become obscure" (Leung 2003c, 383).

When elite physicians did practice external medicine, they still found ways to distinguish themselves from popular healers. Qi Dezhi (ca. 1335), a Yuan court surgeon, criticized healers who specialized in suppurative lesions *(chuang)* for "often bypassing pulse-taking and only treating the external [symptoms]. If a case is doubtful and difficult, they [have to] ask other doctors who take pulse and prescribe to observe and diagnose. This tribe of lesion specialists accepts bearing the reputation of being shallow and negligent" (Leung 2003c, 384–385).

These marginalized specialized doctors—together with anonymous generalists or ritual healers who did not have the full training of scholar-physicians—provided treatment to the populace who could afford to seek medical help. Some complemented the healing methods of elite scholar-physicians who avoided hands-on techniques, as shown in a case of the famous Anhui doctor Sun Yikui (1522–1619). Sun was treating a patient with a huge suppurative lesion that needed puncturing with a needle. In his own words, "I have always been kind *(ren)* at heart in my whole life, and I cannot bear using the needle." His solution was to ask an external medicine specialist to do the puncturing, while he prescribed internal drugs for the patient (Sun 1999, 3:796). Many mainstream doctors strictly observed this "kindness," central in Confucian ethics, making room for specialists. The case of Sun illustrates the hierarchy of specialists who treated different classes of the population. On their general social situation, unfortunately, we have only sporadic information (Xie 2006, 1220–1223).

A CHOSŎN KOREA MEDICAL SYNTHESIS: HŎ CHUN'S *PRECIOUS MIRROR OF EASTERN MEDICINE*

Soyoung Suh

Chinese medical texts had been relied on for understanding health and disease and for guiding healing in Korea since the Sui (581–618) and perhaps earlier. Official envoys of the Koryŏ Dynasty (918–1392) brought back Song medical texts such as the *Taiping Era Formulary of Sagely Grace* (published 992, brought to Koryŏ in 1016) (Miki 1962, 44). This kind of intermittent textual importation was gradually replaced by orderly, planned state production. King Sejong (r. 1418–1450) sponsored a number of scholarly projects to display the cultural authority and confidence of the recently founded Chosŏn Dynasty (1392–1910); these included the *Classified Compilation of Medical Formulae (Ŭibang yuch'wi)* (Kim 2001, 532–535). One of the most important medical works to emerge from Chosŏn was the court-sponsored work *Precious Mirror of Eastern Medicine (Tongŭi pogam)*. The project, begun by a group of court physicians, was disrupted by invasions from Japan (1592–1598). Hŏ Chun (1539–1615) finally completed it in 1610.

Chosŏn society was highly stratified according to inherited statuses, and technical specialists such as physicians and lower-level bureaucrats tended to come from the "middle people" (*chungin*) class of elite but nonaristocratic commoners. Although some aristocratic official (*yangban*) elites were well versed in medical learning, they disdained its practice for profit and did not encourage their sons to pursue careers as doctors. Hŏ Chun, born an illegitimate son to a *yangban* family, had an ambiguous status that made him ineligible for high office but opened to him alternative careers. He educated himself in Confucian classics, mastered medicine, and became a court physician (Kim 2000, 103). In this position, Hŏ gained the trust of King Sŏnjo (1552–1608) by successfully treating the crown prince's smallpox in 1590 and accompanying the king on the royal exodus from the palace during the war with Japan (Shin 2001, 115–116).

In *Precious Mirror of Eastern Medicine* Hŏ drew on earlier Chinese and native works to produce a new synthesis of medical knowledge. He examined more than 230 previous medical texts, favoring the latest medical writings from Ming China, but also gave more detailed accounts of the names and qualities of local botanicals than had ever appeared before. From these sources, Hŏ listed more than 2,000 symptoms, 1,400 medicinal substances, and 4,000 remedies (Shin 2001, 206), and organized them in five major categories: "Interior Landscape," "External Forms," "Miscellaneous Diseases," "Decoctions," and "Acupuncture and Moxibustion." Hŏ's interest in the indigenous environment was further expressed by his intentional use of "Eastern Medicine" *(tongŭi)* in the title. Hŏ argued that since Chinese physicians such as Li Gao and Zhu Zhenheng were taken to represent "northern" and "southern" medicine, respectively, Hŏ's own synthesis deserved another geocultural distinction.

Nevertheless, Hŏ's claim for a distinctive "eastern" medicine was not a simple shift from a Chinese medical tradition to a purely indigenous one. Rather, Hŏ's *Precious Mirror of Eastern Medicine* exemplifies a Chosŏn doctor's skillful integration of local understandings with new knowledge coming in from China, and his participation in trends in medical writing that prevailed across geographic and political barriers. Hŏ's voluminous compilation was welcomed across eighteenth-century East Asia, not only because of its medical efficacy and indigeneity but also because of its well-composed classical Chinese writing style and rational organization.

Hŏ Chun's *Precious Mirror of Eastern Medicine* has received more scholarly and popular attention than any other premodern Korean medical text. Following its first publication in 1613, *Precious Mirror* was printed in Tokugawa Japan in 1724 and again in 1799. Beginning in 1763, dozens of editions were published in China (Shin 2001, 222–228). Celebrating UNESCO's recent recognition of the text as part of its Memory of World Heritage program, contemporary Koreans view *Precious Mirror of Eastern Medicine* as a culmination of indigenous achievement in traditional medicine.

The Transmission of Medical Knowledge

State medical institutions inherited from the Song trained doctors, promoted classical texts, and provided medicines. In many respects the Yuan continued and even expanded these programs, but such efforts declined under the Ming. On the other hand, there was a growing consciousness of doctoring as a trade with its own specific training process, methods, and ethics despite the absence of formal institutions. Guidelines on doctoring as a trade began to appear in printed texts, such as medical books and medical lineage rules. In the latter half of the Ming period doctors also formed local associations.

For seven decades under the Yuan, until 1313, the civil service examination was suspended, and doctoring became an even more attractive career alternative for Confucian scholars. In 1262 the Yuan government established local medical schools (*yixue*), and in 1272 it created a supervisorate (*yixue tiju si*) to oversee them. They enhanced doctors' social status with special Medical Household (*yihu*) registration and state rituals (Shinno 2007; Qiu 2004, 331–332). (See "Medical Schools and the Temples of the Three Progenitors.") However, such public medical institutions soon lost ground after the establishment of the Ming Dynasty. The Song ideal of having central authorities train and legitimize doctors was not taken up again.

Medical Schools and the Temples of the Three Progenitors

Reiko Shinno

The Mongols valued physicians and a range of other specialists during their conquests across the Eurasian continent in the early thirteenth century, and continued to do so as they consolidated their rule. They gave physicians levy privileges, and in China they created the taxation and judicial category "Medical Households." Khubilai Khan and his advisors also reestablished the Jin Dynasty's Imperial Academy of Medicine *(taiyi yuan)* and granted it greater power and prestige. It was mostly Chinese members of this academy who proposed the revival of government-mandated local Medical Schools, and the system was built soon after Khubilai Khan's ascendance to the throne in 1260. The Yuan government expanded the network of local Medical Schools, bringing it to its peak in the imperial period.

Medical School instructors were required to hold a discussion session every ten days, which all the sons of medical households were expected to attend. Educated men from nonmedical households could also participate if they liked. The Imperial Academy of Medicine distributed the topics for these meetings and required instructors to report back on their own answers and on students' performance. These records were used to evaluate both teachers and students and sometimes were made the basis for promotion to higher offices. An instructor's poor performance could result in a cut to his salary and, in the worst scenario, cost him his position.

It was a contemporary Chinese expectation that formal schools should have temples dedicated to role models. Confucian Schools *(ruxue)*, for instance, had Temples of Confucius *(xuansheng miao)*. By the end of the thirteenth century, the Yuan government established Temples of the Three Progenitors *(Sanhuang miao)* for the medical schools. The Three Progenitors—Fuxi, the Subduer of Animals; Shennong, the Divine Husbandman; and Huangdi, the Yellow Emperor—were mythical rulers believed to have made great contributions to medicine. Previous dynasties had enshrined Fuxi, Shennong, and Huangdi collectively or individually as model rulers and founders of civilization, but the Yuan was the first to dedicate official temples to them because of their medical contributions. The temples also housed the Progenitors' wives (a privilege shared by other deities in China) and ten other famous historical physicians.

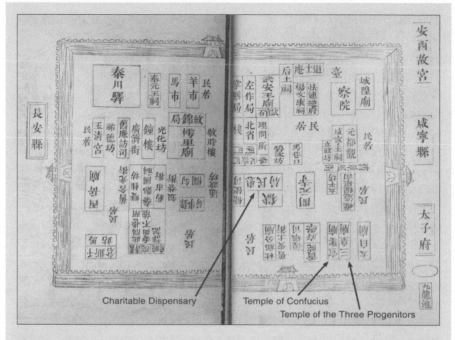

Charitable Dispensary   Temple of Confucius
Temple of the Three Progenitors

Figure 5.2. Yuan period plan of Fengyuan circuit seat. From Li Haowen 1970, *shang*.11b–12a. Courtesy of the Library of Congress.

While some localities, such as Qingyuan circuit, had a building dedicated to the Medical School with the temple as part of the building, other localities, such as Fengyuan circuit (present-day Xi'an city; see Figure 5.2), had just a building for the temple, and Medical School instructors and students simply went there for their regular meetings. The instructor and students were required to pray and burn incense at the temple before their academic discussions.

Many famous literati wrote laudatory essays that were inscribed on the walls of the temples or on nearby stone tablets. Some of these inscriptions argued that the temples were important not only for doctors but also for Confucians in general, because the Three Progenitors were founders of the Way (Dao). In addition, the authors of the inscriptions praised Mongol rulers for their care for people's welfare. In Shangdu, a Yuan capital, a sculptor used western Indian techniques to carve the statues of the Three Progenitors and received lavish rewards from Khubilai Khan, further demonstrating both the importance of the temple and the vigorous cross-cultural interactions common in the period. (Shinno 2007; Allsen 2001, 141–160; Ōshima 1980)

In medical matters, the Ming government was concerned essentially with the selection of palace doctors to care for the imperial household. There was no initiative to establish a centralized medical training or examination program. The system of local medical schools, reestablished by a Ming imperial decree in 1384, was similar to that of the Yuan—in the bottom rung of the bureaucracy. But the great importance that Ming authorities placed on the civil examination as the main channel for Confucian scholars to enter officialdom quickly and substantially reduced the prestige of the physician. Medicine became a second-rate alternative for an otherwise reluctant scholar in the face of repeated failures in the civil examination.

Even though medical bureaucrats recruited by local medical schools were theoretically responsible for training doctors and improving medical service in the locality, such a difficult task was never seriously planned or implemented. Most medical bureaucrats came from local medical lineages or from registered medical households and used the post either to enhance the status of their lineages or as a stepping-stone to more important official jobs, such as palace doctor. By the sixteenth century, with the further decline of the Medical School, most local medical bureaucrats were merely performing perfunctory, petty, and even nonmedical bureaucratic jobs (Leung 1987; Qiu 2004, 327–359). We find a concrete example in Chun'an county in Zhejiang province. According to a sixteenth-century record, the Medical School there had long been deserted:

> One has altogether forgotten when it was abandoned completely. . . . Now the school has no [established] location and the bureaucratic position is not properly filled. Even though there are those who study medicine [in the locality], there is no authority to supervise them. Those who use their vain title to deal with superior authorities are all vulgar persons of the market place. Could one not be perplexed by such a development? (Leung 2001, 223)

The training of doctors during the entire period was thus essentially carried out independent of state institutions. Most doctors of the learned tradition were trained either by masters or by senior family members, especially in medical lineages. To a great extent, there was a return to the classical master-disciple model, established through rituals and the passing on of texts (Sivin 1995, 182–183). With the popularization of printed medical texts, including classics, however, an increasing number of doctors trained themselves, at least at the initial stage of learning.

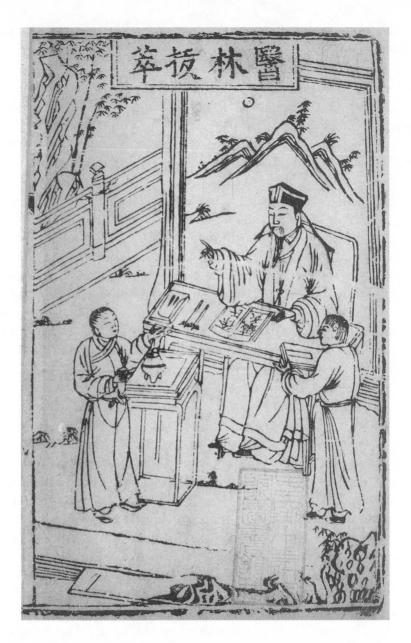

Figure 5.3. Scholar-physician teaching apprentices, one holding acupuncture needles and one holding a text. From Xu Feng, *Mr. Xu's Great Compendium of Acupuncture and Moxibustion: Combined Edition with the [Illustrated] Bronze Statues (Tongren xushi zhenjiu heke).* Courtesy of the Wellcome Library, London.

Among the different channels of transmission of medical knowledge, the most characteristic among literate physicians was the exclusive master-disciple model common in Neo-Confucian teaching. Medicine was also transmitted within families, creating medical lineages. The two patterns contributed to the consolidation of separate medical schools or "currents of learning" *(xuepai)*, especially in the Jiangnan region. For example, after a period of studying on his own, Zhu Zhenheng became a student of Luo Zhiti, who had inherited the tradition of the northern masters. Zhu passed his medical knowledge to his son and nephew (thus founding a medical lineage) as well as to many other disciples in his region. His school of medical thought had important and prolonged influence in the Jiangnan region throughout the late imperial period (Leung 2003c, 388–389; Furth 2006, 430–432).

Even though women were excluded from the master-disciple model of training, they sometimes received training as doctors within clans and lineages so that they could care for young or female family members. Some were even summoned to the palace to treat female members of the imperial household. By the late Ming, we begin to see highly educated women doctors from elite families authoring medical writings of the learned tradition (Cass 1986; Furth 1999, 285–298; Leung 1999, 126–127).

Women were even more active in popular healing traditions. The training of popular healers is difficult to trace, as it mostly occurred orally, and we learn about their activities mainly from the writings of scholars and learned doctors, who often depicted them in a negative light. Elite men viewed women who specialized in healing and other vocations, because they came and went from the inner quarters to which decent women had by this period become confined, as potentially corrupting. A Yuan period scholar coined the epithet "three aunties and six grannies" *(sangu liupo)*, diviners and Buddhist and Daoist nuns being the "aunties," and shaman-healers, medicinal drug peddlers, midwives, brokers, matchmakers, and procuresses being the "grannies," and late imperial men advised respectable families to avoid all nine categories like "snakes and scorpions." Besides the more obvious healing-related vocations, from various writings we also learn that many religious women such as nuns were adept in such skills as acupuncture, moxibustion, ophthalmology, and skin diseases (Leung 1999). (On scholarly alternatives to women healers' knowledge for the care of children care, see "Children's Medicine.")

Children's Medicine

Hsiung Ping-chen

Historically, not all societies have treated children as salient objects of concern, nor as being in some way fundamentally dissimilar to or having needs different from those of adults. In China, however, for many centuries knowledge particular to the care of children was not only an arena of domestic folk knowledge but a prominent subfield of learned medicine as well. Religious and ethical views, often associated with Confucianism but not exclusive to it, powerfully reinforced the love of children and elevated their nurture to a sacred duty of parents, senior family members, and public-spirited and responsible people (Hsiung 2005).

After Qian Yi (1032–1113), the children's "department" or branch of medicine increasingly became a specialty not only for some practitioners but also for entire medical lineages, as in the case of the Wan family. The Wans began practicing medicine in the fourteenth century in Luotian district, Hubei province, in the middle part of the Yangzi Valley. Wan Quan (1499–1582), the third-generation inheritor of the practice, carefully compiled the family's practical knowledge into a concise text, *Family Secrets of Infant Care (Yuying jia mi)*, which quickly achieved wide popularity in the middle Yangzi, Jiangnan, and southeastern provinces. Ironically, not one of Wan's ten sons was interested in carrying on the family vocation, a fact that threatened to consign the family medical expertise to obscurity. This prompted him to compose an additional book, *Elaboration on the Children's Branch [of Medicine] (Youke fahui)*, giving more thorough theoretical background to supplement *Family Secrets*. What had been a duty to maintain and continue family medical traditions thus translated into a broader social mission and contributed to the circulation of medical knowledge (Wan 1986, iii; Hsiung 2005, 40–43).

Similarly, male popular healers appeared in the writings of scholar-physicians. Sometimes disparagingly called "vulgar doctors" *(suyi)* or "luck doctors" *(fuyi)*, they were not well read in medical books and "knew little about pulse and symptoms," but some said their "treatments were always effective" (Leung 2003c, 397). Yuan and Ming society also included a wide array of itinerant healers—"healers with a bell" *(lingyi)* and "healers traveling in bushes and marshes" *(caoze yi)*.

By the late Ming, some officials expressed alarm at what they deemed to be the widespread lack of proper training. The scholar Lü Kun (1536–1618) suggested that the government should revive the functions of the local medical schools, proposing that the Medical Bureau set examinations for all medical practitioners, male and female alike. Those who succeeded with the best results should then undergo further training by reputable doctors; those with mediocre scores should be taught to memorize prescriptions that would improve their practice; and those who failed altogether should be forbidden to treat patients. Unqualified quacks who dared to practice medicine should be permanently expelled from the locality. Even though the central government never considered Lü's proposed reforms, let alone implemented them, his suggestions expressed a common concern over popular healers and a growing idea of creating standards of knowledge and practice (Leung 2003c, 397–398). Nevertheless, the Ming state was not known for any institutional innovation in medical matters, nor did it attempt the regulation or licensing of doctors.

Despite this lack of official interest, a kind of professional consciousness did grow among scholar-physicians. In the early Ming the influential palace doctor Liu Chun (late fourteenth century) wrote and published a set of instructions to students and descendants, providing guidelines on therapy and ethics. He was specific about respecting standard prices, complying with accepted prescriptions, and following standard diagnostic and therapeutic principles (Leung 2008). Later, medical associations produced and published similar sets of instructions. In 1568 in Beijing, for example, the famous Anhui doctor Xu Chunfu, who was then practicing in the capital, established one of the first associations for doctors, called the Medical Society for Harboring Kindness (*zhairen yihui*). Forty-six doctors of the society collectively drew up technical and ethical guidelines and signed a pact agreeing to respect them (Xiang 1981, 144–146).

Similar medical associations appeared in other places with high concentrations of scholar-physicians. The Association of Heavenly Medicine (*tianyi she*), for example, was established in the Qiantang (Hangzhou) region during the Wanli period (1573–1620), grouping together famous local doctors (Leung 2003b, 148). The growing number of medical textbooks for beginners published in the Ming also often included technical and ethical guidelines, crafted to inform the reader about what a properly trained doctor should be like. Doctors of the learned tradition shared a growing agreement about the necessity of drawing a line between fine physicians and quacks or popular healers (Leung 1997; Unschuld 1979). This consensus was not induced by the state or any formal public organizations but grew with the increasing number of scholar-physicians and medical lineages and with the expansion of the market of printed books (Brokaw 2007).

The appearance of a new genre of medical texts around the sixteenth century, the medical casebook *(yi'an),* provided a further indication of the maturing of the doctors' trade during the Ming. Case descriptions in succinct style already existed in early medical literature, but it was only now that entire books devoted to such records began to be published, especially in the Huizhou region, where Confucian scholarship was honored, mercantile and medical culture flourished, and the publishing industry prospered. Often authored by a physician or his disciples, the casebook recorded the condition of the patient as well as how the doctor diagnosed and treated the ailment. Some records also showed intriguing relations between the doctor and the patient or the patient's family. The growing popularity of medical casebooks demonstrated the recognized social status of the scholar-physician. The genre highlighted the superior medical skills and moral power of the doctor and revealed his dense social network, which encompassed both celebrities and lowly workers. These books also deliberately promoted models of professional behavior in a culture where diverse groups—scholars, merchants, and doctors—mixed freely (Furth 2007; Grant 2003; Zeitlin 2007).

Provision of Medicines

While Yuan authorities followed the Song model of distributing free or cheap medicines to the poor through a network of charitable dispensaries *(huimin yaoju),* such efforts were not sustained for long under the Ming. The Yuan dispensaries were established most intensively during the years 1298–1299, making full use of the service of registered medical households. Some seemed to operate on a considerable scale. In Ji'an county of Jiangxi province, for instance, the charitable dispensary built in 1299 was "supervised by well-qualified doctors." The establishment "had an outside tower, leading to the great hall inside. There were side buildings where instruments were kept, and special places reserved for the sunning and storage of herbs, and for the distribution of medicines to the public." The dispensary was also responsible for providing medicines and food to local sick prisoners. The institution seems to have functioned for a long period, and it was renovated in 1350 when bureaucrats and local medical households donated money for the purpose (Leung 2001, 226).

A certain hierarchy characterized the dispensary system in some provinces. The one in She county of Anhui province, also established in 1299, for instance, had the capacity to "produc[e] more than four hundred drugs, with two supervising doctors, five pharmaceutical interns *(yaosheng),* and local Medical Households taking turns to manage [the institution] every year." This dispensary seemed to be at the top of the provincial hierarchy. In 1305, for example, the provincial authorities of Anhui ordered each county to establish a branch dispensary to provide the poor with medicines manufactured at the central provincial dispensary in She county. Such cases of large-scale public dispensaries seem to have been common in southern China during the Yuan (Leung 2001, 226).

Charitable dispensaries continued to exist during the early years of Ming but, as with the local Medical Schools, they soon entered a steady decline. Even though the first Ming emperor ordered the reestablishment of public charitable dispensaries in 1370 and 1374, these never obtained as much institutional support from the authorities as they had during the Yuan. The last imperial edict to demand the restoration of the dispensaries was proclaimed in 1428. After that, the central government seemed to abandon all interest in the institution. Finally, the system of registered medical households inherited from the Yuan became irreversibly lax and its role obscured, and the government lost the last human resources it could mobilize for local public health functions.

The function and efficiency of charitable dispensaries thus depended largely on the will of individual local bureaucrats. During the 1370s, for instance, the dispensary in She county still operated on more or less the same scale as it had in the Yuan, with two medical bureaucrats taking charge, assisted by two pharmaceutical interns. However, it declined in the following years and "people did not benefit from it." After a brief restoration by the local prefect in 1501, it was definitively abandoned. Another example was Hangzhou county in Zhejiang, which had eight such dispensaries in 1370 when the system was revived by the first Ming emperor. The number dwindled to one during the latter half of the fifteenth century. The decline became general after the mid-sixteenth century. Only occasionally did local bureaucrats or philanthropists revive the dispensaries to distribute medicines during epidemics (Leung 1987; 2001, 227).

To some extent, the continuing decline of state interest in medical matters in the Ming was offset by the growth of private charitable institutions. Written sources such as local gazetteers and the writings of literati show that from the sixteenth century onward, retired scholar-officials, well-to-do literati, and even drug businesses became increasingly active in setting up charitable dispensaries in their native places, both in response to increasing need and to enhance their prestige and status as local leaders. An early and famous example was the Society for Broadening Kindness (guangren hui), initiated by the scholar Yang Dongming in his hometown, Yucheng, in Henan province. He organized thirty-one of the richest people of his locality, including some well-known doctors, to form the society and pool donations to purchase medicines for distribution to the poor (Leung 1987, 145; 1997, 38, 59). Similarly, Qi Biaojia (1602–1645), a famous Ming loyalist (resistant to the conquering Qing) and prominent scholar-official of Shaoxing county in Zhejiang province, organized charitable clinics and dispensaries in his hometown several times during epidemics in the 1630s. In 1636, for example, he contracted with ten local physicians to run a dispensary, conveniently situated in a Buddhist temple. Every day a team of two doctors would be in service to give free consultation and medications to the sick. In 1641, he organized an elaborate sick ward for vagrants. Twelve physicians were to take turns at treating the bedridden and providing outpatient consultation for the local poor. Expenses of such enterprises were covered by Qi and his family, as well as by donations from his friends (Leung 1987, 145–146; 2001, 229; Smith 1995).

Peng Qisheng (1584–1646), another Ming loyalist from Haiyan in Zhejiang, organized similar charitable dispensaries, with doctors in service, at the four main gates of his hometown's city wall during an epidemic in the summer months of 1626. He did this mainly at his own expense, with subsidies from the government (Tao, Zhu, and Hong 1988, 20). These were not isolated examples, and they inspired a series of similar local charitable enterprises toward the end of the Ming Dynasty that would continue into the Qing (Fuma 1997; Leung 1997).

In addition to such charitable enterprises, private commercial dispensaries also grew in number and in scale from the fifteenth century onward. The commercialization of herbs and drugs during the Ming seems to have formed a maturing national market, with several regional centers holding seasonal drug fairs: Yuzhou, Huizhou in Henan province, Bozhou in Anhui, Anguo in Hebei, Jinan in Shandong, Chengdu in Sichuan, Zhangshu in Jiangxi, and possibly a few other smaller ones, covering the whole empire. The strengthening of the drug market explains the establishment of major commercial dispensaries that operated on a national scale and continued to grow under the last imperial dynasty and even into the modern period (An et al. 1993; Chen 1996). The worship of various "medicine gods" (yaowang), which partially replaced veneration of the "Three Emperors" established in the Yuan, was another indication of the growth of regional drug markets (Chao n.d.; Zheng 1996; Zhao 2006).

The commercialization of drugs was accompanied by progress in manufacturing technology that tended to reduce drug toxicity and thus potency—a trend that continued during the late imperial period (Zheng 2005, 211). (See Figure 5.4.) Such a development was partly in response to the current development of the drug market. The composition of the most important classic on Chinese materia medica, the Systematic Materia Medica (Bencao gangmu) by Li Shizhen (1518–1593), was thus not only an achievement of the robust intellectual pharmaceutical tradition of Ming China but also one built upon the solid material foundation of the time. (See "Li Shizhen.")

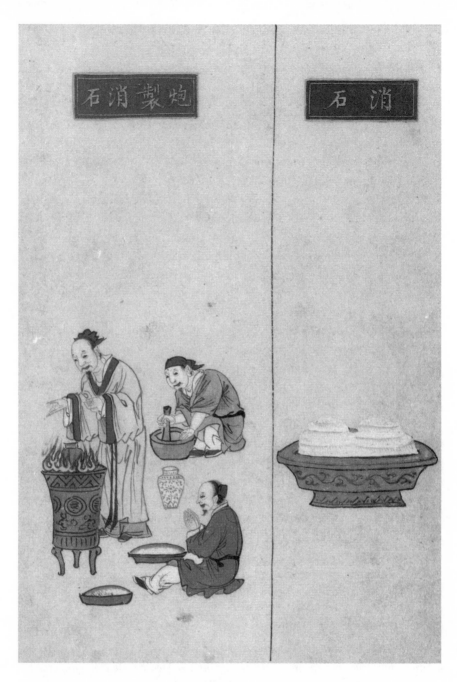

Figure 5.4. *Left:* Processing saltpeter. *Right:* Saltpeter. From *Buyi leigong paozhi bianlan* (1591 palace edition), p. 154. Courtesy of Harvard-Yenching Library, copyright Cishu chubanshe, Shanghai.

Li Shizhen

Kenneth J. Hammond

As a young man growing up in what is today Hubei province in central China, Li Shizhen (1518–1593) belonged to a family with a generations-long tradition of medical learning and practice. Li's family had accumulated sufficient wealth to allow him to be educated in the classical Confucian curriculum in preparation for taking the imperial examinations. Passing even the lowest level of the examinations would have brought the Li family great prestige and enhanced their economic prospects. Li's father, Yanwen, had passed the entry-level exam but had not been able to rise any higher, and had turned his attention to the family's traditional medical livelihood. In 1549 Yanwen was appointed to a position in the Imperial Medical Academy in Beijing and spent a year there studying. Li Shizhen himself passed the county examination as a young man of thirteen but, like his father, never managed to pass any higher level. After 1538 he abandoned the effort, taking his own place in the family business. When his father went off to Beijing, Li was well established in his own right as a local medical practitioner. When his father returned from the capital, Li in turn was able to spend a period of time studying in Beijing as well. This was followed by an appointment as court physician for the Prince of Chu, the local branch of the imperial family in Hubei.

In his work as a doctor Li found himself increasingly frustrated with the existing state of knowledge about the various kinds of medicinal preparations available as treatments. Information about drugs was found in imperially sponsored compendia of medical knowledge dating back to the Song period and earlier (see Chapter 4), but there was also a growing tradition of private scholars and practitioners publishing notes and records of the efficacy of their treatments and prescriptions. Li often found these sources to be vague or simply inaccurate in their descriptions of particular substances and their therapeutic properties. Resolving to remedy the situation, he embarked upon a program of research, both textual and empirical, that culminated in the publication of the *Systematic Materia Medica (Bencao gangmu)* in 1596, three years after Li's death.

In compiling the *Systematic Materia Medica*, Li read and critiqued some 40 earlier pharmacopoeia, plus another 361 medical texts. In addition, he examined and incorporated medical information from 591 more general works, 277 of which had not previously been included in medical collections. But Li's

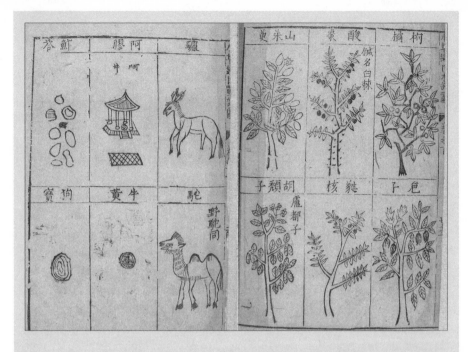

Figure 5.5. *Left:* Top row, from right to left: donkey, donkey-hide glue, horse bezoar. *Bottom row,* from right to left: camel, cow bezoar, dog bezoar. *Right:* Top row, from right to left: trifoliate orange, spine date, dogwood. Bottom row, from right to left: cape jasmine (*Gardenia jasminoides* Ellis), *Prinsepia uniflora* Batal., thorny elaeagnus/*Elaegnus pungens.* From Li, *Systematic Materia Medica,* 1590, 1st ed. Illustrations credited to Li Shizhen's son, Li Jianyuan. Courtesy of the Wellcome Library, London.

investigations took him far beyond examining texts and into the empirical evaluation of evidence, and it is in this regard that he can be seen as part of a broader process of intellectual development in sixteenth-century China. Scholars and researchers in many fields embarked upon the "investigation of things." Li traveled widely across central China, from Sichuan in the west to Hunan, Jiangxi, Anhui, and Jiangsu in the east. He visited the libraries of many scholars and examined collections of plants and other materials used in making drugs. He made drawings and recorded careful descriptions of the items he studied, and these formed the basis for his great compendium. Li also engaged in discourse with other scholars who shared his interest in understanding the natural world, including the brothers Gu Wen (Metropolitan Graduate degree *[jinshi]* 1538) and Gu Que (1528–1613), the geographer Luo Hongxian (1504–1564), and the preeminent literary figure Wang Shizhen (1526–1590), who wrote a preface for the *Systematic Materia Medica.* In these contacts and conversations we can see parallels to the kind of circulation of knowledge and sharing of empirical data that was characteristic of European intellectual discourse around the same time. Corresponding societies such as the Linnaean Academy, founded in 1603 in Italy, brought thinkers from across Europe into contact with one another to share their investigations and insights into the nature of the world around them, just as Li and his circle visited each other and wrote to each other about nature, technology, and the patterns and principles they observed in history and contemporary life.

Even though only well-off (often urban) families had access to the better-quality herbs and medicines sold in commercial dispensaries, the wider circulation of herbs produced inside or even outside the empire also increased the availability of many cheaper drugs sold by itinerant drug sellers. (See Figure 5.6.) We have seen the relatively lax attitude toward these popular vendors under the reform program suggested by the late Ming scholar Lü Kun: those who failed the test designed by qualified doctors would not be allowed to practice as physicians, but they could sell drugs. In other words, Ming society showed a fair degree of tolerance for popular drug sellers. The activities of these peddlers increased the availability of cheap herbs and medicines to the populace despite the decline of governmental dispensaries.

Conceptions of Health, Disease, and the Body

The concept of a cultivable body that could achieve extended longevity was fully revealed in the art of "nourishing life" *(yangsheng)* that matured during the later Ming period. Nourishing life, a part of the literati lifestyle, grew out of the rich material culture of Ming Jiangnan. On one hand, it was a refinement of everyday living, encompassing everything from the design of the habitat and research on clothing to meticulous care taken with food and drink (Clunas 1991; Mote 1977, 225–234; Lo and Barrett 2005). On the other hand, and perhaps more important, nourishing life embodied fundamental concepts of the ideal, healthy, fertile body.

The deep structure of the ideal male "generative body," able to achieve both fertility and longevity, was, as Charlotte Furth aptly puts it, "based on 'inner alchemy' *(neidan),* a sprawling tradition of philosophy and body practice identified originally with the religious Daoism of medieval China, but also long associated with esoteric medical teachings." By the late Ming, "inner alchemy was a multidimensional aspect of upper class philosophical eclecticism

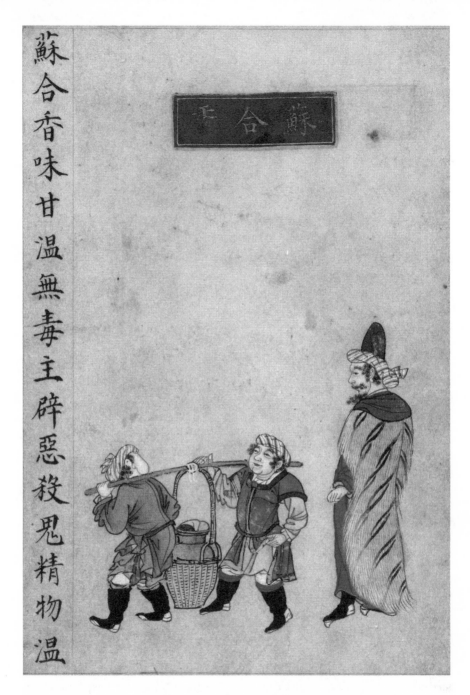

蘇合香味甘溫無毒主辟惡殺鬼精物溫

Figure 5.6. Rose Storax *(suhexiang),* made from the sap of the Turkish sweetgum or *Liquidambar orientalis,* conveyed by a stereotyped Central Asian or Persian trader in tiger-skin cloak, accompanied by his porters. The text lists among the drug's properties the power to ward off malignant and deadly demons. From *Buyi leigong paozhi bianlan* (1591 palace edition), p. 972. Image courtesy of Harvard-Yenching Library, copyright Cishu chubanshe, Shanghai.

and religious syncretism as well" (Furth 1999, 191). This art of nourishing the body's Essence (*jing*), *qi*, and Psyche (*shen*) became an intrinsic part of the literati lifestyle. The art combined physical and spiritual self-cultivation that simultaneously aimed at increasing the male body's fertility. In keeping with Zhu Zhenheng's advice on controlling excessive Yang, or Fire, the ideal male body was one in which anger and other strong sentiments were subdued and desire moderated. Regimens included monitoring one's diet and undertaking regular breathing exercises and meditation (Furth 1999, 199–206).

This ideal male body conceptualized by Jiangnan scholars and physicians contrasted notably with the imagined lustful, undisciplined, and semicivilized body emerging from the southern frontier region of the Empire. In early literature, the Lingnan region was already described as distinctly miasmatic. By Song-Yuan times, increasing cultural and political contacts reinforced views of this region as excessively hot and humid, a place where the local peoples had distinct physical traits and where dangerous, contagious diseases were rampant (Leung 2002, 172).

This imagined contagious southern body now seemed to pose increasingly imminent dangers, best symbolized by the Numbing Wind (*mafeng*) patient or by the victim of Guangdong Sores (Guangdong *chuang*). These ailments strongly resembled, and probably consisted largely of or were related to, leprosy and syphilis, respectively. Medical books of the late imperial period often confused the two ailments, as both had similar external symptoms. While Numbing Wind was the common term used in the late imperial period for a category of ailments that had been known as *li/lai* in earlier periods, the ailment known as Guangdong Sores was considered to be a new disease, appearing first in Guangdong province at the beginning of the sixteenth century. The miasmatic ecology, together with the purportedly undisciplined, lascivious behavior of local peoples, were considered to be the main factors behind the spread of the two diseases, which doctors increasingly viewed as generically close skin ailments. As diseases belonging to the external medicine specialty, both Numbing Wind and Guangdong Sores were discussed mainly by marginal doctors and shunned by most scholar-physicians (Leung 2003a, 2009).

It was these marginal doctors who elaborated on the idea of these diseases' spread through person-to-person contact, including the sharing of living quarters and toilets, contact with the bedding and clothing of the sick, and sexual intercourse. These understandings of contagion first appeared in Daoist ritual texts (Strickmann 2002, 36–39) and were taken up by such Song doctors as Chen Yan (fl. 1161–1176). Chen was the first to identify the *lai* disorder as contagious. But it was essentially marginal doctors—notably Shen Zhiwen of the mid-sixteenth century, who had been greatly influenced by Daoist medical thought—who provided the most detailed descriptions of the various channels of contagion of Numbing Wind. Chen Sicheng of the late Ming Dynasty was another such example. He was the first physician to write a treatise on Guangdong Sores, published in 1632, and closely followed Shen's ideas about the spread of Numbing Wind to explain the contagiousness of the new disease. Chen's text received great attention in Japan, where syphilis became a serious health concern after the seventeenth century. Ironically, it was a Japanese printed edition popularized in China in the early nineteenth century that helped the disease catch the attention of Western missionary doctors (Leung 2009).

The growing visibility of Numbing Wind and the spread of Guangdong Sores, together with a series of epidemics in the later Ming period (Dunstan 1975), stimulated the publication of other new medical ideas. Wu Youxing's (ca. 1561–1661) *Treatise on Epidemics Due to the "Warmth" Factor (Wenyi lun,* 1642) was an outstanding example. Wu, a native of Suzhou, proposed the explanation that these diseases and epidemics were caused by certain impure *qi (zaqi)* in the locality, which infected the victims via the mouth and nostrils. His notion of impure *qi* combined the already current concepts of disease-provoking miasmatic air emerging from the soil of hot, humid regions with theories regarding filthiness caused by stagnant water, decaying plants and corpses, or moral corruption (Leung 2002). Compared with the idea of person-to-person contagion elaborated by Shen and Chen, Wu's idea of disease-provoking *qi* was clearly a conscious revision of the classical explanation that epidemics were caused by Cold Damage *(shanghan),* a theory contained in the Han classic *Treatise on Cold-Damage Disorders (Shanghan lun)* by Zhang Ji. For Wu, disorders caused by the polluted *zaqi* could be caused by contagion, but not Cold Damage. Wu's insistence that specific local environmental and human pathogenic elements composed such *qi* was new and would be further developed by later Qing physicians. (See "The 'Warm Diseases' Current of Learning" in Chapter 6.)

The wide establishment of leprosaria in southern China from the sixteenth century onward amply reveals the impact on society of the idea of disease contagion. Such institutions were found in Jiangxi, Fujian, Guangdong, and Zhejiang provinces in Ming times and would grow in number under the Qing. Unlike medieval Buddhist institutions that accommodated *lai* patients as a demonstration of religious compassion, the government financed these late imperial institutions, setting fixed quotas of patients, for the explicit purpose of separating the sick from the healthy in order to stop contagion. These institutions first appeared in town centers but in the later period were gradually pushed farther and farther outside the city wall into remote hills or islands, clearly demonstrating the populace's increasing fear of contracting the contagion through contact with the sick. These were the first segregated institutions ever set up in China to protect the healthy population, and they continued to exist in the modern period. However, regional differences in disease conceptions should also be noted, as these institutions do not seem to have been established in the northern regions.

The emergence of new medical technology reinforced new ideas of diseases and the body. The development of variolation—the inoculation of a healthy child with human pox under controlled conditions—emerged toward the end of the fifteenth century and became popular especially in the Jiangnan region in the later Ming and Qing dynasties. The inoculation was, ideally, performed at a favorable time (such as during clement weather) in the hope that that the operation would provoke a benign and safe case of smallpox and immunize the child against more dangerous epidemics. The most common form of variolation involved introducing human pox into the child's nostril, in the form of either fresh lymph or dried and powdered scabs. The preparation and preservation of the lymph or powder would be increasingly refined during the late imperial period, to ensure the safety of the artificially induced smallpox (Fan 1953; Leung 1987, 1996). (See "Variolation.")

VARIOLATION

Chang Chia-Feng

Smallpox was a deadly disease that produced pustules and could also spread through them. Variolation was the practice of using smallpox matter to induce a mild case in those as yet uninfected, thus preventing the often disfiguring and even lethal full-blown version of the disease. In the Ming the practice of variolation seems to have spread from the south and was commonly practiced on children. Some have argued that it first appeared in China and then spread to other parts of the world, although it may have emerged in different places independently.

In China, variolation was first practiced in rural areas and was laden with agricultural metaphors: the medical term for smallpox was homophonous with "beans," and the graph was written with the disease radical and a component meaning "bean." Variolation (*zhongdou*, "planting smallpox") techniques relied on using the scab or pustule matter (*miao*, "sprout"), described as a "seed" from which would grow the "heavenly flower" (*tianhua*, another name for small-pox). By way of explaining how variolation worked, practitioners cited the maxim "Plant beans and you will harvest beans" *(zhongdou dedou)*. Variolation methods included wearing smallpox sufferers' clothing or quilts, and transferring pustule matter or moist or dry scabs. Eventually the most popular method came to be inserting cotton sprinkled with dry scabs into the patient's nose and plugging the nose with wax for twelve to twenty-four hours until the inoculation took.

Variolation was initially practiced by "smallpox planting masters" *(zhong-doushi)*, most of whom learned the technique from other masters, often their fathers. They traveled to towns and villages mainly during the spring and autumn. Some worked in teams of several practitioners, or one healer with his disciples or assistants. They usually stayed in a given locale for about a month, because a normal course of variolated smallpox took twelve to thirty days. They visited their young clients every day and performed rituals invoking the blessing and protection of smallpox deities. In rare cases they prescribed medicine to those who developed severe smallpox. As the practice of variolation spread, ethical issues came to the fore. Some variolated patients developed severe cases of smallpox or unexpected side effects, and some even died, raising criticism and doubt. Nevertheless, variolation remained the most popular way to fight smallpox in seventeenth- and eighteenth-century China.

It is not clear whether there was a historical connection with Chinese practices, but smallpox inoculation came to European attention when, around 1717, the wife of the British consul in Constantinople observed Turkish women inserting scab matter into the skin of healthy people. During the last quarter of the seventeenth century, British surgeon Edward Jenner drew on the work of others to popularize inoculation with cowpox, a related virus. As late as the early twentieth century, cowpox vaccination, which by then had become common worldwide, had not completely replaced the older approach in China (Chang Chia-Feng 1996a, 124–159).

In the thirteenth century, doctors explained the effects of variolation through the notion of fetal toxin *(taidu)*. They considered fetal toxin—a poison innate in the fetus, resulting from the lustful intercourse of the parents during pregnancy—to be the cause of a number of serious diseases with skin manifestations. Engendering smallpox by variolation was, in principle, a way to disperse fetal toxin, after which the child would not develop a fatal case of the disease

(Chang 2000, 23–38). The later introduction of new types of variolation and even, in the early nineteenth century, of Jennerian vaccination, rather than prompting alternative explanations, only served to reinforce the theory of fetal toxin.

Conclusion

The Yuan and Ming governments are sometimes stereotyped as autocratic and their literati as conservative, but this was in fact an age of great ferment. The expansion of state-sponsored medical learning in the Yuan did not prevent, and may have facilitated, if indirectly, the proliferation of diverse extragovernmental streams of medical learning. State medical education and relief contracted in the Ming, but practically oriented household healing manuals, medical primers, and collections of medical cases became more widely available, and increasing numbers of men began studying medicine independently through published works. Local gentry became more involved in charitable works, including in medical relief. The growth of the higher-status scholar-physician class did not prevent popular innovations such as variolation from spreading and becoming ubiquitous. Elite women became more restricted to the "inner quarters," but elite men could not block their access to alternative knowledge and healers such as the "three aunties and six grannies." New diseases such as Numbing Wind and Guangdong Sores provoked the reconsideration of old theories, and old problems such as epidemics and contagion received theoretical reconsideration.

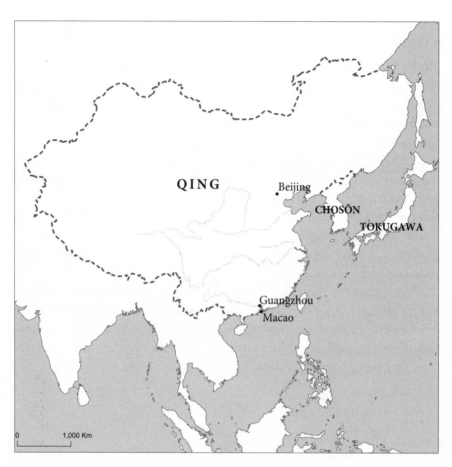

Qing Period

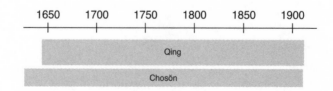

SIX

THE QING PERIOD

Yi-Li Wu

IN JUNE 1644, Manchu forces led by the prince regent Dorgon (1612–1650) entered Beijing, claiming the imperial throne in the name of the Qing Dynasty. Their ancestors, the Jurchens, had once ruled northern Chinese territories as the Jin Dynasty. Dorgon's father, Nurhaci (1559–1626), and elder brother, Hong Taiji (1592–1643), aimed to repeat this feat. During the preceding decades, they had laid the foundations for a new dynasty to rival the Ming by asserting their leadership over the Jurchen tribes of northeast Asia (subsequently renamed the Manchus), conquering territories in China proper, and co-opting Chinese officials and commoners into their administrative and military structures. The Manchus' opportunity came in April 1644, when a native Chinese rebellion led by Li Zicheng (1605–1645) captured Beijing, driving the Ming emperor to hang himself. Securing the support of the Ming general Wu Sangui (1612–1678), the Manchus defeated Li's forces and entered Beijing in the name of restoring benevolent rule. Over the next four decades, the Manchus successfully consolidated their power over all of the former Ming territory, mopping up Li's forces, suppressing local uprisings, defeating Ming loyalist claimants, and quelling armed rebellion by Wu Sangui and other erstwhile supporters. By 1760, the Qing emperors had also expanded their territory until they controlled a multiethnic empire more than twice the size of the Ming's (Peterson 2002).

As during the Yuan, Qing policies were shaped by the challenges of being a vastly outnumbered ethnic minority group trying to rule a huge Han Chinese population. The Manchus preserved the basic social, ideological, and political frameworks of the Ming while also incorporating innovations designed to reinforce Manchu authority. They actively sought to recruit elite Chinese men into government service via the examination system, even as they reserved the top positions for Manchus. Beginning with the Kangxi Emperor (r. 1662–1722), Qing rulers also actively patronized and promoted Neo-Confucian teachings. They thus affirmed the values of the Chinese elite while using these values to bolster the legitimacy of the Manchu emperor, portraying him as a sage ruler and a true Son of Heaven.

As the empire recovered from the trauma of conquest and entered a long period of stability, historical dynamics that had already begun to transform society during the late Ming again came to the forefront, finding ever fuller expression. One was extensive and intensive economic growth, which manifested itself during the Qing in the commodification and commercialization of crops, land, and agricultural labor, as well as in the expansion and monetization of interregional, long-distance trade. The Qing is also known for rapid population increases. Although scholars disagree as to whether the population doubled or tripled over the course of the eighteenth century, it is indisputable that the Chinese population was huge by contemporary standards, reaching an estimated three hundred million (around one-third of the world's population at this time) by 1800 (Lee and Wang 1999; Peterson 2002). The factors that influenced population growth rates in the Qing have yet to be fully understood. However, historians have found evidence for decreased infant mortality and increased life expectancy, themselves linked to well-known developments such as the positive impact of cash-cropping on agricultural production, the spread of new technologies and seeds that increased crop yields, and the introduction of New World plants such as sweet potato and maize that made it possible to grow food on marginally tillable land (Lee and Wang 1999).

FERTILITY CONTROL AND DEMOGRAPHICS

Francesca Bray

Until recently, demographers depicted late imperial China as a society where only war, famine, and disease limited untrammeled population growth. Yet the data from before 1949—drawn principally from state tax records, censuses, and lineage documents—are incomplete and open to interpretation. Some historians (Wolf 2001) maintain that the patrilineal compulsion to maximize the number of sons at any cost determined the macropatterns of the Chinese population throughout imperial history. But many other demographic historians now argue that Qing records demonstrate a different picture: a later start

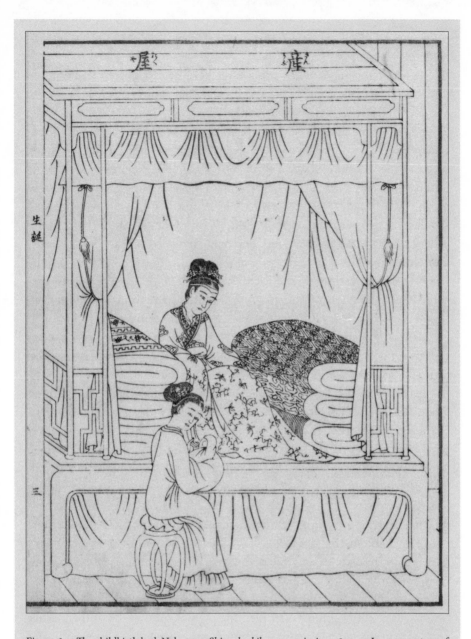

Figure 6.1. The childbirth bed. Nakagawa *Shinzoku kibun,* no. 7 in *juan* 6, 1799. Image courtesy of Harvard-Yenching Library.

of childbearing and lower total marital fertility rate (number of live children) than in most European societies before 1850, and a spacing between recorded births that indicates deliberate fertility control. They suggest that late imperial families exercised preventive fertility checks such as sexual abstinence or selective infanticide (sometimes of boys as well as girls) in order to invest more resources in each child (Li 1994; Lee and Wang 1999; Campbell, Wang, and Lee 2002; Zhao 2002).

The new demographers also point to medical theories that favored limiting procreation, as spelled out in the rubrics of women's medicine *(fuke* or *nüke)* and pediatrics *(erke)* that first emerged in the Song and that, by the mid-Ming, had become flourishing specialties (Furth 1999; Hsiung, this volume). Circulated widely in late imperial society (at least among the affluent and educated), such theories discouraged women from bearing children before the age of eighteen years (twenty *sui* in Chinese reckoning) for fear of damaging their internal organs. Men should wait until thirty *sui,* to ensure firm *yang* energies, and should have sex sparingly, to improve the quality of the conceptus (Furth 1994).

Did such theories translate into practice? Here medical cases provide further clues. Those that note the patient's age and concern pregnancy usually involve women over twenty *sui.* From the more than three hundred cases recorded by Xu Dachun, for example, only one discusses a woman younger than twenty *sui* (Xu 1988, j. 32). Reproductive profiles range from women who were pregnant only once or twice in their lives to one whose twenty-one pregnancies resulted in only five live children; her longed-for son was born when she was thirty-seven (Bray 2008).

Medical cases highlight the vulnerability of pregnant women, fetuses, and infants. They deal not with routine experiences but with anomalous ones, including ghost pregnancies and monstrous births (Wu 2002; Zeitlin 2007). They never mention infanticide, but instead show how medical theory might translate into other, more socially acceptable techniques for regulating reproduction, notably by prioritizing menstrual regulation *(tiaojing)* as the key to women's health and fertility. Amenorrhea signaled a potentially dangerous disorder yet was difficult to distinguish from early pregnancy. Skilled physicians prescribed mild Blood-stimulating drugs to test for pregnancy. Quacks or women themselves might resort to stronger Blood-moving drugs to bring on the menses. Physicians might also use these stronger drugs to terminate a difficult pregnancy, but reluctantly, because abortifacient drugs endangered the mother's health. Reconciling conflicts between the physiological needs of the mother and those of the fetus sometimes required great ingenuity to treat both successfully. When this proved impossible, the mother's needs took priority; sometimes a physician administered abortifacients at an anxious husband's request (Bray 1997, 317–334).

Medical materials provide a cultural context for demographic models but chart quite different dimensions of experience or choice. Generally, however, they support the demographers' argument that affluent families in late imperial China prized quality above quantity where offspring were concerned, and suggest that the ambivalences of pregnancy offered women certain forms of control over their fertility. What we cannot tell is how such practices may have affected demographic patterns.

These economic and demographic developments also transformed society and culture. Cities grew, publishing and print culture flourished, and access to education increased. Greater interpenetration of urban and rural economies helped to popularize scholar-elite values among commoners, even as educated men pursued an expanding set of vocations outside government service. Disenchanted with the speculative bent of late Ming Neo-Confucianism, which they blamed for the fall of the dynasty, many Chinese scholars embraced an influential new intellectual movement that promoted rigorous philological research into classical texts, an endeavor made possible by the growth of wealthy merchants' private libraries and their patronage of scholarship and the arts.

This was the empire that faced the British gunboats in 1839 at the outbreak of the so-called Opium War. The catalyst for the conflict was a Chinese government commissioner's confiscation and destruction of foreign merchants' opium stocks. But the stage for this war had been set far earlier by growing British resentment over Qing refusal to expand trade relations. Great Britain's victory inaugurated an era of intensifying imperialist demands on the Qing state, demands that either accompanied or occasioned new military conflicts. By century's end, foreign powers were competing to acquire territorial concessions and leaseholds in China, provoking Chinese fears that the empire would be "cut up like a melon." To make matters worse, imperialist pressures were accompanied by internal upheavals, most devastatingly the civil war known as the Taiping Rebellion (1851–1864).

In the post–Opium War, post-Taiping decades, however, imperial and local leaders actively confronted these challenges with measures to strengthen and reinvigorate the Qing state and society. During this time, they also integrated Western learning into various new governmental institutions. But in the aftermath of Qing defeat in the Sino-Japanese War of 1894–1895, many elites became deeply disillusioned with the court's inability to resist foreign pressure and its reluctance to enact thoroughgoing reforms. By the beginning of the twentieth century, revolutionary groups called for the overthrow of the Qing, and Sun Yat-sen's slogan "Nationalism, democracy, and people's livelihood" served as a rallying cry for many who wanted to create a new Chinese nation. A revolutionary uprising of Ocober 1911, supported by civilian officials and military commanders eventually left the emperor no choice but to abdicate. China's imperial age had come to an end.

When twentieth-century Chinese reformers looked back at their predecessors, they blamed them for having been shortsighted, mired in tradition, and unwilling to change. This narrative also came to dominate earlier Western-language histories of China, including histories of medicine. Recent studies, however, have promoted a much-needed revision of this picture by showing that the Qing was a period of social and cultural innovation, intellectual dynamism, curiosity, and openness. This will be our starting point, and our goal will be to understand how the distinctive features of the Qing shaped the ways in which people approached illness and healing. Our discussion will revolve around two organizing themes: (1) how social changes during the Qing shaped the ideological and institutional points of reference around which healing activities were constructed, and (2) cross-cultural medical encounters, particularly between the Qing and the West.

Cultural, Social, and Intellectual Trends

Preceding chapters have emphasized the pluralistic and diverse nature of healing activities in China. So too, the Qing period was characterized by fluid boundaries between multiple realms of curative and health-promoting activities (Wu 2010). Existing laws provided for the punishment of physicians and ritual experts found guilty of causing a client's death. Yet no regulations controlled who could provide healing services, and the only practical requirement to become a healer was the ability to attract patients. Consequently, the types of healers varied as much as their methods. While some made their living exclusively as doctors, spirit mediums, or other experts, there were others for whom healing was but one among several income-generating activities. For that matter, when illness occurred, the sick person and his or her family were often the first recourse for diagnosis and treatment. Knowing what foods to eat, what tonics to use, and what charms to hang on one's front door were forms of everyday knowledge exchanged among relatives, friends, and neighbors.

People also consulted "daily use encyclopedias" that had become common beginning in the sixteenth century, providing advice on topics from raising silkworms to interpreting dreams. Medicine and health preservation were also standard topics in these household reference works, which assumed that knowing how to promote good health was as important as knowing how to cure illness after the fact. Similarly, the rubric of "protecting life" and "nourishing life" *(weisheng, yangsheng)* included a variety of practices for regulating, harmonizing, and boosting the body's vitalities. These ranged from rising and sleeping in accordance with the rhythms of the seasons and abstaining from excessive emotional or physical indulgence to meditative and gymnastic techniques (Furth 1999; Rogaski 2004).

Some activities that promoted health overlapped with those claiming to confer immortality. These included "internal alchemy" *(neidan),* in which the adept manipulated and refined the forces of Yin and Yang within his own body, seeking to return to a primordial state of oneness with the origins of the cosmos. In a process analogous to "external alchemy" *(waidan),* in which the practitioner smelted natural substances to produce pills of immortality, the internal alchemist used his own body as a crucible for producing an "immortal embryo" (Robinet 1997). While internal alchemy was historically a male practice, the Qing also witnessed the development of a full-fledged "female alchemy," adapted to the special characteristics of the female body and focused on harnessing the generative powers of female blood (Despeux 1990; Valussi 2008a).

FEMALE ALCHEMY

Elena Valussi

Nüdan (female alchemy) is a tradition of inner alchemy that developed in China from the seventeenth century onward. Directed explicitly at women practitioners, the tradition grew in response to a number of factors. On one hand, a growing number of women were interested in seeking instruction in religious practices. On the other hand, changes in the social climate fostered concern over female involvement in religious (and nonreligious) activities outside the house. The Qing ruling house brought with it a heightened interest in chastity, instituted a more punitive legal code for women, and in general had far more reactionary ideas about the role of women in society. This meant that many religious activities in which women had previously been involved could not be pursued outside the confines of the home (Theiss 2004). The *nüdan* tradition, although developed by men, presented itself as a safe alternative, a practice to be conducted without the presence of male teachers and in the privacy of the home (Valussi 2008c).

The following excerpt from a preface to the 1906 collection *Combined Collection of Female Alchemy (Nüdan hebian)* describes male and female bodies from the point of view of alchemical practice. It reveals contemporary medical beliefs and cultural understandings about men's and women's cosmological, social, and physiological differences.

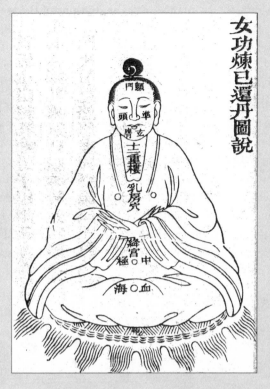

Figure 6.2. A woman sitting in meditation, inscribed with the most important loci for the refinement process. He, ed., "Nügong lianji huandan tushuo," in *Nüdan hebian*, 1906. Courtesy of Elena Valussi.

Just as the man is Yang, and Yang is clear *(qing)*, so the woman is Yin, and Yin is impure *(zhuo)*. The male nature is hard *(gang)*, the female nature is soft *(rou)*. A man's feelings are excitable, a woman's feelings are tranquil; male thoughts are mixed, female thoughts are pure. The man is fundamentally in movement, and movement facilitates the loss of *qi;* the woman is fundamentally quiet, and quietness facilitates the accumulation of *qi.* The man is associated with the trigram *Li* and, like the sun, he can complete a whole circuit of the heavens in one year; the woman is associated with the trigram *Kan* and, like the moon, she can complete a whole circuit of the heavens in one month. For a man, *qi* is difficult to subdue; for a woman, *qi* is easy to subdue.

These are the differences concerning innate nature.

The man has a knot inside the windpipe [i.e., the Adam's apple], the woman does not. The male breasts do not produce liquids and are small; the female breasts produce liquids and are big. A man's foundation is convex *(tu);* a woman's foundation is concave *(ao)*. In the man [the convex organ] is called the essence chamber *(jingshi);* in the woman [the concave organ] is called the infant's palace *(zigong)*. In men the vital force is located in the *qi* cavity *(qixue);* in women the vital force is located between the breasts. In the man, generative power is located in the pelvis; in the woman, generative power originates from the blood. In the man [the generative power] is the essence, its color is white and its name is White Tiger *(baihu)*; in the woman it is the blood, its color is red and its name is Red Dragon *(chilong)*. As for male essence, it is Yin within Yang; as for female blood, it is Yang within Yin. The power of male essence is more than sufficient; the power of female blood is insufficient.

These are the differences concerning Form and Structure.

A man first refines the root origin *(benyuan)*, and only subsequently does he refine the form *(xingzhi)*; a woman, instead, needs to refine her form first, and only then can she refine the root origin. The male Yang leaks downward, whereas the female Yang moves upward. When a man has completed the practice and the seminal essence does not drip away anymore, this is called "subduing the White Tiger." When a woman has completed the practice and the menstrual flow does not drip away anymore, this is called "beheading the Red Dragon." In the man, seminal essence moves against the current and he becomes immortal; in the woman, blood moves upward, ascending toward the heart's cavity. . . . The masculine practice is called "refining the *qi* of the supreme Yang," the feminine practice is called "refining the blood of the supreme Yin." For the man we speak of "Embryo" *(tai)*; for the woman, we speak of "Growing" *(xi)*. When the man has subdued the White Tiger, the stem (*jing*) [i.e., the penis] will retract and become similar to that of a young boy; when the woman has beheaded the Red Dragon, the breasts will retract and become similar to those of a male body [the White Tiger here symbolizes the male spermatic essence, while the Red Dragon symbolizes the female blood]. The man progresses slowly at the moment of the manifestation of the spirit, and he is slow in achieving the Dao; the woman progresses fast at the moment of the manifestation of the spirit, and she is also fast in attaining the Dao. A man can ascend [to Heaven] on his own; a woman needs to await salvation *(daidu)*. Men must meditate facing the wall; women who succeed in going back to emptiness are very few. The man will become an authentic man *(zhenren)*; the woman will become a princess of the origin *(yuanjun)*. These are the differences concerning the methods of practice.

We can say that, as for the principles that regulate Innate Nature and Vital Force, there are no differences [between men and women]. I advise the female adepts first to find out points of contiguity where there are differences, and only then to discover the differences hidden where there is similarity. In most cases, however, the contrasts are to be found before

> the beheading of the Red Dragon, whereas the major analogies emerge
> after the beheading of the Dragon. These are irrefutable and immortal
> arguments.
>
> (Translation adapted from Valussi 2008c.)

People drew freely from this repertoire of beliefs and techniques, often using many strategies simultaneously. By the time they called in an outside expert, they might have already tried various self-help methods. Their choice of expert reflected their own assessment of the problem. Was it something that could be cured by drugs? Would an offering to the gods or an exorcism be more efficacious? Was the illness perhaps caused by some transgression in a past life or by the poor siting of an ancestral grave? The typical pattern, found in medical case records as well as in stories and novels, was that a family would consult all the practitioners they could afford—sometimes sequentially, sometimes simultaneously—and compare, modify, and reject their recommendations based on the family's own sense of what was appropriate. Unlike today's biomedical physician, who deploys diagnostic and therapeutic technologies to which patients have no access, the Qing physician relied on the unassisted powers of human observation and on medicinal substances that were readily purchased in the marketplace. These resources were, in principle, also available to anyone who took the time to study their uses. Thus, the practical difference between the activities of a doctor and a layperson could be a matter of degree, not of kind.

None of these broad features was unique to the Qing. During the late imperial period, however, the fluidity of boundaries between healing practices and practitioners was intensified by historical dynamics that had become increasingly pronounced since the Ming. A greater number of educated men saw medicine as a worthy career or attractive hobby, and they blurred the lines between scholarly doctors and literate medical amateurs. The growth of publishing also made it easier to obtain medical literature or to get one's own medical opinions into print. Meanwhile, the proliferation of popular medical texts reinforced the idea that everyone could be his or her own doctor (Wu 2010). These centrifugal forces were particularly important during the Qing, when the center of gravity for medical initiatives shifted to regional elites.

Government Medicine and Medical Publishing

In contrast to earlier dynasties, promoting medicine was not a political priority for the Qing, nor did its emperors show a personal interest in authoring medical texts or shaping medical institutions (Leung 1987). While the Manchu rulers maintained the official structure of the Ming governmental medical service, they also reduced the scope of its activities. Ming court physicians had counted high officials among their regular clientele, for example, but their Qing counterparts were restricted to treating members of the imperial clan, all the better to prevent possible anti-Manchu collusion between ethnic Han doctors and statesmen (Chang 1998). The Qing also eliminated the practice of legally designating certain households as hereditary medical families who were responsible for ensuring a supply of doctors to the government (Ho 1962). To the extent that the imperial government took initiative in medical matters, it was in situations directly affecting its political legitimacy or ability to rule. A particular concern was controlling smallpox. This disease was endemic in China but not in the Manchu homeland, and it was thus deadly to adult Manchus, who lacked childhood immunity. As a result, the court enacted quarantine and segregation procedures to minimize the possibility that Manchu soldiers, officials, or imperial family members would be exposed to smallpox. The Kangxi Emperor, who had survived smallpox as a child, also promoted variolation among members of the royal family (Chang Chia-Feng 1996b; Chang 2002). Manchu worries over smallpox also inspired the creation of a new department of "pox diseases" *(douzhen)* in the Qing Imperial Medical Bureau. But Qing rulers allowed local officials and elites to take the initiative in mitigating other epidemics, such as the outbreaks of bubonic plague that began to spread from southwest China after the eighteenth century. The central government's response in such cases was modeled on famine relief procedures, focusing on crisis mitigation by issuing free medicines and other similar measures to promote confidence and social stability (Benedict 1996).

THE NINETEENTH-CENTURY BUBONIC PLAGUE EPIDEMIC

Carol Benedict

In 1894, bubonic plague broke out in the southern Chinese city of Guangzhou and the British colony of Hong Kong. Within a decade, steamships carried plague-infected rats to seaports as far-flung as Bombay (India), Cape Town (South Africa), Rio de Janeiro (Brazil), and San Francisco (United States), precipitating a global pandemic that lasted well into the twentieth century (Echenberg 2007).

This modern pandemic originated in southwestern China. Ecological conditions in the mountains of western Yunnan supported an ongoing reservoir of wild rodent plague. After 1750, expanding Qing copper mining brought Chinese settlers into ever more frequent contact with this reservoir. Between 1772 and 1830, the disease moved from Yunnan's western frontier to more populated areas in the eastern half of the province. After 1850, Cantonese traders carried it further eastward, along the overland and river routes that linked remote Yunnan to the coast. Moving first through Guangxi and western Guangdong in the 1860s and 1870s, the disease eventually reached the Pearl River Delta in the 1890s. Plague continued to spread up the Chinese coastline and across the Taiwan Strait, spreading to coastal cities such as Xiamen and Shanghai, as well as Guangzhou and Hong Kong (Benedict 1996).

The 1894 appearance of bubonic plague in Hong Kong brought China's nineteenth-century epidemic to international attention. In the eyes of many Europeans and Americans, plague marked China as a hygienically "backward" country that continued to incubate a "medieval" disease in the modern era. Fearful of the potential impact on their own societies, the governments of Europe, America, and Japan quickly sent scientists to the British colony to investigate. The French microbiologist Alexandre Yersin and the Japanese bacteriologist Kitasato Shibasaburo independently identified the causative agent of plague, *Yersinia pestis* (Cunningham 1992).

Although the Hong Kong epidemic occasioned the identification of the microorganism responsible for plague, biomedical understandings of plague ecology and epidemiology were still evolving. The role of rat fleas as the primary disease vectors, for example, was not widely accepted until after 1900. Many Western doctors working in Hong Kong at the time remained convinced that plague was a "filth" disease caused by the "uncivilized" living conditions of the Chinese. This analysis precipitated invasive plague control policies, including a massive cleanup of lower-class neighborhoods, isolation of plague patients from their families, and imposition of a cordon sanitaire to prevent Chinese from moving about freely. Not surprisingly, these policies provoked resistance on the part of the Chinese community, among both elites and non-elites, and were only partially effective.

Nearly two decades later, when a devastating outbreak of pneumonic plague appeared along the railway lines of northeastern China in 1910–1911, official Chinese attitudes toward forceful Western-style public health measures had changed dramatically (Nathan 1967). With both Japan and Russia pressing for more territory in the northeast, Qing officials were concerned that foreign powers would use plague containment as an excuse to expand into Manchuria. They imposed quarantine and other Western-style plague control measures on

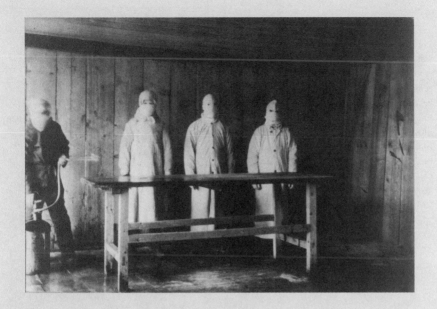

Figure 6.3. The pneumonic plague in China. The autopsy room, Plague Hospital, Mukden. Assistant at the hospital with carbolic spray disinfecting apparatus. Winter 1910–1911. Courtesy of Library of Congress Prints and Photographs Division, Washington, DC.

Chinese populations themselves. The Qing government believed that hygienic modernity—a complex and dynamic group of sanitary practices that incorporated state power, scientific standards of progress, and social Darwinian concepts of the relative fitness of the "Chinese race" for modernity—was essential for national salvation. Consequently, hygienic modernity became the style of public health pursued by all the regimes that governed China across the twentieth century (Rogaski 2004). The nineteenth-century plague epidemics thus proved fundamental to constructing a new vision of the Chinese state and its relationship to society in the modern era.

Insofar as the imperial government sponsored medical text publishing, it was in the larger context of literary projects designed to demonstrate the emperor's benevolent sagacity and thereby enhance the throne's political legitimacy (Hanson 2003). One of these projects was the *Synthesis of Books and Illustrations from Antiquity to the Present (Gujin tushi jicheng)*, a ten-thousand-chapter work commissioned by the Kangxi Emperor and completed under his son and successor, the Yongzheng Emperor (r. 1723–1736). The medical section of this imperial encyclopedia anthologized important teachings drawn from texts dating from the

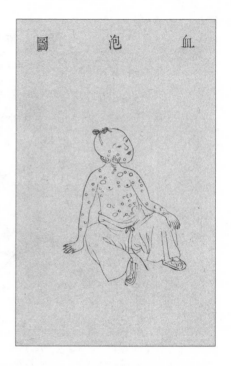

圖　泡　血

Figure 6.4. The Qing period's Manchu rulers were acutely concerned with preventing and controlling smallpox, an undertaking that also required people to differentiate accurately between various pediatric skin eruptions. This image of "blood blisters" is one of forty-two illustrations of different forms of "pox disease" *(douzhen)* published in the government medical textbook *Imperially Commissioned Golden Mirror of Medical Learning.* Wu, ed., *Yuzuan yizong jinjian,* 1742. Courtesy of the Wellcome Library, London.

Inner Canon onward, presented chronologically in sections organized by subfield and topical headings. Medical texts were also included in the massive collection known as the *Complete Books of the Four Treasuries (Siku quanshu).*

In 1772, the Qianlong Emperor (r. 1736–1796) called for the compilation of an authoritative imperial library. Hundreds of scholars collected and evaluated more than ten thousand works gathered from throughout the empire, ultimately copying more than three thousand texts into a final compendium (Guy 1987). A total of seven sets were made, all copied by hand, with four reserved for imperial use and three made available to the empire's subjects in designated library buildings (the entire collection is now available to modern scholars in a digital, full-text searchable form). The *Four Treasuries* project has been criticized as a literary purge, because during its compilation thousands of works judged to be anti-Manchu were identified and destroyed. Nevertheless, the approximately one hundred medical works preserved in this collection provide an invaluable window into the state of proper medical knowledge as defined by influential eighteenth-century scholars.

The *Golden Mirror*

The *Synthesis* and the *Four Treasuries* presented medicine as one among many topics that were integral to human knowledge. The only text that the court sponsored for purely medical reasons was the *Imperially Compiled Golden Mirror of Medical Learning (Yuzuan yizong jinjian)* of 1742. This magisterial ninety-chapter work served as a textbook for court doctors and a standard of best practice in the unhappy event that an imperial physician was accused of incompetence (Chang 1998). While it had no normative power outside the court—indeed, doctors outside the government criticized court practitioners for adhering too slavishly to its guidelines—the *Golden Mirror* is a revealing case study of elite medicine during the eighteenth century. Imperial sponsorship of the *Golden Mirror* embodied the Qianlong Emperor's desire to be seen as a sage-ruler defining the bounds of correct practice for the empire. However, it was not Manchu officials who determined medical orthodoxy in this case. Instead, the editorial board was dominated by Han Chinese doctors from the Jiangnan region, south of the Yangzi River in eastern China (Hanson 2003). Since Song times, this had been China's most economically developed and most culturally advanced region, producing a preponderance of Chinese scholars and statesmen, not to mention doctors.

The Emperor's Physician

Chang Che-chia

The emperor's physician had two roles. One, at least nominally, was to take charge of an empire-wide medical administration system and adjudicate what constituted orthodox medical knowledge. The more important one involved providing the imperial family with health care and carrying out medical assignments from the emperor, such as examining the state of a minister's health. During the Qing period, the office for such functions was the Imperial Academy of Medicine *(taiyi yuan)*. The academy had discontinued its supervision of medical schools *(yixue)* under local government, unlike its predecessors during the Song or Yuan periods, but it still required local branches to send their most outstanding representatives to the court, to ensure the quality of its service. In addition to physicians who rose through official channels, occasionally the emperor might summon well-regarded private practitioners to serve at court. Regardless of how one reached the academy, the individual chosen to be the emperor's physician was considered the best doctor under Heaven.

Folktales arose regarding these physicians. One well-known legend involved a doctor's diagnosing a female member of the imperial family. To preserve propriety, it was said, the physician had to feel her pulses through a silk string wrapped around her wrist as she sat behind a curtain. However, according to

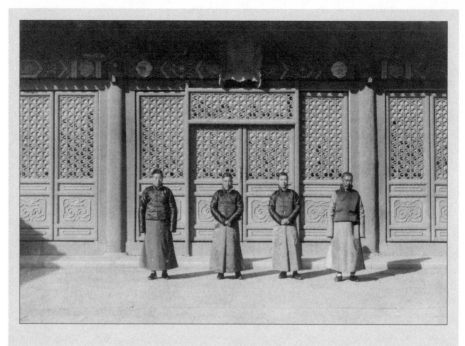

Figure 6.5. Four uniformed men in front of the Office of Imperial Physicians, Beijing, ca. 1920. Becker Medical Library, Washington University School of Medicine.

reminiscences left by private physicians who had served Dowager Empress Cixi, the legend was only a rumor. Reliable sources suggest instead that safe and effective therapy remained the greater concern at court.

To ensure that imperial patients received appropriate treatment, the physician's relevant activities were well documented and monitored. As was common practice at that time, usually more than one physician treated the patient. According to regulation, each physician first drafted his own prescription independently. Then all the physicians—including the grand councils supervising imperial health care—discussed therapeutic options until they reached consensus. By regulation, the resulting official document governed and recorded all subsequent steps—the patient's approval of the plan, preparation of the medicine, and later publicizing of the actual interventions. This procedure ensured that the imperial patient's condition was made known to subjects outside the palace, thereby avoiding sudden conspiracies or murder. It also allowed more people to contribute medical information, in order to review the imperial physicians' performance.

Originally only a limited group of officials had access to these documents. During the last years of the dynasty, however, under the control of Dowager Empress Cixi, the Guangxu Emperor's health records were published daily in the newspaper. Many of these documents still survive in the form of *yongyao dibu,* or "office copy of the records of using medicine."

Many people doubt the veracity of these documents, believing that Cixi had the contents fabricated for her own political ends. However, the diary of imperial tutor Weng Tonghe, along with other sources, corroborates that the documents do have some authenticity, since people involved in imperial treatments drew on them to review and even question the physician's therapeutic approach. To win glory for healing a court patient, a physician had to be able to defend his position from challenge and persuade political authorities to comply with the authority of his medical knowledge.

On the hundredth anniversary of the Guangxu Emperor's death, in 2008 authorities in the People's Republic of China announced that recent analyses of the emperor's hair revealed arsenic levels that supported a theory of poisoning. Questions regarding this claim remain. However, if eventually verified, it would indicate that—although the system of oversight may have prevented malpractice—it may not have been able to protect the imperial patient from murders plotted by political conspirators.

A distinctive feature of the *Golden Mirror* is that it presents Han Dynasty doctor Zhang Ji's (d. 219) *Treatise on Cold Damage Disorders (Shanghan lun)* and *Prescriptions of the Golden Casket (Jinkui yaolüe)* as the foundations of proper medical practice. This choice owed much to attempts by literate physicians to improve the status of medicine by creating an intellectual lineage rooted in antiquity. During the sixteenth and seventeenth centuries, doctors had spoken of Zhang Ji as one of the "four great masters" *(si da jia)* of the Jin and Yuan period. By the eighteenth century, however, scholarly physicians such as Xu Dachun (1693–1771) were arguing that Zhang's status far surpassed that of the other three. More than simply a great master, Zhang Ji should be considered a "sage" whose relationship to medical learning was analogous to that of Confucius for Confucian scholars (Chao 2009).

The *Golden Mirror*'s editorial choices embodied the priorities of "evidential research" *(kaozheng).* This influential intellectual current, also dominated by southern scholars, employed philological analysis and critical comparison of texts to recover the original form and meaning of Han Dynasty works—including Zhang Ji's—that allegedly had been distorted by Song-era commentaries and interpretations. Evidential research scholars thereby hoped to discredit Song Neo-Confucianism and restore the original Han Dynasty classics to central importance in Chinese intellectual life (Elman 1984). Medicine, too, was shaped by these trends. A few decades after the publication of the *Golden Mirror,* the editors of the *Four Treasuries* evaluated books on the basis of whether they employed *kaozheng* methodology, rejecting those works that did not (Elman 1984). The medical sections of the *Four Treasuries* thus further reinforced the relationship between literate medicine and evidential research.

Gentrification of Medicine

The influence of evidential research scholars on medicine was one facet of a broader dynamic that may be described as the gentrification of medicine during the Qing. During the Song era, government officials tried to raise the quality of state medical practice by convincing men from elite families that medicine could be a respectable occupation for a scholar. They likened medicine to state-craft, and described it as a worthy vehicle for expressing the humaneness of the superior gentleman. By the Qing, the scholar-turned-healer had become a mundane figure both in fiction and in fact. While writers still echoed Song-era tropes linking medical knowledge to Confucian virtue, the context for such rhetoric had changed. Now it was integrated into debates over what kind of training a good doctor ought to have, and many used it to assert the superiority of scholarly doctors over other types of practitioners (Scheid 2007; Wu 2010).

Again, this development had its roots in the Ming Dynasty. The founding Ming emperor, Taizu (r. 1368–1398), expanded the educational pipeline by creating a lower tier of county-level examinations that would qualify men to take the civil service examinations at the provincial and then metropolitan levels. Coupled with late imperial population growth, this policy vastly increased the number of men entering an already fiercely competitive system. But the number of available official government posts remained relatively steady, and the pass rates for the highest metropolitan-level degree became minuscule (Elman 2000). The result was a burgeoning number of educated men who needed an alternative livelihood, and one possibility was medicine. On a superficial level, this was reminiscent of the Yuan Dynasty, when the Mongols suspended the examinations and medicine became a career path that could provide access to powerful and wealthy patrons (Hymes 1987). But now it was the examination system itself that created a steady stream of unemployed literati.

The Qing-era doctors showcased in the "skills and techniques" sections of officially compiled local histories typically included many lower degree holders who had taken up medicine as a profession when they were unable to advance in the examinations. One such practitioner was the Fujian native Chen Nianzu (1753–1823). Chen did not manage to pass the provincial-level examinations until he was forty, a relatively late age (Elman 2000). By this time, he had already begun practicing medicine, most likely under the influence of his grandfather, also a scholar-turned-physician. Chen became renowned as a medical popularizer, composing pedagogical works for medical learners. Among the most famous was his *Trimetrical Classic of Medicine (Yixue san zi jing)*, which in title and format mimicked the primers that young boys used to begin their classical Confucian studies. Doctors had first produced these sorts of medical primers in the fourteenth century, but they became a staple of the medical literature during the Qing (Leung 2003a). In addition to providing accessible introductions to medicine for scholars who wished to become doctors, their authors also sought to define the boundaries of legitimate medical knowledge and practice by presenting model curricula. Like Chen Nianzu's *Trimetrical Classic*, these works were regularly modeled after Confucian primers, with their authors drawing explicit comparisons between the practice of medicine and the Way of the scholar. Many relied on mnemonic rhymes to aid absorption of key concepts, a format also used in the imperial textbook *Golden Mirror of Medicine*.

The production of these self-consciously normative works resonated with literate doctors' wider attempts to convince people that scholarly formation was necessary for medical competence. One of their strategies was to reinterpret an old adage, originating in the *Book of Rites (Liji)*, that warned, "If a doctor lacks three generations of medicine, do not take his drugs" *(yi bu sanshi, bu fu qi yao)*. It was widely accepted that "three generations" referred to membership in a medical family, one in which knowledge had been handed down from grandfather to father to son. Indeed, people widely assumed that such hereditary doctors *(shiyi)* had especially efficacious skills and therapies. Beginning in the fourteenth century, however, medical writers began to challenge this interpretation, arguing instead that the three generations referred to mastery of three canonical medical texts (Chao 2000). These debates grew particularly vigorous after the late Ming, and Qing doctors also themselves employed the methods of evidential research to bolster the "three canonical texts" explanation. But the gentrification of medicine meant that many classically trained physicians were in fact from medical families. Thus these debates were primarily about defining medical legitimacy and should not be interpreted as a struggle between discrete groups of "hereditary" and "scholarly" physicians *(ruyi)*.

In sum, it is during the Qing that we find a critical mass of literate practitioners who increasingly viewed themselves as an intellectual community and who were concerned with enhancing their social status and medical authority (Chao 2009). Unlike their contemporaries in Europe or North America, however, these educated Chinese doctors did not pursue legal regulations or form occupation-based institutions to delineate who was qualified to practice medicine. Instead, they constructed their authority in cultural terms, allying themselves with the values of the elite scholar-official class and arguing that medicine could be properly practiced only by gentlemen with a classical education and superior moral cultivation (Scheid 2007). They denigrated their competitors as quacks who parroted the ancients without understanding them, and they deplored the unlettered "grannies" and midwives who drummed up business by ingratiating themselves with the lady of the house (Furth 1999). They also criticized patients who placed more trust in folk remedies or the advice of friends than in the counsel of erudite physicians (Xu 1990).

Ironically, these constant complaints reveal that scholarly doctors were in fact often unable to convince medical consumers of their innate superiority, and that healers from all walks of life continued to be important players in the medical marketplace. Even the most ardent critic of midwives had to recognize that no family would willingly choose to do without an experienced female birthing attendant (Wu 2010). To a great extent, furthermore, complaints about bad practitioners formed part of a broader litany of complaints by upper-class men who worried about threats to Confucian morality. For example, the "grannies" who treated women's bodies might also fill their heads with heterodox or fanciful ideas (Furth 1999). (See Chapter 5.) Such concerns were acute in an era of far-reaching economic and social transformations such as the Qing, especially since elite status was determined by personal achievement, not birth. A man of means could purchase an education or even a government post for his son, while eminent families could easily decline in the absence of sufficiently talented descendants. Population growth only intensified the competition for social and material resources. For upper-class families, Confucian respectability and morality constituted an important marker of elite social identity. It is no coincidence, for example, that the Ming-Qing period witnessed the intensification of "an anti–spirit medium consensus" among literati (Sutton 2000, 13). Both dynasties maintained regulations for punishing spirit mediums who allegedly misled people with their heterodox practices. Some popular versions of the Kangxi Emperor's *Sacred Edict (shengyu),* originally written to promote Confucian ideals among his subjects, also criticized these healers. But even if some elites might disdain spirit mediums, other folk continued to patronize them.

Medical Publishing

Many historians point to the Song Dynasty as the age of the printing revolution in China. However, the growth of print that characterized the commercialized, urban culture of China after the sixteenth century was quantitatively and qualitatively more expansive, not only in terms of the availability of texts and their accessibility but also in the penetration of text-based literate culture into the population at large. The late imperial period was the heyday of the nouveau riche, inspiring the proliferation of handbooks to teach people the accoutrements of upper-class society such as painting, poetry, and tea drinking. The publishing houses of Sibao in Fujian province also flourished during the Qing, churning out cheap texts for the masses, including works on drugs and medicines (Brokaw 2007).

This expanded access to medical literature coincided with increased compilation of medical primers, proving a boon to would-be scholarly doctors. It also gave greater agency to people who were suspicious of doctors, by allowing them to compile household manuals directed at laypeople. For example, some of the most frequently reprinted popular texts in eighteenth- and nineteenth-century China were the handbooks on women's reproductive ailments attributed to the Bamboo Grove Monastery of northern Zhejiang province (Wu 2000). The upper-class men who reprinted these works claimed that they had discovered the monks' secret formulas and wanted to make them more widely available so that people could cure gynecological complaints at home. Other literate men treated medicine as a hobby, compiling and printing their own medical works based on excerpts selected from other texts. In short, while the proliferation of medical texts aided the training of literate doctors, it simultaneously undermined their claims to have privileged knowledge.

Medical Charity and Philanthropy

Dispensing medicine and health care advice to family, friends, and colleagues was part of everyday social interaction, providing a way for both men and women to show concern and care for those around them. When the official Gong Chunpu (fl. ca. 1854) worried that he had no heirs, for example, his colleague Zhu Yun'gu gave him a formula that he personally had found useful (Wu 2000). Zhu himself had originally obtained this remedy from another official, Wang Maocun, whose family had used it for generations.

Women, too, studied medical literature and employed medical books for the benefit of others. A good example is Zeng Jifen (1852–1942), daughter of eminent Qing official Zeng Guofan (1811–1872). According to an account left by her son-in-law, Jifen's medical pursuits were part of the charitable and virtuous activities that patterned her well-ordered and disciplined life. Even in old age, she spent every morning praying, practicing calligraphy, and writing letters. After lunch and a nap, "she attended to clothing materials, medicines, tonics, and such things. She personally operated the sewing machines and made clothing to distribute to the needy. Each year she mixed medicines according to prescriptions. . . . If she heard that friends or relatives were sick, she either presented them with medicine or told them of a prescription" (Zeng 1993, 101). Besides scouring the printed literature for useful medical formulas, Jifen also collected prescriptions from relatives, acquaintances, and medicine shops. One of her references was *A New Compilation of Tested Prescriptions* (*Yanfang xinbian,* first ed. 1846), a handbook compiled by a lower-level literatus from Changsha named Bao Xiang'ao (fl. mid-nineteenth century). This work was itself a compilation of remedies that Bao had gleaned from books and from the experiences of his friends and relatives.

Amateur healing activities were also inspired by the belief that performing good deeds would allow people to accrue karmic merit and obtain worldly rewards. A practical system of collecting and calculating merits was first popularized by the scholar and doctor Yuan Huang (Metropolitan Graduate 1586), and it remained an important practice throughout the Qing (Brokaw 1991). One result was that well-intentioned men and women would print and distribute popular medical works as an act of charity. Merit accumulation was in fact an important factor driving the dissemination of the *Treatise on Easy Childbirth* (*Dasheng bian*) of 1715, one of the most famous and ubiquitous medical works of the Qing (Wu 2010). This brief book written in plain language was authored by a lower-level literatus who identified himself only as "Lay Buddhist Jizhai" (*Jizhai jushi*). Addressing himself to both men and women, Jizhai argued that childbirth was a natural process and that the key to safe delivery was to allow labor to follow its own innate rhythms. Whatever its inherent medical value, the wide circulation of this work owed much to people such as Song Er'rui, a native of the lower Yangzi region, who vowed during a storm at sea to print and distribute three thousand copies if his ship did not capsize. In the appendices to various editions of the *Treatise on Easy Childbirth,* Song and others told of the rewards they had received (or hoped to receive) for reprinting this work: the birth of heirs, success in the examinations, economic prosperity, family harmony, long life, and relief from illness.

Medicine and Secret Societies

The sharing of medical knowledge was also integral to the growth of secret societies and religious sects. The function of these groups ranged from mutual aid and defense to religious study. Many also embraced millenarian beliefs that, in some cases, inspired popular uprisings. To recruit and retain adherents, group leaders promised to initiate their adepts into secret revelations. These revelations notably included esoteric methods for health preservation and longevity: protective mantras, meditation, and martial arts techniques—

"boxing"—that gave adepts practical self-defense skills as well as warding off disease. In fact, many sect leaders were also themselves healers, and they actively recruited grateful patients into their groups. Such dynamics fueled the growth of the White Lotus groups that eventually led an antigovernment uprising in 1813 (Naquin 1976).

The *Jianghu* Performance of Medical and Martial Arts in Late Imperial Vernacular Fiction

Paize Keulemans

Twentieth-century martial arts fiction often depicts Chinese medicine and martial arts as conceptually related through the internal force, *qi* (Schmidt-Herzog 2003). By manipulating and cultivating *qi,* both medical and martial practitioners are said to cure patients or kill opponents with a single touch. More than half of the hundred entries on martial arts techniques in *The Great Dictionary of Appreciating Martial Arts Fiction (Wuxia xiaoshuo xinshang dadian)* involve *qi* (Wen 1994, 941–983). The chapter on *materia medica* observes: "In martial arts novels, *mo* and acupoints are not only crucial to drive out illness and help the wounded. They have developed to become a unique method for learning the highest form of martial arts" (Wen 1994, 559).

In contrast, vernacular martial arts novels from the sixteenth to the nineteenth centuries have no such emphasis. Neither the earliest (the sixteenth-century *Outlaws of the Marsh [Shuihu zhuan])* nor a last late-imperial example (Wen Kang's [fl. 1823–1866] *Tale of Romance and Heroism [Ernü yingxiong zhuan]*) mentions using *qi* as a martial arts technique (Wang 2002, 419). Instead, they describe outer forms, magical amulets, poison, and strategies based on battle arrays. Consequently, scholars of the medicine of this period turn to novels such as *The Dream of the Red Chamber (Hong lou meng)* (Idema 1977; Schonebaum 2004), which represent the domestic realm.

Late-imperial martial arts literature does connect medical and martial arts in a peripheral world known as *jianghu* (literally "rivers and lakes"), an alternative to regular society in two ways. Existing outside of the primary social structures of family and officialdom, it is set instead in inns, on street corners, at temple fairs, or in wild forests. Second, unlike the more rigidly stratified

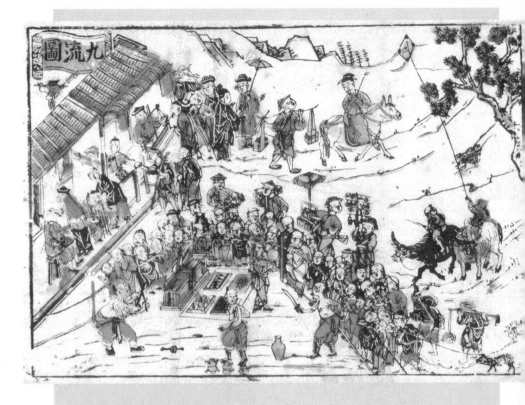

Figure 6.6. "The Nine Streams" (*jiuliu tu*), an early Qing-period New Year's print. Courtesy of Wang Shucun (private collection).

structures of regular society, the *jianghu* is always in flux, inhabited by itinerant outcasts: monks, martial arts masters, street peddlers, thieves, and medical practitioners who drift from town to town. As a marginal domain, it eluded regulation and could, at times, even fall under suspicion (Kuhn 1990).

Late imperial novels frame *jianghu* medical/martial arts not as interior cultivation but as an exterior performance amidst circulating bodies, money, and social energies. For example, an early Qing-period New Year's print, *The Nine Streams (jiuliu tu)*, shows the nine occupational classes of society, who "stream" together. A circular flow begins with the scholar on horseback, moves toward a child on a water buffalo, and arrives at martial artists striking agile poses. Three bare-chested martial artists perform, one gripping two daggers, another brandishing a sword, the last leaping lightly from one crockery pot to the next. Holding a small drum, another troupe member stands next to assorted medical supplies (Wang 1991, 407), amidst scholars on horseback and lowly book peddlers, children and old men, beggars and merchants. A scene from *Outlaws of the Marsh* illustrates how late imperial fiction imagined such moments:

They came to a bustling market town. Attracted by a crowd, Song Jiang pushed his way through and saw that they were watching a wandering medicine seller putting on a display with weapons.... The man first showed his skill with a lance. Then, he set that down and gave a demonstration of unarmed combat. "Excellent," Song Jiang exclaimed. The man picked up a tray and addressed the crowd. "I've come to your honorable town from afar to ply my trade," he said. "There's nothing startling about my talent. I rely entirely on your good will. Though I've been praised in distant places, you can see that I'm a mere juggler. I'm selling plasters for injured muscles and bones. If you've no need for them, bestow a few silver coins or coppers, so that my journey here will not have been in vain." (Shi and Luo 1993, 574; Chen, Hou, and Lu 1998, 1:671)

Actual medical matters involve only the sale of "plasters for injured muscles and bones"—items eminently reasonable for a martial artist. Yet this example also illuminates connections between medical/martial practices in a popular social stratum often overlooked in texts by the literati elite.

The affinity between healing and secret societies also played a key role in the formation of the so-called Boxers United in Righteousness (yihe tuan), whose antiforeign attacks in 1898–1900 proved an important turning point in Qing history. The Boxers' distinguishing practices were an amalgam of healing and health preservation techniques espoused by various secret societies active in northern China at this time: martial arts, qi manipulation exercises, charm-swallowing practices, and healing via spirit possession. In addition to conferring health, these practices were supposed to make the adept's body impervious to weapons (Cohen 1997). Boxer violence against foreigners was originally inspired by resentment against German missionaries and Chinese converts who used their connections to the foreigners to gain an upper hand in local disputes. In 1900, these attacks expanded into a direct assault on foreign legations in Beijing and on foreigners in other cities. The uprising was encouraged and endorsed by Empress Dowager Cixi (1835–1908), who hoped that the Boxers could drive the imperialists out of China. But the Boxers were defeated by a joint expeditionary force from eight foreign countries: Japan, Russia, Great Britain, the United States, France, Italy, Germany, and Austria-Hungary. The victors imposed the so-called Boxer Protocol of 1901, which wrested a staggering indemnity from the Qing government and gave foreign powers the right to station troops in Beijing. This defeat shook the court out of its conservative complacency while intensifying anti-Qing sentiment among elite reformers. A decade later, these tensions would culminate in the overthrow of the imperial house.

Global Medical Exchanges

As we saw in earlier chapters, the repertoire of health-related beliefs and practices in China historically had incorporated elements from the cultures of China's neighbors as well as of non-Chinese peoples in the imperium. At the same time, Chinese classical medicine was adopted by Japanese, Vietnamese, and Koreans as part of a larger ensemble of philosophical and technological borrowings. Throughout the late imperial period, Chinese medical knowledge continued to circulate throughout Asia. Medical texts were a commodity distributed along regional trading networks, and Li Shizhen's (ca. 1518–1593) encyclopedic compendium, *A Classification of Materia Medica (Bencao gangmu)*, was a famous example of the Chinese works that one could purchase in Korea, Japan, Vietnam, and communities in Southeast Asia (Elman 2005). The tribute system that structured Chinese relations with other kingdoms also provided a conduit for medical exchange. Medicinal substances were among the goods commonly exchanged as state gifts, and foreign envoys in China and Chinese envoys abroad also carried medical books back to their home countries.

In 1738, for example, the Chosŏn court bestowed a copy of the magisterial *Precious Mirror of Eastern Medicine (Tongŭibogam, Chinese Dongyi baojian)* on a visiting Chinese emissary (Cui 1996). Produced by Chosŏn court physicians and first published in 1613, this twenty-five-chapter work subsequently circulated widely in the Qing. Similarly, two Chosŏn officials dispatched to Beijing in 1790 acquired a text on Chinese smallpox variolation, which they formally presented to King Jeongjo (r. 1776–1800) and used to disseminate the technique among their fellow subjects (Cui 1996; Li and Lin 2000). In sum, there was a long history of international circulation of medical ideas to and from China. What distinguished the Qing was the expansion of a previously minor arena of medical exchange, namely, that between China and Europe and North America. These exchanges, furthermore, would eventually have significant impact on the events of the dynasty.

Since the time of Marco Polo, European travelers to China had written reports that included information about health-related practices, but these accounts were relatively sketchy and sporadic. Beginning in the fifteenth century, the quest for overseas riches and possessions and the concomitant expansion of maritime trade by Spain, Portugal, and later Holland, Britain, and France intensified European interest in Asia. After the founding of the

Society of Jesus in 1540, Asia also became an important mission field for European Catholics seeking to combat the rising influence of Protestantism. The growth of these exchanges allowed detailed information about Chinese healing techniques to reach Europe (Barnes 2005b). The earliest known European-language work on Chinese medicine was a treatise on pulse lore and prognostication, compiled in 1671 by an anonymous French missionary who reportedly had served in China. Another missionary observer was the Polish Jesuit Michael Boym (1612–1659), who went to China in 1645, reporting to the Ming loyalist court just after the Manchu conquest. Boym authored a work on the medicinal uses of Chinese flora and fauna (published in 1656) and a work on pulse lore (published posthumously in 1686).

But the three most influential accounts of Chinese practices were written by doctors and scientists who learned about Chinese medicine while living in other parts of Asia, their travels and activities made possible by Dutch commercial networks. One was Andreas Cleyer (1634–1697), a German physician who served as surgeon general with the Dutch East India Company in Batavia (now Jakarta, Indonesia) from 1665 to 1697. Between 1680–1682, Cleyer produced two works on Chinese pulse lore and medical doctrine, both of which relied heavily on unpublished material compiled by Michael Boym. The Dutch physician Willem Ten Rhijne (ca. 1647–1700) studied acupuncture and moxabustion in Tokugawa Japan for two years before also relocating to Batavia. His 1683 exposition on the treatment of gout included a discussion of how the Japanese used acupuncture and moxabustion to treat this condition. Similarly, the German naturalist and doctor Engelbert Kaempfer (1651–1716) spent two years in Tokugawa Japan with the Dutch East India Company. His detailed account of Japanese history and culture, compiled in 1694, also described the use of acupuncture and moxabustion. All three works circulated in Europe and were considered standard references for those interested in Chinese medicine (Barnes 2005b).

The history of these texts attests to the diffusion of Chinese medical knowledge throughout Asia and the fascination it held for Europeans. Besides acupuncture and moxabustion, Europeans were also eager to learn more about Chinese drugs. This was a natural extension of long-standing European commercial interests in Asian spices, many of which had medicinal applications, but it was also stimulated by new accounts of Chinese wonder herbs (Barnes 2005b). One was ginseng, long used in China as a Yang tonifying drug to replenish and increase *qi*. Europeans appear to have known about ginseng by the mid-seventeenth century, and Chinese enthusiasm for ginseng also spurred enterprising North Americans to look for an indigenous equivalent. Having found it, the Canadians and Americans made healthy profits exporting ginseng to China and Europe before the ginseng trade tapered off in the nineteenth century.

Westerners also regularly imported an herb from China known as "China root," "China wood," or simply "China," most probably the fungus *fuling (Poria cocos)*. Introduced to Spain by the Portuguese in 1535, China root was credited with curing Spanish King Carlos V of his gout. This was but one of many medicinal and health-promoting substances that Europeans purchased from China, a list that included diverse products such as alum, ginger, star anise, cardamom, camphor, and galangal. Two other significant imports were rhubarb and, of course, tea. By the eighteenth century, however, British and American enthusiasm for tea was exacerbating a worrisome Western trade deficit with China, especially troubling because China seemed indifferent to most products that the foreigners might sell in return.

The Qing empire was thus part of a global trading network in pharmaceutical herbs, minerals, and animal products. But the drug that came to dwarf all others in importance was opium. Introduced to China by Arab traders by the eighth century, the opium poppy was valued initially as an ornamental plant and subsequently for its medicinal properties (Su 1997; Li 1986). Opium's ability to alleviate diarrhea, coughing, pain and fever meant it was regularly used for treating the symptoms and aftereffects of infectious and epidemic diseases, including what biomedicine would identify as dysentery, malaria, smallpox, and cholera (Dikötter, Laaman, and Zhou 2004; Su 1997; Xu 1986). Around the mid-seventeenth century, the habit of smoking opium mixed with tobacco was also introduced into China from Southeast Asia, likely through Dutch traders. Over the next century and a half, recreational smoking of pure opium itself became an activity widely enjoyed by all social classes.

Such was its popularity that opium became the one commodity sufficiently enticing to Chinese consumers to redress Western trade imbalances in China. Revenues from importing Indian opium to China also became the financial linchpin of British imperialist expansion (Brook and Wakabayashi 2000; Blue 2000). Foreign imports of opium to China thus grew even in the face of intensifying Qing government bans on the drug after 1729. British imports of opium to China were a relatively modest 200 chests in 1729, but by the turn of the century averaged between 4,000 and 5,000 chests per year. Thereafter, the numbers quickly soared, with more than 7,000 chests imported in 1823, more than 20,000 chests in 1833, and more than 34,000 chests in 1838 (Zhou 1999, 14; Spence 1999, 130). These imports also competed with a lucrative trade in domestic Chinese opium grown in western regions such as Yunnan and Sichuan.

Opium smokers included those who used it primarily as a leisure activity, as a social lubricant, or for specific therapeutic purposes. Wealthy connoisseurs showed off by smoking high-quality opium, using implements that were also objects of art. Poor laborers could smoke leftover dregs to dull the pain of hunger or fatigue. However, during this period, opium addiction also emerged as a widespread social problem of immense import. Contemporary observers blamed opium for destroying individual health, family prosperity, social morals, and the preparedness of the empire's military (Brook and Wakabayashi 2000; Blue 2000). The outpouring of Chinese silver into the pockets of foreign opium traders also threatened the health of the Chinese economy. In 1839, when the imperial commissioner Lin Zexu (1785–1850) confiscated and destroyed more than twenty thousand chests of foreign opium in Guangzhou, he was complying with the Daoguang Emperor's orders to halt the opium trade once and for all. But this short-term victory was quickly canceled out by the armed British response that ultimately opened China to many more decades of imperialist intrusions.

The Jesuits and the Introduction of European Medicine

Global trading networks allowed information about Chinese medicine to travel to Europe. They also facilitated the dissemination of European medical knowledge to East Asia. In the case of Tokugawa Japan, it was the Dutch East India Company that served as the primary vehicle of transmission. Fearing the potentially subversive influence of foreign merchants, missionaries and Japanese Christians, the Tokugawa shogunate severely restricted Japanese interactions with other countries. After 1639, the government limited all foreign trade to the island of Deshima (off the coast of Nagasaki) and forbade any Europeans except the Dutch from trading there. It was thus through Dutch-employed doctors and traders on Deshima that information about Western medicine entered Japan.

In seventeenth- and eighteenth-century China, by contrast, Jesuit missionaries served as the chief transmitters of European medical knowledge. Their strategy was to convert Chinese elites, and they deliberately employed European science as an aid to evangelization, using it to impress educated Chinese men with the achievements of Western civilization (Standaert 2001). Through this means, they did successfully convert some prominent Chinese officials, also gaining imperial favor because of their knowledge of mathematics and astronomy. They received official appointments in the imperial Astro-Calendric Bureau and helped to resolve the late Ming calendar crisis. From 1644 to 1664, Adam Schall von Bell directed the Qing Astro-Calendric Bureau, until his Chinese rivals succeeded in having him imprisoned on charges of spreading heterodox and seditious religious teachings. In 1669, however, the Jesuits' demonstrated ability to make more accurate astronomical calculations allowed Ferdinand Verbiest (1623–1688) to regain directorship of the bureau (Standaert 2001).

The Jesuits also introduced aspects of European medicine. Information about anatomy, physiology, and pharmacology appeared in their works on natural science and religion. The Jesuits also composed specialized medical works to expound European teachings (Standaert 2001), the earliest of which originated as a draft manuscript on anatomy composed around 1625 by the Swiss Jesuit and physician Johann Schreck (1576–1630). In 1634, Schall showed the work to the Chinese scholar-official Bi Gongchen (Metropolitan Graduate 1616), who was so impressed with it that he revised and expanded it and published it under the title *An Overview of Western Doctrines of the Human Body (Taixi renshen shuogai)* (Hummel 1943; Standaert 2001). A second text, composed during the 1630s, was the *Illustrated Treatise on the Human Body (Renshen tushuo)*, a translation of a treatise on anatomy by the celebrated French surgeon Ambroise Paré (1510–1590). This text was primarily the work of Italian Jesuit Giacomo Rho (ca. 1593–1638), who worked on it in collaboration with the Jesuit Nicolò Longobardo (1559–1654) and Schreck (Standaert 2001). The subsequent circulation and dissemination of these two texts among Chinese readers remains to be fully understood, but we know that at least some doctors and scholars in the eighteenth and nineteenth centuries were able to obtain and discuss them (Hanson 2006; Wang 1851).

Within the Qing court, the Kangxi Emperor had an active interest in European therapeutics and drugs, including "snakestone" for curing poison. In response, Verbiest and Joachim Bouvet (1656–1730) composed essays and texts on these subjects for the emperor's edification. In 1685, the emperor had even asked Verbiest to arrange for additional European physicians to be sent to his court. The emperor's interest in Western medicine was further stimulated in 1693 when Jesuits used Peruvian cinchona bark (containing quinine) to cure him of a debilitating febrile illness, most likely malaria. Subsequently, the Kangxi Emperor ordered the French Jesuit Dominique Parennin (1665–1741) to compile a Manchu-language work on Western anatomy, now known as the *Manchu Anatomy*. Its contents notably included William Harvey's (1578–1657) discovery of the circulation of blood (Asen 2009). Nine versions of this text are extant today, with the most expansive containing 135 anatomical plates adapted from European works (Walravens 1996; Hanson 2003). However, the text was apparently intended for consultation only by the imperial household, and no attempts were made to disseminate this information to practitioners at large.

Acupuncture in Europe

During the eighteenth century, European attitudes toward China and Chinese medicine were generally positive. Although European observers disdained what they saw as Chinese ignorance of anatomy, they admired Chinese drugs and the seemingly wondrous efficacy of acupuncture and moxabustion (Barnes 2005b). In fact, the 1820s and 1830s witnessed a kind of acupuncture craze in Europe and the United States. The first French doctor to use acupuncture on his patients was Louis-Joseph Berlioz (father of the composer Hector Berlioz). In 1816 Berlioz published an account of his successful experiences and advocated that acupuncture be more widely adopted. Despite criticism and skepticism from some quarters, experiments by French surgeons allowed acupuncture to become popular in France and other parts of Europe. By the 1820s, practitioners in England, Italy, Ireland, Scotland, Spain, and Germany had published accounts of their experiences with the technique in important medical journals. The presence of American medical trainees in major European cities, as well as the overseas circulation of these journals, stimulated American interest in acupuncture and influenced some American physicians to test the procedure themselves. These included Franklin Bache (great-grandson of Benjamin Franklin), who published a well-known account of acupuncture's effects in 1826.

Eighteenth-Century European Views of Gongfu (Kungfu)

Linda L. Barnes

Gongfu refers generally to self-cultivation skills, but today the term is recognized around the world in its Cantonese pronunciation, "kung fu" or "kungfu," as denoting certain styles of martial arts. Long before movies, television, and music popularized gongfu's applications to martial training, though, Europeans commented on the wider range of gongfu practices. In 1779 Jesuit missionary Jean-Joseph-Marie Amiot (1718–1793) wrote from Beijing complaining that the Chinese had long been deceived into viewing these "singular postures" as a religious exercise that cured infirmities, released the soul from the power of the senses, prepared one to interact with spirits, and opened the doors to immortality. According to the Chinese, Amiot added, the body's mechanism was hydraulic, with health residing in a dynamic equilibrium. Gongfu practitioners attended to sympathetic correspondences between parts of the body, the actions and reactions of the organs of circulation, the secretion of humors, and the digestion of food. Amiot proposed that European doctors "examine whether the medical part of the daoshi's gongfu is really a practice of medicine of which one might make use, for the relief and cure of some ill-

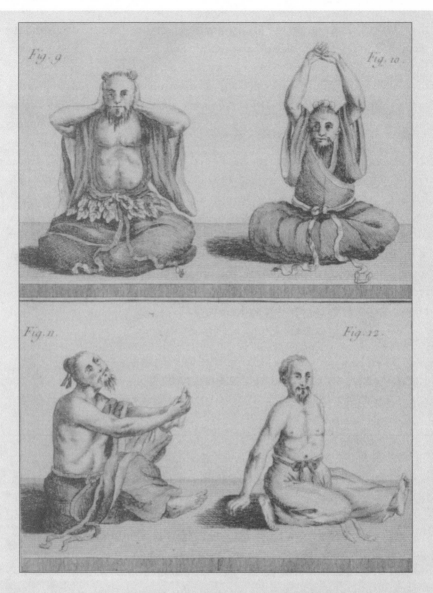

Figure 6.7. Gongfu of the Daoist monks. Amiot, *Mémoires concernant l'histoire, les sciences, les arts, les moeurs, les usages, &c. des Chinois*, vol. 4, 1779. Widener Library of the Harvard College Library.

nesses." If so, he would feel compensated for the trouble he had taken with the subject.

Yet in 1783, having learned about Anton Mesmer's theory of animal magnetism, Amiot had changed his mind, writing, "I already glimpse, as though through a cloud, that it could as well be of Chinese *gongfu,* as of Mesmeric medicine" (Huard and Wong 1968, 62–63). He equated Yin and Yang with magnetic theory:

For animal Magnetism and its two Poles, I substitute very simply *Tai-Ki* [*Taiji*], *yin*, and *yang*. . . . The order that reigns in nature, its power—of which our weak constitution does not know the limits—its marvelous fecundity, the astonishing variety of its productions . . . is only the effect of the conjunction of *yin* and *yang* combining with each other, following the rules of harmony. (64–65)

Excess or deficiency in either Yin or Yang led to false harmonies and disorder, resulting in illness. To restore harmony and health, one rectified the surplus or lack. Mesmer's practice, Amiot suggested, was equivalent to knowing the state of Yin and Yang:

What perhaps seems to you an unintelligible jargon, is for me a language as luminous as that of your Newtonian and other philosophers when they speak of principles of attraction, of Electricity, of the movement of Magnetism, of the turning of planets etc. etc. . . . . For thirty years, I have only heard *qi*, *yin*, and *yang* spoken about; I should be familiar with these terms which are the key to all the sciences here. (67–68)

He speculated that *gongfu* dated back to the (mythical) emperors Shun, the Yellow Emperor, and the Divine Husbandman, and that some doctors must still practice it. "If there were only two or three in the vast precinct of Beijing," he added, "I would unearth them, and I would render you an account of their operations, of their manner of operating and the principles upon which they are based" (63).

In 1784, he suggested that the Chinese had predated Mesmer's theory of animal magnetism by four thousand years with Yin-Yang. "This fluid which is universally spread out and contained in a way so as not to suffer any vacuum, whose subtlety does not permit any comparison, and by its nature is susceptible of receiving, propagating, communicating all the impressions of the moment, is none other than the yin-yang of the Chinese" (Huard 1968, 81–82). Those who learned to attune themselves to the Yin and Yang within themselves could direct both through "the fluid of the same nature that fills space," extending out to distant phenomena and returning to transmit an awareness of what they had touched upon at a distance. Such men seemed able to know what occurred far away, "as though it were happening before their eyes" (83). Nor did Amiot dismiss that possibility (Adapted from Barnes 2005b).

By contrast, the influence of Western medicine on Chinese therapeutics during this period was minimal. Jesuit influence notably waned by the end of the eighteenth century. When the pope tried to forbid Chinese converts from performing ancestral and Confucian rituals, the Kangxi emperor expelled all missionaries who refused to accommodate these Chinese practices. Although the Jesuits remained, these tensions persisted, and the pope subsequently ordered the Society of Jesus to disband in 1773. It was only in the nineteenth century, when Protestant missionaries began going to China, that deliberate efforts were again made to plant Western practices in Chinese soil.

Protestant Medical Missionaries

During the early nineteenth century, missionary activities were restricted to the southern outskirts of the empire: the Portuguese enclave of Macao and the city of Canton (Guangzhou), the latter the sole Qing port where foreign trade was permitted. In 1807, the first Protestant missionary arrived in China, sent under the auspices of the London Missionary Society. This was the British missionary Robert Morrison, who had also worked for several years as an interpreter for the British East India Company. In 1820, British East India Company surgeon John Livingstone recruited Morrison to help him open a dispensary in Macao. They outfitted it with a Chinese medical library and stocks of Chinese herbs and employed a Chinese physician to attend to clients (Wong and Wu 1932). At this point, however, medicine had not yet been explicitly recruited as a handmaiden to Christian evangelization. This was to change with the mission of the American physician and minister Peter Parker, sent to China by the American Board of Commissioners for Foreign Missions. In 1835, Parker opened a hospital and dispensary in Canton, where he made a name for himself as a curer of eye diseases. Parker and his sponsors believed that Western medicine would show the superiority of Western culture, and the physical proximity to Chinese patients in the clinic would provide ample opportunities for proselytization. Parker also trained Chinese students in Western medicine so that they could work alongside him.

Britain's victory over Qing in the Opium War (1839–1842) opened five ports to Western residence and trade. After losing the Arrow War of 1856–1858 to Britain and France, Qing was forced to open another ten ports and grant foreigners the right to travel throughout the country. Inspired by religious revival movements at home, and now granted unprecedented access to the Chinese multitudes, the number of European and American missionaries surged. They also continued to employ medicine as an aid to evangelism, setting up dispensaries, hospitals, and medical schools. In absolute terms, the missionaries, their converts, and the number of Chinese trained in Western medicine never constituted a numerically significant group. Nevertheless, they were a major conduit for the modernizing ideas that would take center stage in Chinese reform movements during the late nineteenth century.

Chinese Views of Western Medicine

Interested in science and technology, and eager to learn new ideas, Chinese thinkers approached Western teachings "on their own terms," utilizing them in the service of distinctly Chinese intellectual aims (Elman 2005). For example, the Jesuit introduction of European science came at a time when the indigenous Chinese tradition of "investigating things and extending knowledge" *(gewu zhizhi)* was already undergoing a transformation and revival. Prominent literati such as Fang Yizhi (1611–1671) sought to accumulate verifiable facts about natural phenomena to explain the observable patterns of the cosmos. Fang thus embraced those portions of Jesuit science that seemed useful to his own endeavor, including astronomy, anatomy, and physiology (Standaert 2001). At the same time, he rejected unverifiable teachings that required leaps of faith, notably the foreign idea that the universe's structure proved the existence of a creator God (Elman 2005).

Likewise, existing Chinese practices and concerns shaped Chinese responses to nineteenth-century Euro-American medicine. The Western therapies that attracted Chinese patients included treatments for diseases that indigenous healers could not cure or did not treat. This included tumors, which Chinese doctors generally treated with poultices and orally ingested drugs designed to regulate disharmonies of *qi*. Missionary doctors removed them surgically, giving relief to Chinese men, women, and children who sometimes had suffered for years from massive and disfiguring growths. Peter Parker and other missionaries documented their more spectacular cases in paintings and etchings designed to depict the fortitude of Chinese sufferers and their willingness to go under the knife in the right circumstances (Heinrich 2008). Chinese patients also patronized Western therapies that appeared to be more effective versions of existing Chinese techniques. For example, missionaries in China developed a reputation for curing eye diseases—including cataracts—making these procedures a staple of Protestant medical dispensaries and hospitals (Wong and Wu 1932). Although Westerners expressed amazement at the willingness of Chinese to have eye surgery, Indian methods for needling cataracts had been part of the Chinese therapeutic repertoire since Tang times (Andrews 1996; Kovacs and Unschuld 1998).

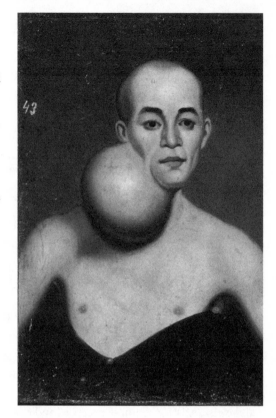

Figure 6.8. This image of a man with a tumor comes from a collection of more than one hundred oil paintings that the famous Chinese portrait artist Lam Qua (1801–1860) made of patients treated by American medical missionary Peter Parker. Parker displayed some of these paintings in the waiting room of his hospital in Canton to show the curative powers of Western medicine to prospective Chinese patients. He also exhibited these paintings to foreign audiences during fund-raising tours to illustrate the need for Christian charity in China. Courtesy of Yale University, Harvey Cushing/John Hay Whitney Medical Library.

Similar dynamics shaped the Chinese reception of Jennerian vaccination against smallpox. Beginning in at least the sixteenth century, the Chinese had practiced variolation using scabs or pustules from smallpox sufferers. The idea that one could create immunity to smallpox by inducing a controlled form of the disease was thus a familiar one. In 1805, the East India Company surgeon Alexander Pearson (1780–1874) introduced vaccination with cowpox in Macao. Working with Chinese assistants, Pearson reportedly vaccinated thousands of local Chinese by the end of 1806 (Wang and Wu 1936, 279). While Chinese variolation practitioners viewed this as unwelcome competition, many elites promoted vaccination as a superior form of variolation and established philanthropic organizations to provide free vaccinations and train practitioners (Chang 1996). These included a dispensary set up in 1815 by the wealthy "hong merchants" of Guangzhou, the only Chinese businessmen authorized by the Qing to trade directly with the West. Another early adopter was the merchant Qiu Xi (ca. 1733–1851), vaccinated as an adult soon after hearing of Pearson's work. Qiu became an active advocate of vaccination, promoting it in his *Outline on Inducing Pox (Yin dou lue)* of 1817.

Many Chinese readers were also fascinated by Western works on anatomy, such as the *Outline of Anatomy and Physiology* (*Quanti xinlun*, first ed. 1851) by English surgeon and missionary Benjamin Hobson (1816–1873). Hobson was the first Protestant missionary to publish Chinese-language texts on Western medicine, which he compiled in Chinese with the aid of Chinese scholars. But although Hobson wished to reform Chinese medical knowledge, his readers had no reason to abandon the conceptual body of Yin-Yang in favor of European models. In fact, Chinese thinkers interested in Hobson's works primarily used them to improve their understandings of *qi*. These included practitioners of inner alchemy, who relied on diagrams of the body's "inner landscape" to guide their visualization of *qi* as they directed its flow through the body (Despeux 1994; Andrews 1996). Prominent Chinese physicians also argued that one could not understand the generation and circulation of healthy and pathogenic *qi* in the body without understanding the true forms of the organs and internal structures, their relative positions in the body, and their physical connections to each other (Wang 1999).

Such concerns had in fact motivated the Chinese physician Wang Qingren (1768–1831) to conduct his own observations of exposed corpses and the bodies of executed criminals. Wang criticized existing medical texts for their incorrect depictions of internal organs, and presented his revised findings in *Correcting the Errors of the Doctors* (*Yilin gaicuo*) in 1830. Wang's work attracted considerable attention (both negative and positive) and was reprinted numerous times (Andrews 1996). In this intellectual environment, Western anatomical texts could also prove a valuable resource. For this reason, in 1853 Ye Zhishen (who used the sobriquet Suiweng), father of the then viceroy of Liangguang, republished the illustrations from Hobson's *Outline* in the form of eight hanging scrolls. These illustrations of bodily structure, he explained, could help doctors better apply the classical diagnostic techniques of "looking, inquiring, listening/smelling, and palpating the pulse" (Hobson 1851b; "Obituary" 1873; Hummel 1943).

Some doctors also made comparisons between Western anatomical knowledge and that found in Chinese forensic medicine texts. The earliest specialized treatise on forensic medicine published in the world was Song Ci's (1186–1249) *Collected Writings on the Washing Away of Wrongs* (*Xiyuan jilu*, 1247), which became the basis of official Chinese forensic practice in subsequent centuries (Needham 2000). In 1694, the Qing government produced a new version that melded Song Ci's original text with specialized writings by Yuan- and Ming-era authors, promulgating it as the official guide for all subsequent death investigations. In 1770, the imperial government also issued an official set of skeleton charts for magistrates to use when recording signs of trauma found on the body of the deceased. Although the government's objective was to standardize and improve forensic practice, many of the officials and legal experts who had to use these materials complained that they contained serious errors. Beginning in the late eighteenth century, therefore, some of these men published private, unofficial forensic handbooks and case collections intended to rectify the shortcomings of the official guides (Will 2007).

County magistrates dealt with dead bodies and oversaw forensic examinations, while medicine was the province of doctors trying to save the living. Nevertheless, there were intersections between the two realms: Qing forensics authors read the medical classics to better understand the processes by which death occurred, while doctors consulted forensic works to improve their knowledge of the skeleton and thus of bodily structure (Despeux 2007; Will 2007). The latter group included the Hangzhou physician Wang Shixiong (1808–1868), who wrote an essay comparing accounts of the skeleton derived from Jesuit texts, Hobson's *Outline*, Chinese medical and forensics works, and the observations that a magistrate friend had made while supervising death investigations (Wang 1999).

It was natural that Chinese thinkers should explain new Western ideas in terms of what was familiar. Missionary translators also reinforced such tendencies by using modified versions of existing Chinese medical nomenclature to render English terms. For example, Benjamin Hobson and his Chinese assistants drew on the concept of *qi* to convey the Western concept of "nerves," which they translated with the term "brain *qi* sinews" *(nao qi jin)*. Similarly, to convey the idea of pulmonary consumption (i.e., tuberculosis), they resorted to an ancient Chinese disease called wasting illness *(laozheng)* to create the term "lung wasting illness" *(fei laozheng)*. In so doing, they blurred the intellectual boundaries between the two systems (Andrews 1997; Shapiro 2003; Chan 2012).

These types of cultural accommodation also appeared in the institutional arena. Chinese willingness to patronize foreign-run dispensaries and hospitals owed much to the existence of analogous Chinese charitable institutions that provided medical and economic aid to the poor and indigent (Renshaw 2005). However, Western hospitals also had to make provisions to accommodate Chinese sensibilities. In deference to Chinese norms of gender propriety, they provided separate waiting rooms for male and female patients and employed a relatively high number of female medical personnel. Western doctors also knew they needed to integrate Chinese practices into their examinations in order to gain patients' confidence, so they made sure to palpate pulses and examine the tongue (Renshaw 2005).

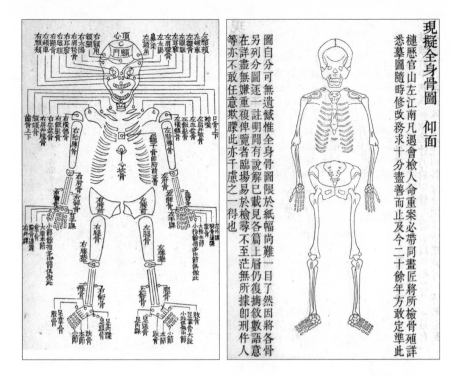

Figure 6.9. *Left:* This front view of the skeleton appeared in an 1818 edition of Qian Xiuchang's *Supplemented Essentials on the Treatment of Injuries,* originally compiled in 1808. It is a copy of the government-promulgated "bone investigation charts" that Qing officials used when conducting forensic investigations. Qian Xiuchang discussed a wide range of topics, including wounds caused by weapons or bites, internal injuries and broken bones caused by falls or beatings, and burns from fire or boiling water. He explained that he was providing front and back views of the skeleton because doctors needed to understand the forms of joints and bones in order to effectively treat dislocations and fractures. Qian, *Shangke buyao,* 1955 (1818). *Right:* During the late eighteenth and early nineteenth centuries, a number of government officials and legal experts wrote treatises that aimed to correct errors in the government-issued forensic guides, including the official skeleton charts. This front view of the skeleton comes from *An Explanation of the Meaning of the Washing Away of Wrong,* compiled in 1854, one of the most influential of these new treatises. Its author, the scholar-official Xu Lian (Metropolitan degree 1833), explained that he had an artist accompany him on his forensic investigations to record the forms of bones, and that his revised images were based on more than twenty years of personal observation. Xu, *Xi yuan lu xiangyi,* 1856 ed. Courtesy of Linda L. Barnes.

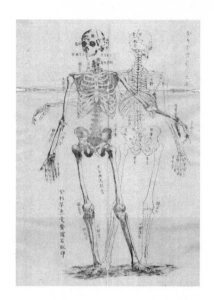

Figure 6.10. The English medical missionary Benjamin Hobson (1816–1873) made the first systematic effort to compile books on Western medicine for the training of Chinese medical personnel. Hobson's works were also an important reference for later missionary medical publications. This double illustration of the front and back view of a skeleton comes from the first edition of Hobson's *Outline of Anatomy and Physiology,* the earliest of four medical works he composed directly in Chinese with the assistance of Chinese scholars. Hobson, *Quanti xinlun,* 1851 edition. Courtesy of the National Library of Australia.

Hobson also tried to introduce Western surgical techniques, requiring a detailed knowledge of anatomy, to his Chinese readers. Additional research is needed to understand how his readers viewed these techniques. Hobson's intended audience of literate practitioners was striving to make medicine more scholarly. In diagnostic terms, this meant refining one's learned discernment of *qi* and its dynamic transformations and manifestations in the body. In therapeutic terms, it meant crafting an appropriate combination of plant, animal, or mineral drugs that would restore the body's innate harmony. These trends thus privileged pharmacological remedies over manual healing. In 1822, the Qing Imperial Medical Bureau even eliminated its department of acupuncture, removing this manual therapy from the realm of scholarly medical practice at court (Andrews 1996; Li 2011).

Yet it must be emphasized that surgical interventions on the skin and flesh were historically a standard part of the Chinese healing repertoire, recorded in medical texts and other writings throughout the late imperial period. Common therapies included lancing boils and needling cataracts, stitching up wounds, and cutting away injured flesh (Andrews 1996; Li 2011). A well-known treatment for epidemic ailments, including cholera, was to pierce the skin at designated points in the crook of the arm or back of the knee to induce bleeding and rid the body of "toxic blood" (Wang 1851). Historians have hypothesized that ancient forms of bloodletting or lancing may even have influenced the development of acupuncture (Epler 1980; Harper 1998). So even if hands-on healing did not constitute a prestigious field of practice or study, minor surgical techniques remained a familiar feature of the Chinese medical landscape.

Western Medicine and Chinese Self-Strengthening

Alongside their healing activities, missionaries sought to disseminate knowledge of Western medicine in China in their newspapers, journals, textbooks, and other translations. After 1860, their efforts were aided by reformist Qing officials who established schools and arsenals designed to strengthen the empire and enhance its ability to negotiate the pressures of Western imperialism. Under the slogan of "self-strengthening," these officials encouraged the dissemination of Western science and technology, including medicine, and often hired missionaries and other foreigners as administrators, instructors, and translators. For example, the Tongwen Guan in Beijing, which the government originally established as a translator's school in 1862, soon expanded into a college that also offered instruction in science and medicine. In 1871, it hired Scottish missionary doctor John Dudgeon as professor of anatomy and physiology. Dudgeon translated and compiled texts on Western medicine, most notably *A Complete Investigation of the Entire Body (Quanti tongkao)*, which the Tongwen Guan published in sixteen fascicles in 1886. The core of this text was a translation of Henry Gray's (1827–1861) *Anatomy, Descriptive and Surgical* (Gao 2009).

The Jiangnan Arsenal, established in 1865, also boasted a prolific translation bureau. Its best-known translator was the Englishman John Fryer, who produced 129 texts on Western science and technology during his twenty-eight years at the arsenal, from 1868 to 1896. Fryer's output included works on anatomy and physiology, *materia medica*, medical jurisprudence, and X-rays (Bennett 1967, 37, Appendix 2). In 1884, Fryer also established the Scientific Book Depot, which sold translations and other "useful literature" to the general public. A catalog dated 1896 lists seventeen translated Western medical works for sale, on topics ranging from anatomy to fevers, eye diseases, and syphilis (Bennett 1967, Appendix 5).

During the late Qing, therefore, detailed knowledge about Western medicine was relatively accessible to interested Chinese. These included the Sichuanese scholar Tang Zonghai (1851–1897), whom modern historians see as a seminal figure in early attempts to assimilate Western medicine into Chinese practices. In response to his father's death from illness in 1873, Tang began a concerted study of classical medicine while also making his way through the examination system (he gained the Metropolitan Graduate degree in 1889). He read Wang Qingren's *Correcting the Errors of Doctors*, and his sojourns in the treaty port of Shanghai also facilitated his access to Western medicine. During the 1880s and 1890s, Tang wrote a number of texts in which he assessed the relative utility of Western knowledge and how it might be integrated into Chinese medicine (Scheid 2007; Pi 2008).

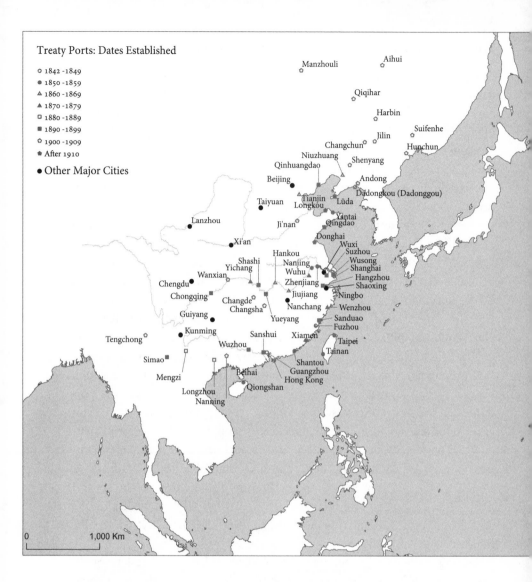

Manzhouli Aihui

Qiqihar

Harbin

Suifenhe
Jilin
Changchun Hunchun
Niuzhuang Shenyang
Qinhuangdao
Beijing Andong
Dadongkou (Dadonggou)
Taiyuan Tianjin Lüda
Longkou
Lanzhou Yantai
Ji'nan Qingdao
Xi'an
Donghai
Wuxi
Hankou Suzhou
Shashi Nanjing Wusong
Yichang Wuhu Shanghai
Wanxian Zhenjiang Hangzhou
Chengdu Shaoxing
Jiujiang
Chongqing Changde Ningbo
Changsha Nanchang Wenzhou
Guiyang Yueyang
Sanduao
Kunming Sanshui Fuzhou
Tengchong Wuzhou Xiamen
Taipei
Simao Tainan
Shantou
Mengzi Beihai Guangzhou
Qiongshan Hong Kong
Longzhou
Nanning

0   1,000 Km

In this period as well, Western medicine was patronized by diplomat and statesman Li Hongzhang (1823–1901), one of the most powerful officials of the late Qing. A leading advocate of self-strengthening, Li had personally promoted numerous initiatives to adopt Western science and technology, most notably in the area of industrial and military modernization. As viceroy of Zhili, Li helped fund the establishment of a missionary hospital and medical school in Tianjin after Western doctors cured his wife of an unspecified dangerous ailment in 1879. In 1888, Li took control of these institutions in the name of the Qing government, intending that they would now train Chinese doctors for his Beiyang

Army and Navy. The school's professors included French doctor René Depasse, who also served as Li's personal physician (Rogaski 1996).

And yet the influence of Western medicine on Chinese healers and sufferers during this time was relatively limited overall. The number of foreign and Chinese personnel trained in Western medicine was just too small to have much of a direct impact on the vast Qing population. More generally, however, Chinese observers had no obvious reason to see nineteenth-century Euro-American medicine as wholly superior to indigenous Chinese medical frameworks. In the last years of the Qing Dynasty, Western medicine would acquire great symbolic value as a tool for nation building, championed by social and political reformers. Prior to that, however, it was evaluated on its therapeutic merits. During the early decades of the medical missions, the great triumphs of Western medicine—germ theory, safe abdominal surgery, vaccines, antibiotics—were still years or even generations away. Western anatomical science, in other words, did not necessarily improve day-to-day medical care. For many acute, chronic, and contagious illnesses, in fact, Western methods were neither more nor less effective than Chinese ones.

Epidemic cholera provides a good example of this dynamic. The disease reached China around 1820, transmitted from India via maritime trading routes (Macpherson 1998). Caused by the bacteria *Vibrio cholerae,* cholera attacks the small intestine and prevents it from absorbing fluids. The result is uncontrollable watery diarrhea that rapidly strips the body of its fluids, leading to severe dehydration and circulatory and organ failure. Left untreated, fatality rates are as high as 40 to 50 percent. During the nineteenth century, cholera pandemics rampaged through Europe, the Middle East, the Americas, and Asia, becoming the pressing global medical problem of the day. In the pre-germ-theory age, Western and Chinese doctors alike drew on environmental and constitutional explanations to manage this horrifying disease. The conventional European view blamed factors such as miasma (foul air) or contact with people who had the disease. Today it is accepted that the only reliable treatment for cholera is intravenous fluid replacement. But standard Western remedies of the nineteenth-century included bloodletting, strong laxatives and purgatives (including calomel, a compound of mercury), and opium.

Chinese doctors, seeking solutions, mined ancient texts and contemporary medical writings, expounding their explanations in a flurry of publications. Cholera seemed to resemble the known maladies of *huoluan* (lit. "sudden turmoil") or *sha* (an umbrella term for a diverse ensemble of illnesses attributed to noxious miasmas). However, there was no consensus as to whether it was a new variant of these old illnesses or an entirely new disease.

Among the most famous of these texts on cholera was Wang Shixiong's *Treatise on Sudden Turmoil Disease (Huolan lun)* (Wang 1851). Wang affirmed that the outbreaks were *huoluan*, but he rejected older teachings that attributed such epidemics to pathogenic invasions of cold. Instead, he drew on an innovative corpus of writings on "warm diseases" to argue that cholera was caused by excessive heat. Wang thus recommended the use of cooling drugs, as well as the regulation of diet and living conditions to minimize exposure to pathogenic heat (Hanson 2011).

The "Warm Diseases" Current of Learning

Marta E. Hanson

Through recorded history, the prevention and treatment of seasonal outbreaks of disease were an ongoing concerns for China's physicians, and sometimes for its governments. During the Qing period, doctors took earlier writings on Warm Diseases *(wenbing)* and transformed them into an influential new etiological framework for explaining epidemics. Yet like many Chinese disease concepts, the notion of Warm Diseases changed meaning over the two thousand years since the concept was first defined. For example, the chapter "On Heat Diseases" ("Rebing lun") in the *Inner Canon: Basic Questions* (first century B.C.E.) gave two key definitions: (1) a range of acute-onset febrile disorders caused by external pathogenic *qi,* and (2) a specific type of Cold Damage *(shanghan)* acquired in the winter, but whose dormant *qi (fuqi)* only transformed into high fevers and Yin-impairing dryness during the spring and summer. Zhang Ji (150–219 C.E.) later adopted this second meaning of Warm Diseases as a subclass of Cold Damage, characterized by excessive heat, in his *Treatise on Cold Damage and Miscellaneous Disorders.*

In 1065, the Northern Song imperial government published a separate *Treatise on Cold Damage.* This work went on to become the main source from which subsequent interpretations of *wenbing* branched in new directions, as later thinkers elaborated on different facets. Key points of contention included the etiological relationship between pathogenic Cold and Heat, as well as the relative significance of these factors in seasonal and epidemic diseases. For example, Liu Wansu (b. 1110) argued that diseases due to Fire and Heat had become more common and problematic in his own day than Cold Damage. Wang Andao (ca. 1332–1391) first proposed that *wenbing* not be classed with Cold Damage. Wang Ji (1463–1539) further differentiated between dormant *qi*-

induced *wenbing* and its newly contracted form. Wu Youxing (1582–1652) argued that a specific pestilential *qi*—rather than unseasonable *qi*—caused
Warm Diseases and that they were a type of "febrile epidemic" *(wenyi)*.

On the basis of these earlier writings, doctors of the mid-seventeenth through
the nineteenth centuries changed the meaning of Warm Diseases from a sub-
set of Cold Damage to a separate class of diseases that merited specialized
monographs and new compilations. These examples illustrate how a core concept can undergo variations in definition and classification—a process not
uncommon in medical history. Twentieth-century Chinese historians have
since identified Warm Disease writers from the Qing period as a "current of
learning" *(xuepai)* (Ren 1980; Scheid 2007; Hanson 2011). The fluid-related
term "current" is apropos, because physicians who focused on Warm Diseases
never became so cohesive a group as to constitute a distinct "school." They
usually came to their interest through some other connection, such as kinship
ties, master-disciple relations, or regional affiliation, or on the practice side
through shared doctrinal preferences or clinical styles. Warm Disease approaches to treatment continued to develop during the twentieth century and
are still debated today. Contemporary doctors continue to find these frameworks clinically useful, notably using them to treat patients in mainland China
during the 2003 SARS epidemic.

Medicine and Modernization

As of 1893, there were a reported seventy-one hospitals and 111 dispensaries run
by twenty-six mission groups from North America and Europe, all working to
address what missionaries called "China's appalling need of reform" (American
Presbyterian Mission 1896, 34, 327). A few years later, the state of indigenous
medicine and health care started to became a salient concern for Chinese intellectuals and statesmen as well. The catalyst was China's humiliating defeat
in the Sino-Japanese War of 1894–95. The war grew out of the competition between Qing China and Meiji Japan to assert dominance over Chosŏn. When
armed conflict first erupted, popular opinion favored China, whose modernized
navy was far larger. Japan's stunning victory over Qing forces, which were crip-
pled by infighting at the highest levels of command, led to a reversal of conventional wisdom (Elman 2005). Now Japan became the symbol for successful
Asian modernization, and reform-minded Chinese youth traveled there to
study Western sciences, including medicine. The most famous of these students

was the author Lu Xun (1881–1936), who went to Japan in 1905 to become a doctor before deciding that the pen was mightier than the scalpel.

During this era, many Chinese thinkers came to see medical modernization along Western lines as a prerequisite for national strength, although they held different ideas as to what that modernization might look like. In the process, Yan Fu's (1854–1921) translations of Thomas Huxley's writings on social Darwinism became an important influence. By 1898, the year of the Guangxu Emperor's abortive attempts to make sweeping social, political, and economic reforms, leading thinkers such as Kang Youwei (1858–1927) and Liang Qichao (1873–1929) took it for granted that the quality of the Chinese race had to be improved if China was to survive. This eugenic rhetoric drew in part on the indigenous Chinese practice of "fetal education" *(taijiao)*, which sought to produce excellent sons in order to ensure a lineage's success. Now, however, the Chinese people were envisioned as a single, racially defined national lineage, engaged in a struggle with the white, black, brown, and red peoples of the world in which only the fittest would survive (Dikötter 1998).

Concerns about racial fitness also inspired efforts to improve the status of Chinese women and the quality of maternal and infant care. Those who saw women's health as a vehicle for female empowerment and national strengthening included Shi Meiyu (1873–1953, also known as Mary Stone), daughter of a Chinese Methodist pastor, and Kang Aide (1873–1931, also known as Ida Kahn and later in Chinese as Kang Cheng), adopted as an infant by the American missionary Gertrude Howe. They were the most famous of a small handful of Chinese women of this era who obtained medical training abroad. Both graduated from the University of Michigan medical school in 1896 and returned to China as medical missionaries. They subsequently promoted Western medicine as a way to improve the health of women and children as well as to create a corps of Chinese female medical professionals equal to men (Shemo 2011). Male intellectuals who saw Western medicine as a tool of reform notably included the Shanghainese doctor Ding Fubao (1875–1952). During the first decade of the twentieth century, Ding emerged as a leading advocate for the scientization of medicine in China, which included reforming Chinese practices as well as promoting Western medicine. Ding's numerous activities included establishing a Sino-Western Medical Research Society *(Zhong xi yixue yanjiu hui)* and an affiliated journal (Andrews 1996).

By this time, the belief that public health constituted the cornerstone of modernity and national prosperity had become a standard view in Europe and Japan. Foreign observers in China were appalled by what they saw as a total lack of governmental concern for hygiene and sanitation and by what they perceived to be the miasmatic squalor of Chinese communities. In the territorial concessions under their control, foreign leaders endeavored with various degrees of speed and efficacy to establish public health infrastructures and, where the opportunity presented itself, to extend them to the Chinese population. After suppressing Boxer forces in the treaty port city of Tianjin, for example, the eight-nation force that occupied the city made public health a priority and refused to hand the city back to the Chinese government unless it agreed to continue these policies (Rogaski 2004). Such views also resonated with the growing number of Chinese who had studied Western medicine, especially those who had been in Japan. The suppression of the Boxer uprising also shocked even the conservatives at court into implementing drastic changes, carrying out reforms to enhance the dynasty's political legitimacy.

In 1902, the empire's first municipal health bureau was created in Tianjin and given a broad remit to "protect the lives of the people" (Rogaski 2004). A few years later, the Qing created the national-level Ministry of Civil Affairs *(minzheng bu)*, which encompassed both police and public health work (Rogaski 2004; Renshaw 2005). When pneumonic plague erupted in Manchuria in 1910–1911, the court charged the Malayan-born, British-educated doctor Wu Lien-teh (Wu Liande, 1879–1960) to deploy modern epidemiological and public health measures to manage the epidemic, including autopsies and cremation of the dead. To bolster its international legitimacy, the government subsequently trumpeted Wu's apparent success in bringing the plague under control (Andrews 1996). Several months later, however, the dynasty was overthrown.

The revolution of 1911 did not create the new China that revolutionaries had hoped for. In the intellectual and political turmoil that followed, medicine continued to be an important target for reformers. Their concerns were driven by genuine admiration for advances in biomedicine as well as a conviction that only a thorough modernization of Chinese culture would save the nation. These sentiments would eventually coalesce in a movement to outlaw indigenous medicine altogether. In response, defenders of Chinese medicine argued that it was an inalienable part of China's national essence. However, their efforts to preserve this cultural patrimony in a world dominated by biomedicine would also inject new institutional and epistemological dynamics into indigenous Chinese health care practices.

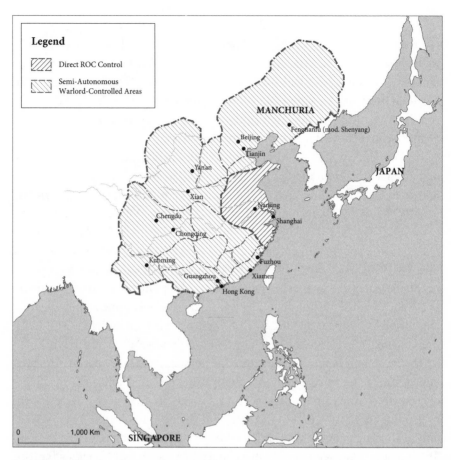

Republic of China (Nanjing Decade, 1928-1937)

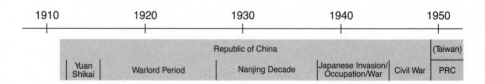

SEVEN

The Republic of China

Bridie J. Andrews

Introduction: The Spectrum of Medical Practice in the Early Twentieth Century

Medicine in China was at its most eclectic during the period of the Republic of China (1912–1949), ranging from folk healing practices to some of the most advanced biomedical facilities in the world. At the most prestigious end of the scale, the (American) Rockefeller Foundation established a state-of-the-art hospital and medical college on the premises of the former Peking Union Medical College (PUMC), originally a missionary medical school. The new PUMC, which opened in 1921, employed prominent Western physicians, was equipped with the best available technology, and trained elite Chinese students to be the future leaders of the (bio)medical profession in China (Bullock 1980).

Other institutions of Western medicine included smaller missionary-run hospitals and clinics; multidenominational "union medical colleges" that pooled missionary resources in order to provide more modern and expensive Western-style facilities; the military hospitals of the Chinese, Japanese, and Russian armies; foreign-run medical facilities in the colonial treaty ports; Chinese Customs Service quarantine stations; and a growing number of privately funded hospitals alongside a few that were run by regional and national governments. There were Western-trained physicians in private practice in major cities; there were other practitioners who claimed an education in Western medicine, but since licensing regulations were seldom enforced, they could have acquired their knowledge from books or from working as hospital porters as well as by studying in one of the many small colleges of medicine (Balme 1921; Wong and Wu 1932). Pharmacies and drugstores often employed or were

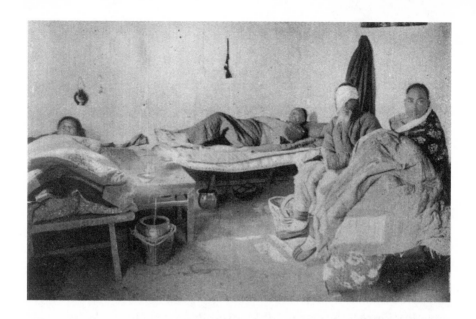

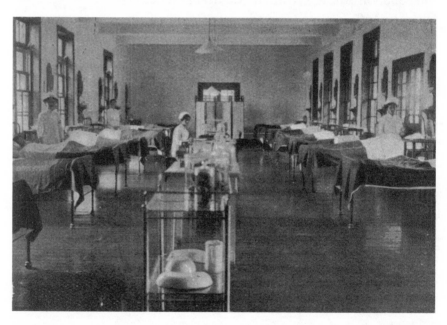

Figure 7.1. A ward in an old-style mission hospital; a ward in a modern mission hospital. Balme, *China and Modern Medicine*, 1921. Francis A. Countway Library of Medicine.

run by a medical practitioner who might prescribe Chinese-style medicines, Western-style drugs, or both.

Within what we may loosely refer to as "Chinese medicine," there were scholarly physicians who had inherited their knowledge from family members or by apprenticeships and who practiced in their own clinics or in the homes of their patients; graduates of the new colleges of Chinese medicine; specialists such as the famous Bamboo Grove monks who specialized in gynecology, martial artists who specialized in orthopedic manipulation, and those who specialized in minor surgery; acupuncturists, who were often not members of the scholarly elite and might even work as itinerant doctors; itinerant peddlers of Chinese drugs; people who gave medical advice in temples, ranging from selling prescriptions to telling fortunes to conducting prayers; massage therapists, often blind; and dentists who would pull a troublesome tooth for a fee, adding the extracted tooth to the mound that advertised their occupation.

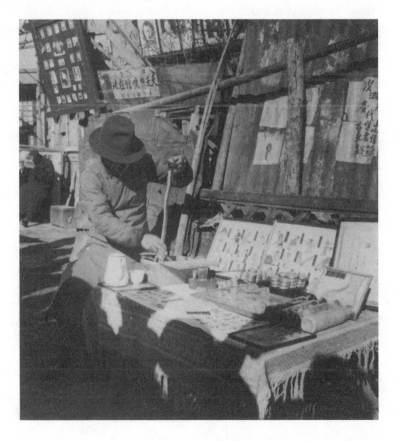

Figure 7.2. Street doctor holding a snake at his stand displaying medicines and posters picturing ailments, Beijing municipality, ca. 1933–1946. Hedda Morrison Collection, Harvard-Yenching Library. Copyright © President & Fellows of Harvard College.

In addition to these predominantly male practitioners of medicine, women healers were active as midwives; as specialists in pediatric care, especially using moxibustion and massage; and as smallpox variolation specialists. These variolators—who also included men—came to a family's home and supervised the careful preparation of an entire family's prayer and diet regimen as an important part of the dangerous ritual of infecting a child with dried, powdered smallpox scabs. Smallpox was regarded as "the gate to life or death," and it was so important to pass through the gate successfully that matchmakers insisted on seeing pox scars as a regular part of their examination of potential brides or bridegrooms. During the twenty to thirty days it took the smallpox material to incubate and the disease to run its course in what was hoped would be a mild case of this "hot" disease, the entire family kept to a vegetarian diet, thereby avoiding the heating qualities of meat. Prayers and offerings were made to the goddess of smallpox, Dou Zhen Niang Niang (and often to other deities also), at home, at altars set up for the duration of the procedure, and at Buddhist and Daoist temples. The entire household was expected to keep clean and pure, both in its physical cleanliness and avoidance of bad language, frivolity, and sex (Chang 1996a).

In the early nineteenth century, when Jennerian vaccination with cowpox was first adopted by Cantonese philanthropic societies in south China, many

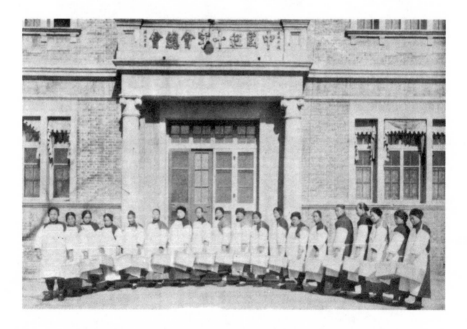

Figure 7.3. A group of traditional midwives after training in sanitary delivery methods, 1929. Training courses were designed by Dr. Marion Yang, director of the Midwifery Commission. Wong and Wu, *History of Chinese Medicine*, 1936. Francis A. Countway Library of Medicine.

of these rituals were retained. The practice of vaccination took longer to be accepted in the central and northern provinces, and in the early twentieth century, the large treaty port cities under foreign control resorted to compulsory vaccination drives whenever epidemics threatened to spread there. Although vaccination seems like a safe and necessary public health measure today, at the time it carried several risks. Early batches of vaccine, imported from Britain, France, and India, often lost their efficacy en route, and so those who were vaccinated might still catch smallpox and die from it. Even worse, in those pre-refrigeration days, some batches became contaminated with bacteria and caused blood poisoning. Lastly, because cowpox left no scars, it became impossible to tell whether a young person had survived the "gate of life and death," which caused some problems during marriage negotiations (Summers 1995).

If we consider only the elite, literate practice of medicine in the first half of the twentieth century, we find many competing currents and medical lineages. Some of the more popular included followers of the Four Famous Physicians of the Jin and Yuan Dynasties, other physicians who specialized in Warm Diseases (wenbing); and yet others who favored the prescriptions of Zhang Ji's Han Dynasty classic Treatise on Cold Damage Disorders. Other currents based themselves on a family lineage, in which knowledge was passed down from father to son or nephew and occasionally to trusted outsiders. Still others, such as the tradition centered on Menghe in Jiangsu province studied by Volker Scheid, created a medical identity based on regional origins, which could then be advertised and developed in the major urban centers, in this case Shanghai. Less literate practitioners were more likely to base their expertise on secret family knowledge, leading to further diversity in medical theories and healing practices (Scheid 2007; Sivin 1995).

Popular responses to epidemics (whether considered the results of Cold Damage or Warm Diseases) might include the collective organization of large processions in the streets to expel the "demons" causing the disease. These processions featured loud, frightening noises from drums, cymbals, and fire-crackers. Some participants wore animal costumes or bore effigies of tigers, lions, and even elephants; others dressed as the imperial officials of the celestial afterworld, bearing placards and banners inscribed with instructions such as "Drive out evil and expel pestilence," "Unite the region in peace," and "Disperse calamity and bring down blessings" (Benedict 1996; Katz 1995).

In the course of the twentieth century, and particularly under the Communist People's Republic (see Chapter 8), this cacophonous medical marketplace was eventually harmonized into a single medical system in which modern biomedicine became the model against which acceptable versions of Chinese medicine were measured. Although it was not until after 1949 that this change was completed, the period of intense state building during the Republican era forced supporters of Chinese medicine to create new standards of theory and practice that could be defended as "modern" and "scientific." Anything less risked making Chinese medicine (and, by extension, all of Chinese traditional culture) the laughingstock of the international community, which China was newly attempting to join (Lei 1999).

Public Health and the Modern State

Responsibility for public health is a function of the modern nation-state. The idea that the state should assume responsibility for providing a healthy environment for all its citizens emerged first in Britain. It grew out of the English Utilitarians' program for greater worker efficiency in the newly industrialized cities, justified with the slogan "The greatest happiness of the greatest number." This program led to the creation of a medical bureaucracy, in which each town had medical officers of health, and the further professionalizing of physicians, who contracted to maintain standards of education and conduct for the government in return for a monopoly on the right to practice (Rosen 1958; Porter 1994).

In China, although some ancient texts describe how physicians ought to be graded according to their ability to heal, in practice examinations were required only of students at the Imperial Medical Academy, which trained physicians for the emperor's household. No general system of medical licensing existed before the twentieth century. At the same time, the people's health was viewed as part of the state's responsibility, leading to the periodic compilation and distribution of state-sponsored medical texts. It led as well to a long tradition of free distribution of medicines by local magistrates—the local representatives of national government—during epidemic outbreaks. During the course of the Qing period (1644–1911), however, responsibility for donations of medical relief during epidemics (and also for famine and flood relief activities) was increasingly left to the charitable activities of the local elites, the so-called gentry (Leung 1987).

It was the events of the tumultuous decade between 1895 and 1905 that brought about the beginnings of modern state building in China, and eventually an increase in government responsibility for the health of the Chinese population. During this period, the Chinese defeat by the Japanese in the Sino-Japanese War of 1894–1895 was seen by many as the consequence of Japan's more efficient and thorough assimilation of Western military technology. China suffered not only humiliation but also territorial loss and the imposition of a large war indemnity. The foreign powers exacted a further huge indemnity after suppressing the Boxer Rebellion of 1900, during which the central Qing government also lost control of several central and southern provinces along with their tax revenue. The foreign indemnity payments exacerbated the loss, finally prompting a period of modernizing reform known as the New Policies of 1901–1909.

The new reforms included (1) the establishment of a new, Western-style army; (2) the abolition of the civil service examinations in order to encourage enrollment in a new school system that included sciences and Western language training; and (3) a commitment to establish representative assemblies as a prelude to a planned constitutional monarchy on the model of Japan's 1868 Meiji Restoration. New fiscal reforms were just as significant, with the establishment of modern banks, the promotion of industrialization, and reform of the taxation system. In general terms, the last years of imperial rule focused on the selective adoption of Western methods for achieving military strength and fiscal health, in the hope of enabling China to keep the Western and Japanese imperialists at bay. As discussed in Chapter 6, Qing use of modern quarantine and sanitary policing methods to control the 1910 outbreak of pneumonic plague in Manchuria succeeded in depriving the Russians and Japanese armies of an excuse to encroach further on Chinese territory. And, as we shall see, Dr. Wu Lien-teh, the Cambridge-educated physician who ran the plague prevention efforts, went on to organize most of the national public health initiatives for the Republican government.

In 1908, this newly modernizing Chinese state sent out the first tangible signals that Chinese medicine would also be subject to reform. The following year, Duanfang, the reform-minded Manchu governor of the Shanghai and Nanjing area, revived an old legal statute that allowed provincial authorities to examine and license medical practitioners. He decided that all doctors who hung out a sign or charged a consultation fee must pass an examination or be fined if they failed to gain a license by examination. The questions set were remarkable in that they demanded considerable knowledge of both Western and Chinese medicine. For example:

1. Describe the advantages and disadvantages of Chinese and Western pulse taking.

2. Describe the similarities and differences between Chinese and Western pharmacy.

3. Discuss the use of anaesthetic drugs in ancient times. [Clearly an invitation to discuss the legendary physician Hua Tuo's anaesthetizing powder *(mafeisan)*, composition unknown.]

4. Discuss the properties and uses of X-rays. [In its full form, this question referred to Hua Tuo's ability to see through bodies and asked for a comparison with modern X-ray technology.]

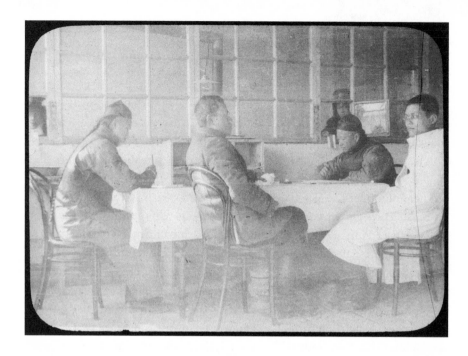

Figure 7.4. Dr. Wu Liande receiving reports at headquarters, Fuchiatien, Harbin, Heilongjiang, 1911. An ethnic Chinese, he was born in Malaysia as Gnoh Lean Tuck. At the age of thirty-one, he was appointed the first director of the Manchurian Plague Prevention Service, going on to achieve international recognition as an expert on infectious disease, the opium trade, and medical education, and receiving a nomination for the Nobel Prize in Medicine in 1935. Papers of Richard Pearson Strong. Courtesy of The Harvard Medical Library in the Francis A. Countway Library of Medicine.

5. Discuss Chinese and Western needling techniques.

6. Discuss the cause and treatment of rat-borne plague. [Again, an invitation to note that bubonic plague had been identified with a seasonal epidemic in China that was known as "rat epidemic" many years before the route of transmission via rat fleas had been elucidated in the West.]

The phrasing of these questions clearly required candidates to be familiar with large chunks of classical medical literature. They also had to be up to date with such Western medical developments as X-rays, which had only been discovered by Wilhelm Röntgen in late 1895, and serum therapy ("Western needling techniques") against infectious diseases such as diphtheria, still very much a new development in the West (Andrews 1996).

This examination is the first recorded attempt in China to enforce the medical licensing of *all* practicing physicians in any area outside of the imperial bureaucracy. It preceded the formation of the Chinese Medical Association (for doctors of biomedicine) by seven years. Not surprisingly, some influential figures in the Chinese medicine world found it distressing. He Lianchen (1861–1929), one of the founding editors of the *Shaoxing Journal of Medicine and Pharmacy (Shaoxing yiyao xuebao)*, wrote in 1908:

> The greatest pity in all this is that those [practitioners] who have diagnosed very many [patients], and whose experience is refined and profound, or whose manual skills are precise and skillful, but who are unable to express themselves in writing, will on this account fail the exams and so the government will stop them from practicing.

He Lianchen used social Darwinian terms to compare the examination to a violent struggle for existence, in which "the superior vanquish and the inferior perish," and urged his colleagues not to join the battleground of the struggle for existence. His support for unlettered practitioners and those who practiced hands-on forms of therapy such as massage and acupuncture was unusual, however. Many more elite doctors were concerned to differentiate themselves from lower-class healers, who represented competition in the medical marketplace.

Republican-Era Politics

When Sun Yat-sen's Revolutionary Alliance succeeded in forcing the abdication of the last Manchu emperor in 1911, it interrupted the late Qing process of gradually assimilating Western political and cultural forms. The new Republic of China, formed in 1912, aimed to remake China into a modern democracy. However, because North China remained under the military control of Yuan Shikai, a former Qing army general, the new regime's aims were compromised. Yuan agreed to support the Republic on the condition that he become its first president. Sun Yat-sen, the provisional president, accepted these terms to avoid war. Yuan Shikai allowed elections to be held in February 1913 (about 5 percent of the population was entitled to vote) but failed to respect the elected parliament. Instead, he had opponents dismissed and even assassinated. By 1915, he had decided to reestablish imperial China and make himself emperor. However, overwhelming opposition to this new dynasty forced Yuan to abandon the attempt three months later, and he died in June 1916.

With Yuan gone, there was no single military power able to hold the new Republic together. The years from 1916 to 1927 became known as the "warlord period," with regional commanders governing their own administrations, taxing local people on their own authority, running their own armies, and even minting their own currencies. Taxation of the largely rural population escalated under the burden of maintaining so many militia. At the same time, revenues from the government salt monopoly and from foreign customs tariffs had to be handed over to foreign powers to pay war indemnities carried over from the nineteenth century, starving the central government of tax funds. By contrast, industrialization proceeded apace in the foreign-held treaty ports (such as Shanghai, Canton, and Tianjin), leading to rapid urbanization and the formation of a small but influential urban wage-labor force.

It was in one such treaty port, Shanghai, in 1921, that the Chinese Communist Party was officially founded. Initially under orders from the Communist International or Comintern, directed from the new Soviet Union, the CCP cooperated with the Nationalist Party, the Guomindang (GMD). Sun Yat-sen, who had established a political base in southern China after Yuan Shikai's death, presided over this policy of cooperation. After Sun's death from cancer in 1925, Chiang Kai-shek emerged as the Guomindang's new leader, a position he cemented in 1926 by beginning his "Northern Expedition," an attempt to reunite the country by military force.

The Communist-led General Labor Union in Shanghai enthusiastically supported the reunification. In contrast, the expedition alarmed China's bankers and industrial capitalists, who favored national unification but not a socialist revolution. China's capitalist class turned to Chiang, funding his reunification efforts and encouraging his anti-Communist leanings. In April 1927, Chiang broke the cooperative agreement by initiating a massacre of Communists in Shanghai and going on to direct bloody suppressions in other cities. The surviving members of the CCP and the unions were forced to disband and regroup in the rural hinterlands.

In 1928, Chiang Kai-shek's Northern Expedition succeeded in taking Beijing. Although warlord control of northern China was not eradicated until the Communist revolution in 1949, Chiang garnered their cooperation enough to declare a new Nationalist government with its capital in Nanjing. The period from 1928 to 1937, when Japan invaded China, is thus known as the "Nanjing Decade." It proved to be a period of rapid state-building activity in medicine, as in many other spheres.

Creation of the New Chinese Medicine

The Republican government was much more uncritically scientistic than its Manchu predecessor and drew up a new set of regulations for the national education system. Chinese medicine received no official support, not even in the form of a nominal class in government medical schools (unlike medical training for doctors attending the imperial court, as had been the case in the late Qing).

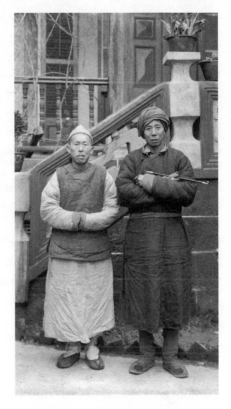

Figure 7.5. "My Chinese Collectors,"
February 15, 1911. The man to the left
was a local doctor of repute in Yichang, Hubei,
who was part of a group of about a dozen men
who assisted botanist Ernest Henry "Chinese"
Wilson (1876–1930) in collecting specimens
from 1910 to 1911. Wilson later served as the
director of the Arnold Arboretum. Photograph
by Ernest Henry Wilson, Arnold Arboretum/
Horticulture Library. President and Fellows of
Harvard College.

So in late 1913, a confederation of several regional medical associations, the All-China Medical and Pharmaceutical Association *(Shenzhou yiyaoxue zonghui)*, organized representatives of Chinese medicine associations from nineteen provinces across China. They sent a delegation to Beijing to plead for the inclusion of Chinese medicine in the national education system and for Chinese medicine schools to qualify for government licenses. This is the famous occasion on which the education minister, Wang Daxie (1860–1929), retorted, "I have decided in future to abolish Chinese medicine and also not to use Chinese drugs."

Wang had been an ambassador to Britain and Japan under the Qing and was therefore well versed in foreign ways. His remark has often been taken as the beginning of an official campaign to abolish Chinese medicine. However, in his pathbreaking study of medical polemics in China, Zhao Hongjun cites other documents describing this encounter and suggesting that, whatever Wang's personal position may have been, the government's refusal to include Chinese medicine in the national education system did not imply any intention to abolish Chinese medicine as such. In fact, the Ministry of State *(guowuyuan)* issued a statement explicitly rejecting this idea. Chinese medicine was to be left pretty much to itself (Zhao 1989).

What is clear is that the status of Chinese medicine certainly suffered from comparisons with Western medicine. During the Qing period, when the Guangxu Emperor and Dowager Empress Cixi died on the fourteenth and fifteenth of November 1908 (Western calendar), respectively, several palace physicians were sacked. A new department of Western medicine, complete with a Western pharmacy, was installed in the Imperial Medical Academy alongside its traditional counterparts. This symbolic act demoted Chinese medicine from its official monopoly position at court; the new Republic deprived Chinese medicine of any official role at all.

Many of the new, foreign-trained, urban intelligentsia of this period were openly antagonistic toward Chinese medicine, particularly during the May Fourth period, which started on May 4, 1919, and set the tenor of cultural reform for the next decade. In 1915, Chen Duxiu, chief editor of the journal *New Youth (Xin qingnian)*, the leading organ of the Chinese "New Thought Tide," wrote the first of a series of articles entitled "My Solemn Plea to Youth," in which he stated:

> Our men of learning do not understand science; thus they make use of yin-yang signs and beliefs in the five elements to confuse the world and delude the people.... Our doctors do not understand science; they not only know nothing of human anatomy, but also know nothing of the analysis of medicines; as for bacterial poisoning and infections, they have not even heard of them. (Croizier 1968, 71)

DISSECTION IN CHINA

Larissa Heinrich

It is a truism of Chinese medical history that dissection was never systematically performed in China before the twentieth century. Nineteenth-century Western medical missionaries initially blamed this lack of medical interest in dissection (and their own frustration with the impossibility of obtaining bodies to dissect) on what they characterized as Chinese "superstitions" about violating the bodies of the dead. As the missionary doctor John Kerr wrote in 1867, "The want of opportunities for dissection has been much felt, and the superstitious regard of the Chinese for the dead would seem to be an insurmountable obstacle to the prosecution of this important branch of study" (Wong and Wu 1932, 392). To circumvent these perceived cultural prohibitions,

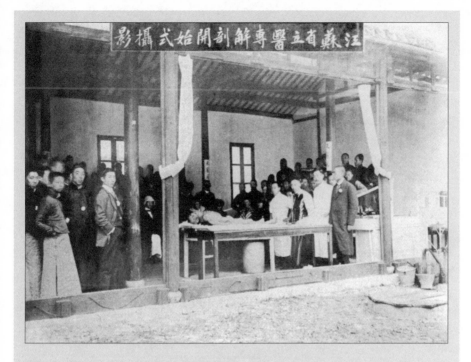

影攝式始開剖解專醫立省蘇江

Figure 7.6. The first public dissection in China occurred in a converted cafeteria at the Jiangsu Provincial Medical School on November 13, 1913. *Jiangsu Public Medical Professional College School Magazine,* 1914. Courtesy of Professor Wang Yangzong.

Western medical missionaries devised ingenious ways of introducing what they believed to be the foundational element of practical medicine: they imported anatomical specimens, dissected animals, built anatomical models, and published illustrated textbooks in Chinese outlining the principles of dissection-based anatomy.

But what many Western missionaries failed to realize was that the roots of Chinese objections to dissection in the late nineteenth century ran deeper than simple superstition. Like European opponents of dissection before them, some Chinese doctors expressed doubt that studying the dead body (with its changed postmortem physiology) would be medically relevant to the living. They also wondered what immediate therapeutic contributions dissection could make to China's rich medical traditions. Moreover, in the case of the illustrated anatomical textbooks, some Chinese doctors noted (consistent with some understandings of "race" at the time) that the bodies represented therein were not, after all, Chinese—and thus of limited use for those working with Chinese bodies. Despite such objections, views about dissection shifted along with changes in policy and rhetoric during the various reform and national advocacy movements of the late Qing period. By the first part of the twentieth century, advocates of the practice had begun to equate support for dissection with support for Chinese political and cultural reform. In some cases, the decision to donate one's body to science was even characterized as an act of selfless support for one's nation, and dissections in medical schools were performed from time to time on an ad hoc basis. After 1911, Chinese and Western advocates alike placed increasing pressure on the new administration to legalize dissection.

The first public dissection in China took place in a converted cafeteria at the Jiangsu Provincial Medical School on November 13, 1913, only eight days before dissection was made legal by presidential mandate. More than a hundred people attended the event, including a representative of the governor of Jiangsu, numerous local officials, doctors, medical students, and a handful of foreign men and women. Considering it a great coup for the advancement of medicine and for Chinese nationhood itself, the organizers made sure to commemorate China's first public dissection by posing for a group photograph. The photograph featured the distinguished guests, the doctors and students, and, of course, the corpse itself.

Faced with such criticisms, leaders of the Chinese medical community responded with attempts to make Chinese medicine appear scientific. For many, the first step was to achieve internal consistency within Chinese medicine. They edited new textbooks of Chinese medicine that obscured contradictions between different medical "classics" by just quoting short passages. This habit persists in the Chinese medical textbooks of today. Many of these reformers also saw the dependence of Chinese medical theory on Yin, Yang, and the Five Phases as a liability, since these concepts had come in for special scorn and derision from the younger generation of Western-trained intellectuals. Many of the new textbooks especially avoided referring to them. The view that Five Phase theory is incommensurable with a "scientific" formulation of Chinese medicine reappeared immediately after the Cultural Revolution of 1965–1976, when some editions of the national textbooks of Chinese medicine deliberately removed all references to it.

Disputes about Yin-Yang theory and Five Phase theory from the 1920s and 1930s are compiled in the "Philosophical Principles" (Zheli) chapter of Wang Shenxuan's Collection of New Discussions about Chinese Medicine (Zhongyi xin-lun huibian, 1932), where they are mainly reinterpreted rather than discarded. For example, the famous Shanghai physician Yun Tieqiao (1875–1935) considered the Five Phases to be metaphors for the seasons. In contrast, many modernizers—including Lu Yuanlei (1894–1955), who led the project to "scientize" Chinese medicine at the Institute of National Medicine *(Guoyi guan)*—dismissed Five Phase theory as mere superstition (Lu 1931, 1–3). The first (1978) and second (1985) editions of the higher-level basic theory text for students of pharmacy *Foundations of Chinese Medicine (Zhongyixue jichu)* differ markedly in that the first edition discusses Yin-Yang theory but not the Five Phases. In contrast, the second edition reinstates Five Phase theory in its own chapter and also as an organizing principle. (As a student of Chinese pharmacy in the late 1980s in Nanjing, I asked about this discrepancy, and was told by China Pharmaceutical University faculty, "In the 1970s, Five Phases were considered unscientific.")

Others resisted these measures strongly, arguing that they would result in Chinese medicine no longer being Chinese. Xie Guan (1880–1950), for example, accused these drastic reformers of "starting off as masters and emerging as slaves" (he meant slaves of Western culture, of course). His own strategy lay in resisting all attempts to assimilate the two medical systems, favoring instead the promotion of Chinese medicine as an elite, scholarly discipline in its own right. To this end, he edited a four-volume *Encyclopedic Dictionary of Chinese Medicine (Zhongguo yixue dacidian)*, which was published by the (Chinese-owned) Commercial Press in Shanghai in 1921. This may seem late for the publication of the first-ever dictionary of Chinese medical terms. However, viewed in the context of the time, it makes sense. The introduction of Western steam-powered printing presses made the production of books cheaper, with the Shanghai-based Commercial Press earning most of its money from the sale of reference works and textbooks for the new school system. (For instance, it also published the *Dictionary of Chinese Etymology [Ciyuan]* in 1915.)

Xie Guan deliberately excluded any Western medical terms in Chinese from his dictionary. His aim, instead, was to promote Chinese medicine as part of the nationalistic National Studies *(guoxue)* movement, in clear opposition to those who promoted Westernization *(xihua)*. His dictionary remains an important landmark in early twentieth-century Chinese attempts to standardize Chinese medicine and is regularly reprinted even today. Xie Guan used technologies of the time to create a modern reference tool that would contribute to a reevaluation of Chinese medicine as a modern—but distinctively Chinese—medical profession.

Another prominent Chinese physician and publisher directed his attention to the voluminous case literature in Chinese medicine, deciding to use the format of Western case histories to standardize these records of actual Chinese medical practice. He Lianchen (the same person who had incited people to resist the 1909 medical licensing exams) reorganized the discursive and unstandardized style of Chinese case records under the new rubrics of "patient," "ailment," "cause," "symptoms," "diagnostics" (procedure and results), "treatment method," "prescription," and, importantly, "results." He came from Shaoxing in Zhejiang province, where he was one of the founders of the Shaoxing Medical and Pharmaceutical Association. He argued that by following the example of Western medical case histories, Chinese physicians would be able to strengthen their case for Chinese government support. Far from giving ground to Western medicine, this strategy would help Chinese medicine to retain its unique character. By standardizing Chinese medicine, he believed, one could define it. Once clearly defined, it could then be effectively defended and propagated. Like Xie Guan's dictionary, this kind of innovation not only helped to create a new Chinese medicine but also tended to "fossilize" that new discipline once it had been created. This is one sense in which the new Chinese medicine represented an example of "invented tradition" (Hobsbawm and Ranger 1983).

Perhaps the most prominent figure in the reform of Chinese medicine in this period was Ding Ganren (1864–1924). Originally from the Menghe area in the lower Yangzi River basin, not far from Shanghai, Ding succeeded in synthesizing the styles of several hereditary medical families from Menghe. He propagated the resulting eclectic style as "Menghe medicine," a literate and scholarly blend that borrowed from the extensive libraries of the region's physicians. It drew from both the Cold Damage and Warm Diseases traditions, from classical Han Dynasty sources and also from post-Song traditions. It strove for refinement in the composition of precise herbal formulas.

As such, Menghe medicine was a good candidate for modernization within Chinese medicine, insofar as its relatively nonpartisan approach to traditional texts made it easy to adapt to the rhetoric of science—the use of experience in the service of empirically observed efficacy. Thus, Ding Ganren was happy to allow He Lianchen to rewrite and publish Ding's own case records in the new, standardized case history style. Ding's efforts to raise the standards of Chinese medicine focused on medical education. By establishing and teaching in a modern-style school with a defined curriculum, respected teachers, and clinical training, he too helped to create a respectable medical discipline out of the diversity of Chinese medicine (Scheid 2007).

Ding's college, the Shanghai Technical College of Chinese Medicine (Shanghai zhongyi zhuanmen xuexiao), was founded in 1915 and admitted its first students in 1917. Although the education minister in the first Republican government had refused to allow Chinese medicine into the state education system, the period between 1915 and 1927 was one of great political instability and little central control. There were, for example, about fifty different "cabinets" during this thirteen-year period. Ding Ganren and his colleagues took advantage of the political situation by appealing to a minister sympathetic to the cause of Chinese medicine (and to the cause of "national studies" and Chinese cultural values in general) to have their new college awarded a government school license. Their success raised a howl of protest from the biomedical community in China, even as theirs remained the only government-licensed school of Chinese medicine for several years. The curriculum was organized into a preparatory period of two years, followed by three years of specialist training *(benke)*. Among the subjects taught, there is the surprising appearance of a Western medical term for one of the classes—physiology *(shenglixue)*. The complete omission of any training in acupuncture is also noteworthy.

The 1920s and 1930s saw the founding of many other new schools of Chinese medicine. Their curricula often included anatomy (in the Western sense) and physiology among the compulsory subjects to be taught in the preclinical training. Some went further and taught pathology *(binglixue)* or even bacteriology *(xijunxue)*. Increasingly, these subjects were considered essential to a properly "scientific" education in any kind of medicine, Chinese or Western.

The Movement to Abolish Chinese Medicine

Such efforts were not enough for many educated Chinese, who viewed Chinese medicine as one part of the corrupt and superstitious feudal culture holding back China's modernization. Once the Republican government reestablished a national government in Nanjing in 1928, it set up China's first Ministry of Health, which was dedicated to advancing the cause of modern (Western) medicine in China. At its first national conference on public health, Yu Yunxiu (1879–1954)—a Japanese-educated doctor of Western medicine—proposed a motion to "abolish old-style medicine in order to clear away the obstacles to medicine and public health." His proposal, modeled on the medical reforms of Meiji Japan, was even more draconian. It gave Chinese medicine doctors just three years to obtain a modern medical degree or be barred from practice. Sean Hsiang-lin Lei has called this conference the occasion when "Chinese medicine encountered the state," as it was the first time the national government had considered enforcing standards on *all* practice of medicine (Lei 1999).

The First National Public Health Conference, attended almost entirely by delegates with biomedical degrees, unanimously approved the motion. Alarmed, the Chinese medical community drew on all its new social organizations—journals, societies, and schools—as well as the regular press to mobilize in opposition. A national conference of Chinese medicine was held in Shanghai starting on March 17, 1929, a date later declared National Medicine Day. Two hundred and seventy-two delegates attended, representing more than a hundred medical associations from all over China. To show their support, Shanghai pharmacies went on strike for the day, declaring that the movement to abolish Chinese medicine would deprive an entire native industry of its livelihood. It would, they argued, play into the hands of Western imperialists by making it necessary to import Western drugs in place of far cheaper Chinese herbal medicines. The primary outcome of the conference was the formation of a new national association, the National Union of Medical and Pharmaceutical Organizations, which then appointed a delegation to lobby the government directly. The five-member delegation was headed by Xie Guan, the same reformer of Chinese medicine who had edited the first dictionary of Chinese medicine in 1921 and who had helped Ding Ganren establish the first government-approved college of Chinese medicine.

Chen Cunren, the editor of the journal *Health News (Jiankang bao),* and Zhang Zanchen, editor of *Spring and Autumn of the Medical World (Yijie chunqiu),* were the moving forces behind the congress and subsequent delegation. When they reached the government offices in Nanjing, Xue Dubi, the minister of health, met them in person. Chen records that the minister looked rather embarrassed, which Chen attributed to the fierce opposition the abolition resolution had already encountered even within the government. After Xie Guan delivered the delegation's address, the minister replied: "The Ministry of Health has absolutely no intention of abolishing Chinese medicine, and as for the resolution of the national health congress, it is awaiting a decision from the Ministry's Executive Committee. Please be reassured, and convey this to your colleagues nationally, so that there will be no misunderstanding."

That evening, Xue took them for a meal of Chinese food (the table had Western place settings). He had also invited a prominent foreign geographer, Dr. Harding. Xue hinted to the delegates that it would not be helpful to criticize the abolition resolution over dinner, as it might incite the foreigner's ridicule. After dinner, Dr. Harding rose and delivered a lecture on his geographical researches in Tibet and western China. He described the origin and historical courses of Chinese rivers, illustrating his talk with slides. When he had finished, Xie Guan rose and politely filled in some of the gaps in Dr. Harding's knowledge, citing Chinese maps and sources as he went. He specifically repudiated a prior claim for the discovery of the Jiangchuan River's source, showing that it had been recorded in a particular Qing Dynasty work. Harding was surprised and impressed by this display of knowledge and replied that he had as yet met few Chinese who knew much of the geography of China, and none so well informed as Xie Guan. According to Chen Cunren's account, this praise from the foreign guest cheered and relieved Xue, whose attitude toward the Chinese medicine delegates improved markedly (Zhang 1954, 56–60).

This anecdote reveals much about the value of Xie Guan's involvement in the struggle to reestablish Chinese medicine as a high-status occupation. The minister of health wanted to present China as a modernizing world power at a time when the most influential Chinese were those returning from overseas study, preferably with foreign qualifications. The continued existence of Chinese medicine could prove to be a source of potential embarrassment to these people in their dealings with Westerners. Xie Guan, by contrast, represented the best of the native tradition of scholarship and was even able to employ his home-grown expertise to correct foreigners' rather arrogant assumptions that their findings were completely new.

Xie Guan continued to be prominent in the ongoing struggle to develop Chinese medical education, despite strong opposition from the Westernizing faction in government. The latter persistently opposed including Chinese medicine in any government-sanctioned activity on the grounds that it was unscientific and an obstacle to national progress. Yet Xie was consistently elected to the executive committees (sometimes as chair) of the national organizations that spearheaded the opposition. By the time of his death in 1950, the Shanghai Municipal Sanitary Bureau had carried out licensing examinations for Chinese medicine physicians eleven times. Each time, Xie had served on the examination committee.

Neurasthenia (shenjing shuairuo) in China

Hugh Shapiro

In the history of the body in twentieth-century China, there may be no malady more intriguing than neurasthenia *(shenjing shuairuo)*. Neurasthenia, or nervous weakness, has flourished in China as nowhere else in the world. The contemporary prevalence of neurasthenia is all the more striking when compared with its total absence from the past. Before modern times, the idea of nerves did not exist in the medicine of China. In Europe and America, by contrast, the history of nerves dates to the third century B.C.E. (Staden 1989; Kuriyama 1999). In 1869, the American electrotherapist George Beard posited that the stresses of urban life, the intensity of industrialized existence, and the viciousness of the marketplace conspired to overburden the body's economy, sapping its vital power and depleting its nervous energy (Beard 1869). By 1890, neurasthenia defined Gilded Age American identity. "American nervousness" suggested that modernity itself was pathogenic, that neurasthenia afflicted the modern person (Beard 1881). The more developed a country, the argument went, the higher its rates of *shenjing shuairuo*.

In China the idea is quite new. An instructional poster from 1933, "The Nervous System" *(Shenjing xitong)*, aims to popularize the imported perspectives of foreign medicine, such as the brain's division into compartmentalized faculties.

This new vision of the body shaped new ways of experiencing distress. And once the new ideas of nerves and nervousness did take root, it would seem as though they had always been there. So from this perspective, the spread of neurasthenia to China from the United States, England, France, Germany, Russia, and Japan could be seen as a corollary to the spread of modernity to China.

However, when the concept of neurasthenia first appeared in China in the 1910s, self-consciousness about national development magnified its popular image not only as a modern disease but also a disease of modern people. Over the course of the century, it became the most common diagnosis for psychiatric outpatients. As Arthur Kleinman's pioneering work shows, it is not merely a technical term used by psychiatry and neurology; outside of clinical settings, *shenjing shuairuo* became a routine idiom of suffering, widely used in self-diagnosis (Kleinman 1986). In daily life, neurasthenia is blamed for insomnia, memory lapses, dizziness, anxiety, or anger (Kleinman 1995). Indeed, despite its foreign origins, neurasthenia has thrived in China long after the category was abandoned in the countries of its origin and first popularity.

On the surface, then, *shenjing shuairuo* looks like a classic case of the dissemination of Western medical knowledge into popular Chinese consciousness. But unlike in Europe and the United States, where the concept was abandoned in the 1920s, the idea of neurasthenia in China resisted efforts by academic psychiatry to discredit it, down to the late twentieth century (Lee 1999; Lee and Kleinman 2007). Today, however, in China's major cities and leading medical centers, the term *shenjing shuairuo* has entirely dropped out of medical discourse, and educated youth in such places as Shanghai and Beijing find the term "neurasthenia" alien and puzzling (Phillips et al. 2009; Lee 2011; Kleinman et al. 2011). Yet the idea lingers on, appearing in self-help manuals and often tied to insomnia. Some clinicians still publish articles on the condition.

How are we to understand the extraordinary popularity of neurasthenia and *shenjing shuairuo*'s remarkable longevity in twentieth-century China? China and the West share intuitions regarding corporeal and emotional depletion. The constellation of ideas that emerged as neurasthenia in nineteenth-century America, fin-de-siècle Europe, and Japan of the late Meiji, Taisho, and early Showa eras grew from deeply rooted notions about sexuality, depletion, and vital energy. Sources for the prevalence of *shenjing shuairuo* in China, too, emerged from similar ideas regarding the body's vital forces. Neurasthenia in China, then, might have less to do with the modernity that gave birth to this particular category of distress and more to do with underlying intuitions regarding how the body works.

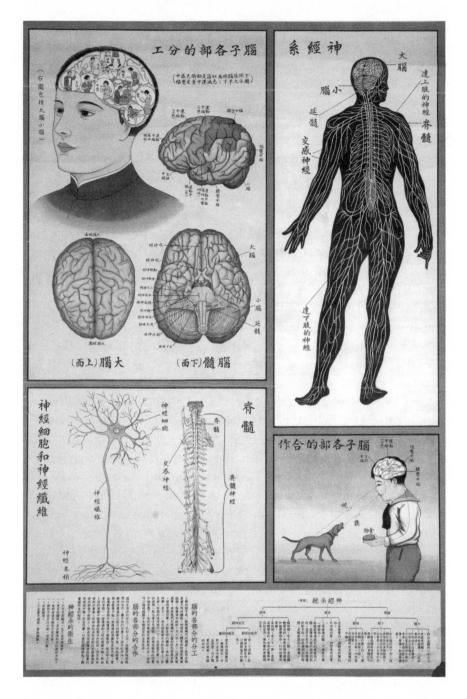

Figure 7.7. Chinese public health poster: "The Nervous System" *(Shenjing xitong)*, 1933. The poster consists of four images of the anatomy of the nervous system, including the brain, spinal cord, and peripheral nervous system. The very bottom part of the poster has texts explaining the nervous system and function of the brain. Courtesy of the National Library of Medicine.

Formation of the Institute of National Medicine

One of the more successful defensive moves made by Chinese medicine physicians during the scientistic years of the 1910s and 1920s was to ally Chinese medicine with the National Studies movement. Widely perceived as conservative, even reactionary, the National Studies movement maintained that Chinese culture was vital to China's continued existence in the modern world. To this end, even modern education should insist on a substantial component of national studies, including classical language and literature, music, art, and Chinese medicine. In reality, most National Studies enthusiasts were also modernizers and agreed that there was a need for a modern school system and the creation of a national vernacular language. They favored comparative folklore studies and shared similar attitudes with Westernizers as to the relative merits of "high" and "low" culture. Medicine posed a problem, however: should "national medicine" be preserved merely because its formulas and remedies encapsulated the wisdom and therapeutic experiences of generations of healers, or should it be regarded as an indigenous healing "science"? Opinions varied along this spectrum, as became painfully obvious in disputes arising over the work of the National Medicine Institute, formed in 1931.

The Chinese medical community was initially jubilant when the Republican government finally legitimized Chinese medicine by establishing the state-financed Institute of National Medicine only two years after the failed initiative to ban Chinese medical practice. However, the function of the institute was to "scientize" and "rectify" Chinese medicine. What exactly would this involve? Some took it to mean that Chinese medicine could be validated only by defending classical theories such as Yin-Yang and the Five Phases and giving them scientific interpretations. Others, such as Lu Yuanlei (1894–1955), one of the first members of the Institute of National Medicine, viewed classics such as the *Inner Canon of the Yellow Emperor* as so much "philosophical speculation." He turned instead to the relatively empirical style of Zhang Ji's *Treatise on Cold Damage Disorders* as a repository of effective therapies that could be investigated scientifically.

Indeed, since the 1880s Japanese scientists had tested many of the drugs listed in the *Treatise on Cold Damage Disorders* for pharmacologically active chemicals. To many in the Western medical profession, this reduction of Chinese medical culture to a potential repository of the raw materials for new Western-style drugs was the only acceptable use for Chinese medicine. This was the position, for example, of Yu Yunxiu, the Japanese-educated physician who had first proposed abolishing Chinese medical practice altogether. Therefore, many supporters of Chinese found it offensive that members of the Institute of National Medicine were effectively promoting the same attitude.

Key to the argument about how to make Chinese medicine acceptable was the concept of experience *(jingyan),* understood particularly as clinical experience. Originally deployed by figures such as Yu Yunxiu, who favored abolishing Chinese medicine, such experience was seen as the only thing of worth in the classical medical literature. It could provide a shortcut to new pharmacologically active (Western-style) drugs that would first be analyzed and then tested clinically before being introduced into modern pharmacopoeias. Faced with a culture in which science was the arbiter of truth, doctors of Chinese medicine clearly could not object to scientific investigations of their medicine. Experience, however, was more than just accumulated clinical observations of the effects of different drugs and formulas. Rather, they argued—following Japanese author and practitioner of Sino-Japanese *(huanghan)* medicine Yumoto Kyushin—that experience included the body and its responses as well as the actions of drugs and formulas. Moreover, the experience of the body and *its* experience of the actions of different treatments could not be neatly separated. In this sense, experience was embodied in the practitioner. It might be separable from theories such as Yin-Yang and the Five Phases, but one could not subtract it from personal interaction. Doctors of Chinese medicine argued that this connection differed from Western medicine's use of laboratory animals to accumulate a disembodied version of experience.

The downside of this argument, as Yu Yunxiu was quick to point out, was that Chinese medicine appeared to be saying that humans were—or at least had been—its laboratory specimens. If the key to effective practice lay in embodied experience, how was Chinese medicine to be taught and transmitted in schools and colleges (Lei 2002)? To some degree, these debates remain with us. For many decades scientism prevailed, promoting the view that scientific explanations of phenomena trump explanations provided by philosophy, religion, or the humanistic disciplines. More recently, opinion in biomedicine has started to swing back toward accepting the role of embodied experience in healing, as many recent studies of placebo effects and the importance of positive patient-healer interactions suggest (Harrington 1999; Kradin 2008). Healers in Republican China might have been familiar with such effects, but the terms of the debate were dictated by what could be represented as scientific.

Advertising Hygienic Modernity

Ruth Rogaski

This 1937 newspaper advertisement shows a young woman demurely bathing in a modern, Western-style bathtub, her slippers on the tiled floor, a curtain only partially shading her naked form. Beneath her, an anthropomorphized bottle of Lysol routs three little horned "devils," representing the germs of contagious disease. The ad encourages the reader to add a few drops to her daily bath, to exterminate *(shamie)* disease-causing bacteria on the skin. According to the ad, Lysol's disinfecting power even penetrated the body's orifices to attack germs, including odor-causing bacteria lurking within the vaginal canal. Lysol promised to be an "excellent companion for women's personal hygiene" *(funü geren weisheng)*.

Lysol-as-douche advertisements were also common in the United States during the first half of the twentieth century (Tone 2001), but the content and context of the Chinese advertisement differed significantly. Faced with the threat of foreign invasion and civil war, China turned to hygiene *(weisheng)* as a central theme in the nation's quest for political autonomy. Even as individual women were encouraged to perform disinfection to achieve a hygienically modern lifestyle, China as a country struggled to adopt techniques of *weisheng* to ensure its survival in the modern world.

China had long possessed its own techniques for individual health preservation (Harper 1998; Lo 2001b), such as ingesting certain foods for their healthful effects, performing various forms of exercise, observing behavioral and dietary taboos, and meditating. Known collectively as *yangsheng* (nurturing life) or sometimes *weisheng* (guarding life), this hygiene drew from the Yin-Yang cosmology of learned medicine, bodily disciplines related to Buddhism and Daoism, and popular knowledge about the body and the environment. It placed responsibility for health with the individual, rather than social groups or the state.

In contrast, the new hygiene drew on the laboratory sciences of physiology and bacteriology and the recent revolutionary growth in the scope of governments in Great Britain, France, and Germany. It applied not only to the individual body but also to groups, cities, and even the nation, requiring governments to measure, monitor, and control the health of their populations, and especially to contain contagious disease. In the eyes of imperial powers such as Great Britain, Japan, and the United States, the ability to stop the spread of germs was the measure of a nation, making the ability to avoid germs the measure of a people. If a national government proved incapable of stopping epidemics, it could lose its sovereignty, leading imperial powers to step in and enforce control (Andrews 1996).

This *weisheng* required tactics such as house-to-house inspection, quarantine, and vaccinations—highly invasive measures alien to Chinese ideas of governance during the imperial period. While many Chinese embraced this new orientation, some saw the obsession with germs as part of a foreign plot to depose Chinese medicine and weaken the Chinese nation. As one Chinese physician writing in 1934 put it, "Western medicine is drunk and has fallen into a vat of germs; it swims in a veritable world of germs . . . and now it dares to invade this land of the Yellow Emperor?" (Rogaski 2004, 249).

Ironically, this advertisement depicting one woman's personal fight against "devilish" germs was published only days after the beginning of Japan's invasion of China on July 7, 1937. Indeed, during the war, the Imperial Japanese Army's Epidemic Con-

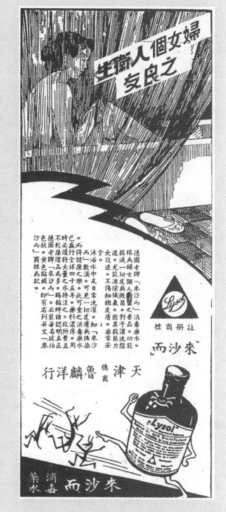

Figure 7.8. "An Excellent Companion for Women's Personal Hygiene." Advertisement for Lysol. *Da gong bao* (L'Impartial), Tianjin, July 26, 1937. Courtesy of Ruth Rogaski.

trol Unit, otherwise known as Unit 731, would use germ warfare against Chinese troops and civilians. This juxtaposition of Lysol and war illustrates how, under the rubric of *weisheng*, new ideas of health and hygiene reflected one aspect of China's complex experience of modernity in the twentieth century.

The Reinvention of Acupuncture

When Westerners say "Chinese medicine," acupuncture comes to mind. Yet even when the Chinese Nationalist government first published national regulations to govern the licensing of doctors of Chinese medicine in 1936, it left acupuncture out of the subjects required for qualification. This omission by those who wanted to make Chinese medicine into a respectable, secular modern discipline was deliberate. While the practice of acupuncture is as old as Chinese medicine itself, by the late Qing Dynasty it had become an artisan-class activity. Moreover, the practice of acupuncture did not consist simply of needling with the fine needles we know today. Rather, acupuncture "needles" came in several shapes and sizes, from bodkins to straight and curved scalpels. Indeed, Chinese illustrations of the "nine needles" indicate that late imperial acupuncture was actually a kind of minor surgery. As such, it was associated with street tradesmen and itinerants rather than with the literate elite. In 1822, the teaching and practice of acupuncture and moxibustion had even been banned from the Imperial Medical Academy. By the early 1930s, several authors complained that the classics of medicine were either vague or mutually contradictory about the exact positions of the acupuncture points.

Cheng Dan'an (1899–1957) brought Western anatomy to the rescue. In his pathbreaking book *Chinese Acupuncture and Moxibustion Therapeutics (Zhongguo zhenjiu zhiliao xue)*, first published in 1931, Cheng noted that acupuncture and moxibustion had virtually disappeared from China. He proposed to revive them. His formula for revival had much in common with earlier Japanese reforms of acupuncture, including the use of Western anatomy to redefine acupuncture points. In 1934, three years after the first publication of his book, Cheng visited Japan, spending a year learning Japanese and attending the Tokyo College of Acupuncture. Drawing on Western anatomy and physiology to create a new understanding of how acupuncture worked, he concluded that the acupuncture tracts or meridians constituted a functional system that encompassed the nerves, blood vessels, and lymph glands of Western medicine. His preface explains:

> The pathways of acupuncture points recorded by our forebears are mostly lacking in detail. There is even less recorded about the contents of the acupuncture pathways. This book employs scientific methods to correct this. Each acupoint must be elucidated anatomically. . . . In manipulating acupoints, although our forebears needled into arteries, this was still nee-

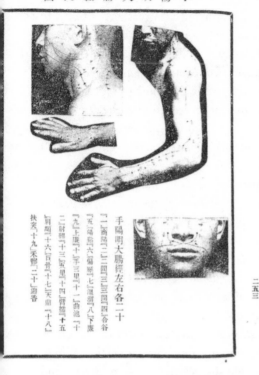
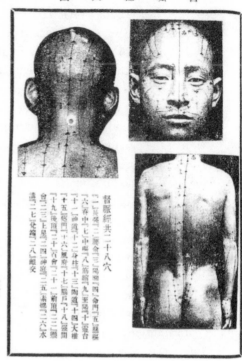

Figure 7.9. A remapping of acupuncture points and channels in 1932 by Cheng Dan'an. Cheng, *Revised Acupuncture Therapeutics*, 1932. Courtesy of Bridie J. Andrews.

dling the nerves of that area, and certainly not [primarily] rupturing the artery.... However, when they did needle them (arteries) the objective was [to reach] the nerves at that spot. (Cheng 1932)

Cheng did not reinvent the acupuncture points at will, however. He started with the ones described in the Song dynasty court-produced *Illustrated Canon of Loci for Acupuncture and Moxibustion for Use with the Bronze Instructional Statues*, which had been republished in a high-quality edition in 1909. Wang Weiyi was a court medical official who wrote his book with much the same agenda as Cheng Dan'an had—to compile a definitive guide to the correct position of the acupoints as a result of the prevailing profusion of alternatives. (See Figure 4.2.)

Cheng depicted his redefined acupuncture "pathways" using photographs of human subjects with the acupuncture tracts marked on the skin. This photographic representation echoed the trend toward realistic photographic illustrations in contemporary textbooks of biomedicine and was much praised by the book's reviewers. Cheng says that he used Western anatomy to ensure that no points were placed near major blood vessels. Yet this approach marks a major shift in acupuncture theory and practice. Before Cheng Dan'an, acupuncture had frequently been used to let small amounts of blood, in order to clear a perceived obstruction to the free flow of blood and *qi*. However, after Cheng argued that acupuncture acted through the nerves, the drawing of blood at an acupuncture point started to be viewed as an indication of the practitioner's clumsiness and lack of experience—a view that still often persists.

The demand for Cheng's new, scientific acupuncture was so great that a revised edition of *Chinese Acupuncture and Moxibustion Therapeutics* appeared only a year after the appearance of the first. The new edition of 1932 was honored by congratulatory inscriptions from twenty-two prominent Chinese physicians, and included laudatory prefaces from another eleven. By May 1937, the book had gone into its eighth edition. Prominent mainland Chinese medical historians describe it as "the most influential work on acupuncture of the last hundred years" (Zhen and Fu 1991, 453).

In addition to employing Western anatomy to create a "scientific" acupuncture, Cheng rejected the idea of strictly timing acupuncture treatments according to astrological and divinatory formulas. He also rejected divisions of days and parts of days into Yin and Yang. He condemned as a remnant of past superstition the idea that men should be treated on their left side and women on their right.

In practical terms, Cheng recommended that moxibustion not be used to cauterize the skin, as it led to ugly and traumatic scars. A prevailing idea that acupuncture and moxa should not be used at the same spot seemed, to Cheng, a product of using thick, coarse acupuncture needles, which caused such damage to the skin that combining them with moxa cautery was likely to leave a considerable wound. If moxa were not allowed to burn the skin and only filiform needles were used, the two treatments could be combined to great effect. Such revisions heralded major changes in the practice of acupuncture that have survived to the present day. Virtually all acupuncture is now carried out with filiform metal needles of varying lengths. The minor surgery or boil lancing with small scalpels and crude bodkins that were once part of the acupuncturist's stock in trade have largely disappeared.

There is no doubt that Cheng was hugely successful in his attempts to make acupuncture "scientific." In the Chinese historical literature on acupuncture, his activities are by far more widely reported than those of any other acupuncture specialist of the Republican period. Indeed, he seems to have been the moving force behind the rehabilitation of acupuncture into elite, learned Chinese medicine. In addition to founding China's first acupuncture correspondence college in Wuxi in 1930 and to setting up a network of affiliated acupuncture research societies from the same date, he also founded the first acupuncture journal, *Journal of Acupuncture (Zhenjiu zazhi)*, in 1933. In earlier chapters we have encountered the names of some of the people he recruited to direct the teaching of the research society: Jiao Yitang, first director of the Institute of National Medicine; Xie Guan, editor of the *Encyclopedic Dictionary of Chinese Medicine;* and Zhang Zanchen, Xie's student and one of the leaders of the antiabolition campaign. By 1935, the society had at least fourteen branches in ten different provinces as well as in Hong Kong and Singapore. By 1937, Cheng's school in Wuxi was running two different courses—a research course, consisting of 150 hours a month of study and teaching for a year, and a specialist course, consisting of 175 hours a month for two years. That same year the school built a library and obtained a government license to teach as the China Technical College of Acupuncture *(Zhongguo zhenjiu zhuanmen xuexiao).*

In 1938, as a result of the Japanese invasion of China, Cheng fled Wuxi for Chongqing. On his return in 1947 he found his school destroyed. After the Communist revolution in 1949, he reestablished the China Acupuncture Research Society and recommenced his publishing activities. In 1954, he chaired the Jiangsu Provincial Congress of Chinese Medicine, and was also elected to the Provincial People's Congress. In November 1954 he was made director of the school that was soon to become the Jiangsu College of Chinese Medicine. In 1955 he was made a member of the Chinese Academy of Sciences and elected vice chairman of the Chinese Medical Association. He died in 1957. The society he founded is still active today.

It should be noted that Cheng Dan'an's work was not without its critics: other revisions and explanations of acupuncture were proposed (Taylor 2005). However, he was the first to successfully superimpose a Chinese medical physiology upon an unambiguously Western anatomy. This composite body is represented most clearly in the modern-day equivalents of Wang Weiyi's bronze figures. Nowadays, leading schools of acupuncture in China, and particularly those that run courses for foreigners, have life-sized models of the human body made of transparent plastic, so that the internal organs are visible on the inside. The acupuncture points and the paths of the tracts are then also clearly visible, even where they are conceived as lying beneath the surface of the skin. Just like the first translations of Dutch anatomical texts into Japanese, these models do not show the musculature, which in Chinese medicine is of little theoretical importance.

It is nicely ironic that the specialty of acupuncture—arguably the most questionable part of their medical heritage for most Chinese at the start of the twentieth century—has become the most marketable aspect of Chinese medicine. Indeed, for many people, acupuncture *is* Chinese medicine. Yet acupuncture as we know it today has hardly been in existence for sixty years. Moreover, the fine, filiform needle we think of as *the* acupuncture needle hardly featured in the repertoire of those itinerant acupuncture specialists who operated at the start of the twentieth century.

EIGHT

The People's Republic of China

Volker Scheid

Communist victory in the Civil War of 1945–1949 and the proclamation of the People's Republic in October 1949 did not augur well for the future of Chinese medicine as an independent medical tradition. Under the slogan "cooperation of Chinese and Western medicine" *(zhongxiyi hezuo)*, the Chinese Communist Party (CCP) in Yan'an had utilized Chinese medicine to gain the support of the rural population and to meet health care needs in settings where Western drugs and technological resources were scarce. Ideologically, however, the party's leadership was committed to establishing a health care system modeled on that of the West, in particular the Soviet Union, in which there was little room for a medicine considered to be a remnant of feudal society and its irrational superstitions. In Nationalist-controlled areas, meanwhile, the Chinese medical infrastructure created during the 1920s and 1930s had been all but dismantled (Deng 1999, 176–191). Yet less than ten years later a large-scale effort was underway to rebuild Chinese medicine as a modern tradition that would make a unique contribution to the health care of China and even the world. On October 11, 1958, Mao Zedong famously declared Chinese medicine to be "a great treasure house" and demanded that its resources be forcefully developed. Another quarter of a century later, in 1982, the principle of "paying equal attention to Chinese and Western medicine" was enshrined in the constitution. Ever since, the country has enjoyed the fruits and problems of an officially plural health care system. (For foundational accounts of Chinese medicine in contemporary China, see Cai et al. 1999; Meng 1999; Taylor 2005; Wang and Cai 1999; Zhang 1994; and Zhen and Fu 1991.)

The process that led to the creation of this system was neither linear nor the outcome of a well-thought-out master plan. Rather, it was "the product of an

239

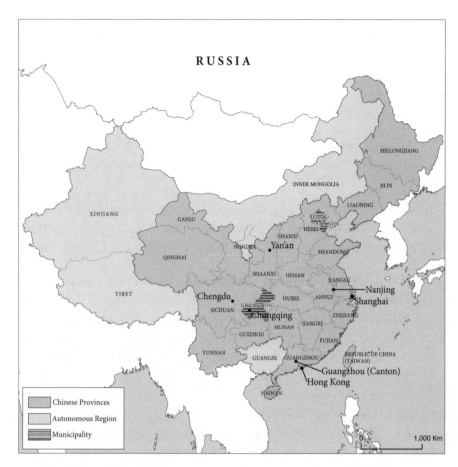

RUSSIA

HEILONGJIANG

INNER MONGOLIA

JILIN

LIAONING

XINJIANG

GANSU

BEIJING

TIANJIN

HEBEI

SHANXI

NINGXIA   Yan'an

SHANDONG

QINGHAI

SHAANXI   HENAN

JIANGSU

TIBET

Chengdu

HUBEI   ANHUI   Nanjing

Shanghai

SICHUAN   CHONGQING

Chongqing

ZHEJIANG

JIANGXI

HUNAN

GUIZHOU

FUJIAN

YUNNAN

GUANGXI   GUANGZHOU

REPUBLIC OF CHINA
(TAIWAN)

Guangzhou (Canton)

Hong Kong

HAINAN

Chinese Provinces

Autonomous Region

Municipality

0   1,000 Km

People's Republic of China

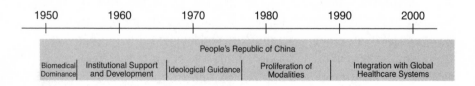

1950	1960	1970	1980	1990	2000

People's Republic of China

Biomedical Dominance	Institutional Support and Development	Ideological Guidance	Proliferation of Modalities	Integration with Global Healthcare Systems

undetermined and piecemeal process" that owed more to "a careful manipulation of [Chinese medicine's] value as a 'cultural legacy'" than to "any consideration of its actual therapeutic value" (Taylor 2004, 151). The emergence of plural health care in contemporary China thus might be said to mirror the tortuous, painful, and frequently contradictory path the country itself has taken into the present: from early dreams of fashioning a revolutionary "new medicine" blending Western modernity with essences distilled from distinct Chinese experiences to current efforts at inserting a commoditized Chinese medicine into the technocultural networks spanning global markets. For this reason alone, narrating the history of Chinese medicine in contemporary China is best accomplished by linking that history to that of the wider body politic of the country.

This narrative can be divided into five periods, although no fixed boundaries exist between them: (1) the period from 1949 to 1953, which was characterized by attempts to subsume Chinese medicine into a biomedically dominated health care system; (2) the period from 1954 to 1965, during which the CCP, under the direction of Mao Zedong, switched to a policy of supporting the development of Chinese medicine and its institutional infrastructure; (3) the period from 1966 to 1977, which includes the Cultural Revolution, when activity in the field of Chinese medicine contracted under the guidance of ideological simplification; (4) the immediate post-Maoist era, which lasted from Mao Zedong's death on September 9, 1976, to the Tiananmen Massacre in 1989, spanning the feverish decade of the 1980s, when the field of Chinese medicine (among others) exploded once more into a myriad of options and possibilities; and (5) the period from 1989 to the present, during which Chinese medicine has been guided toward integration into the technoscientific networks of a global health care system.

As shown in Chapter 7, the biomedical body and ideologies of science had become inescapable points of reference for Chinese medicine during the Republican era (Andrews 1996; Karchmer 2004; Lei 1999). Yet, inasmuch as the political drive in Maoist and post-Maoist China has been to fashion modernity with distinctly Chinese characteristics, a medicine defining itself as essentially "Chinese" has also been allocated an institutional space into which it could retreat in order to survive. In this sense, each of the five periods discussed in this chapter outlines different solutions to the challenge that has confronted Chinese medicine physicians and their supporters throughout the twentieth century: how to reconfigure tradition in relation to the modern, and how to be Chinese in relation to the world.

The twentieth century, and in particular China after 1949, thus saw Chinese medicine involved in entirely new struggles for legitimation. While in late imperial China the status of scholar-physicians as members of the elite had never been entirely secure, they at least shared with that elite the same cultural outlook and sensibilities, as well as an understanding about how their medicine might achieve its effects. Magical, ritual, and religious healing practices represented ever-present alternative pathways in the personal quest for health, including that of physicians themselves. They did not, however, present a real challenge to the cosmological foundations of a common culture, of which medicine was a long-standing part. Science and Western claims to embody an alternative and even more evolved universal culture changed all that. Yet it would be too simplistic to see the history of Chinese medicine in contemporary China as merely an effort to survive this assault. It was that, but it was simultaneously much more besides.

Viewed against the development of Chinese medicine over a longer period, modernization after 1949 did not merely continue trends set in motion during the Republican era. Rather, it also offered a chance to find solutions to problems endemic to the tradition. For example, how to safeguard a medical orthodoxy that would support the identity of the system as a whole and, by implication, access to status and power within that system. At the same time, it would have to grant individual practitioners the necessary freedom to adjust practice to local contexts. This combination of orthodoxy and freedom would make it effective as both a medicine and a tradition. From this perspective, the most noteworthy feature on which to focus in narrating Chinese medicine's development in contemporary China is not its ongoing encounter with the West but rather the fact that, for the first time since the Song, the state now assumed direct and deliberate responsibility for regulating the field of medicine. In so doing, it fundamentally transformed the alignment of all other agents on this field, as well as curtailing the degree of latitude available to them.

1949–1953

When Mao Zedong proclaimed the establishment of the People's Republic on October 1, 1949, he did so as a figurehead of a movement able to project its will and its dreams onto the entire country. From this position of strength the CCP set out to deliberately shape both the overall structure of the health care system and the roles and relations of its individual components. In practice, these efforts were oriented by "four great guiding principles" formulated during the First and Second National Health Conferences in 1950 and 1951: (1) medicine had to serve the working people; (2) preventive medicine programs were to be given priority over curative ones; (3) Chinese medicine was to be united with Western medicine; and (4) health programs were to be integrated with mass movements (Cai et al. 1999, 6). How these principles were to be translated into practice was not specified, however. As a consequence, concrete policies were shaped by complex power struggles among political factions in the CCP and the Ministry of Health over such translations. Broadly speaking, while the Ministry of Health was dominated by biomedical physicians who favored modernization along Western—specifically Soviet—models of professional health care, the CCP under the leadership of Mao Zedong favored prevention, mass campaigns, and the subordination of professional knowledge to revolutionary ideals (Lampton 1977; Taylor 2005).

PROPAGANDA AND HEALTH

Stefan R. Landsberger

The Communist Party's experiences with mass movements in Yan'an before 1949 generated useful tools for mobilizing change that spanned politics, production drives, and literacy campaigns (Cell 1977, 44–46). To rouse the masses to action, the party deployed a broad arsenal of media and methods—both indigenous and inspired by Soviet practice, and including newspapers, handbills and leaflets, songs and poems, skits, and slogans. Campaigns made wide use of the propaganda poster, a tool imported from the Soviet Union. Initially painted on city walls, village houses, or huge cloth banners, these images were later distributed through work units and bookstores. Soldiers, workers, and local people excelling in production or other commendable behaviors served as the models, which others were to emulate.

Posters explained abstract ideological principles to a largely illiterate population, providing the knowledge and expertise needed to achieve political goals, production quotas, or other results. They illustrated, for example, the specific behaviors being promoted, or the types of slogan required over the course of an unfolding movement. Yet posters never played a freestanding role. Instead, they visually complemented and reinforced messages conveyed through print or broadcast media. In this supporting role, they helped interpret, organize, and confirm developments taking place (Lupher 1995, 324).

Once the party took control over all of China, it loosed mass campaigns on a regular basis well into the 1980s. This "flow of campaigns," organized at both national and local levels and in rural and urban areas, addressed national, international, moral, and social topics. It was intended to strengthen support for the party, deepen understanding of its ideology, and promote economic production. Education campaigns related to health increased after 1949, often as hygiene movements, reflecting the central leadership's philosophy that both hygiene and physical fitness were part of the modernization agenda. Physical preparedness and well-being were construed as essential to a revolutionary China that would no longer accept being bullied by others.

The first Patriotic Hygiene Campaign occurred in 1952 and was linked directly to the Korean War. It highlighted prophylactic inoculation drives to reduce the potential effects of alleged U.S. bacteriological warfare. At the same time, it provided detailed information about crop contamination and other health threats caused by disease-spreading insects. While this and later movements were less confrontational than campaigns against evil feudal landlords and enemies of the state, their more general aims and methods were more difficult to convey. The task of these campaigns was to combat what the party viewed as centuries-old ways of thinking about cleanliness and hygienic behavior. The party, for example, targeted spitting in the street for eradication (Rogaski 2002; Yang 2004, 172).

To convey images realistically, poster artists employed simple forms and lines, flat colors, and a sparing use of black (Hung 1994, 263–266). The design depended on the campaign aims. Inoculation drives, for example, used bold designs with a clear, single message. Hygiene education called for a more detailed and overtly instructional approach involving the detailed depiction of pests and their detrimental effects. Both types served a pedagogical function; it is unlikely that these posters found their way into private homes for purely decorative purposes.

The government organized one of the most spectacular campaigns in the late spring of 1958, aimed at eliminating the "Four Pests": flies and mosquitoes as carriers of disease, and rats and sparrows as destroyers of grain. Previously, rats had been singled out as potential carriers of purported American bacteriological warfare; this time the party mobilized the people to eliminate them altogether (Rogaski 2002, 393–394, 408). The large scale of the movement is often seen as an overture to the subsequent Great Leap Forward (1958–1960).

Enterprises, government agencies, and schools held pest-eradication contests, giving nonmaterial rewards to those who handed in the most rat tails, dead flies, mosquitoes, or sparrows. The movement became something of a sport, with particular appeal to children. Eyewitnesses recalled how, as youngsters, they would bang pots and pans so that sparrows could not rest on tree branches and would fall from the sky, dead from exhaustion (MacFarquhar 1983, 21–24). However, the campaign became a disaster, as the leadership realized too late that destroying pests actually upset the ecological balance. Eliminating sparrows, for example, gave worms and other crop-threatening insects free play.

Figure 8.1. Health-related posters.

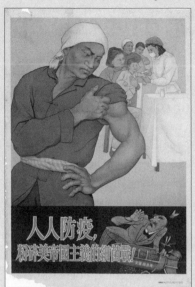

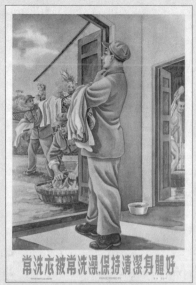

Poster 1. Ye Shanlu, *Renren fangyi, fensui Mei diguo zhuyide xijunzhan!* [Everybody must take precautions against epidemics to smash the germ warfare of American imperialism!] Renmin meishu chubanshe, June 1952, print no. 0421. Courtesy of IISH Stefan R. Landsberger Collection.

Poster 2. Zhang Danian, *Chang xi yi bei chang xizao, baochi qingjie shenti hao* [Regularly wash clothes and bedding, bathe often, maintain cleanliness for good health]. Hygiene Department of the East China Military Region Logistics Department, Shanghai, early 1950s. Courtesy of IISH Stefan R. Landsberger Collection.

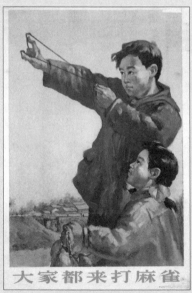

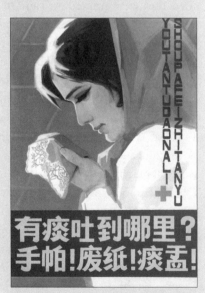

Poster 3. Bi Chen, *Dajia dou lai da maque* [Everybody comes to kill sparrows]. *Chaohua meishu chubanshe,* September 1956, print no. T8082.1060. Courtesy of IISH Stefan R. Landsberger Collection.

Poster 4. Jin Futang, Yang Jingzhi, *You tan tu dao nali? Shoupa! Feizhi! Tanyu!* [Where do you spit your phlegm? In a handkerchief! In wastepaper! In a spittoon!] Chinese Red Cross Association, February 1983. Courtesy of IISH Stefan R. Landsberger Collection.

So, in 1960, catching bedbugs replaced hunting sparrows. From 1955 to 1959, the various schistosomiasis eradication campaigns targeted snails, with the aim of wiping out "big belly" disease. They were generally seen as more successful, although later discredited (Horn 1969, 94–106; Cell 1977, 54; Rogaski 2002, 408; Wang 2000, 270–271). Posters and related visual materials were designed to raise "snail awareness."

Despite the striking visual imagery supporting the hygiene campaigns, their overall longer-term success is debatable. Even now, injunctions against spitting in the street appear regularly, indicating that the challenge remains. More recently, educational television commercials have superseded the use of posters.

The new slogan "Unify Chinese and Western medicine" *(zhongxiyi tuanjie)*—coined by Mao Zedong, but flexible enough to accommodate different interpretations—thus governed health care policy involving Chinese medicine in the early 1950s. Pragmatically, it allowed the sizable manpower of the Chinese medicine sector—estimated at around 300,000 physicians in 1949—to be recruited into the official health care system, specifically to the mass action programs favored by Mao. For this purpose, Chinese medicine physicians were taught to administer vaccinations and provide other basic medical care. In return, they were granted the right to practice, provided they could demonstrate some basic proficiency in biomedical knowledge. There was no intention, however, to extend this right indefinitely, or to create a separate space for Chinese medicine within the overall health care system. Rather, it was to be assimilated into a "new medicine" *(xinyi)* that would once and for all remove existing divisions on the field of medicine (Wang and Cai 1999, 5–10).

Utopian visions of a "new medicine" that would arise from the fusion of East and West, science and tradition, had constituted a recurring theme in the writings of a wide spectrum of reformist physicians from the late 1920s onward (see Chapter 7; Lei 1998). At the conservative end, scholar-physicians such as Qin Bowei and Ding Zhongying thought of "scientization" as systematization (Qin 1929; Ding 1936). For them, making Chinese medicine more "scientific" meant uniting the many competing currents within Chinese medicine into one medical system while, at the same time, effectively enhancing the value of its core doctrines. More radical modernizers such as Lu Yuanlei and Zhang Cigong, on the other hand, were critical of what they viewed as the unscientific and mystical nature of Chinese medical learning (Lu 1934; Zhu 2000). For them, the real value of Chinese medicine lay in the experience *(jingyan)* of generations of physicians, embodied in classical formulas, diagnostic techniques, and styles of medical practice, all of which might be analyzed by and integrated with scientific (that is, Western) medicine (Lei 2002; Li 2003).

In the political climate of the early 1950s, it was this latter position that resonated most closely with the thinking of leading Ministry of Health bureaucrats at the time—including He Cheng (1901–1992), the vice minister at the time (Yu and Zu 2006). It also came close in many respects to that of Yu Yunxiu, chief ideologue of medical revolution in Nationalist China, who had maintained an active interest in the scientization of Chinese medicine and who now was well positioned to make a political comeback. In 1950, both Lu Yuanlei and Yu Yunxiu were invited to the First National Health Conference in Beijing, reflecting clearly the direction of modernization at the time.

This direction also became apparent in the focus on acupuncture and Chinese medicinals that came to dominate medical research during this period. Acupuncture was perceived as being both uniquely Chinese *and* explainable by Pavlovian neuropathology—a Soviet and therefore politically correct way to do science. Chinese medicinals, on the other hand, could be framed in nationalistic terms as constituting the concrete embodiment of the Chinese people's experience in their struggle against disease. Furthermore, strategies for translating such experience into biomedical practice and thereby separating it from traditional doctrines had been underway since the 1930s.

Working outward from such concrete research efforts, it was decided to apply the same strategies to Chinese medicine as a whole. Leading strategists within the Ministry of Health deemed it "not too late" to "train large numbers of new physicians possessing both adequate levels of scientific training and experience as replacements" of traditionally educated physicians once the latter had outlived their pragmatic usefulness (Cui 1997, 218). Between August 1950 and December 1951, the new government thus passed a series of laws that redefined entitlements to practice Chinese medicine. Licenses were granted only to those physicians who had graduated from a college in Republican China or who had passed one of the national licensing examinations that had been sporadically offered during this period. The new laws thereby prevented all self-trained physicians, as well as those educated within traditional master-disciple relationships, from continuing to practice.

In 1952, a new licensing examination was introduced. Because it tested mainly Western medical knowledge, the failure rate was so high that it excluded the majority of Chinese medicine practitioners (Wang and Cai 1999, 8). In many cases physicians were able to exploit legislative loopholes and carry on as before. But a significant number did give up their practices. As a consequence, in a city such as Shanghai, which still had the most vigorous Chinese medical infrastructure, the number of Chinese medicine physicians decreased by around 11 percent between 1949 and 1953 (Wang 1998, 68; Zhang and Shao 1998, 137).

At the same time, the government began to organize the large-scale reeducation of practicing Chinese medicine physicians through what were called "Chinese medicine improvement schools" *(zhongyi jinjiu xuexiao)*. The purpose of these schools, which continued to function until the end of the decade, was to raise the level of biomedical knowledge and political awareness among Chinese medicine physicians. Although from a later perspective the biomedical training offered by these schools was woefully inadequate, they did succeed in familiarizing many physicians who previously had no understanding of Western medicine with its main concepts and ideas. In addition, a number of young but already established physicians were selected on the basis of competitive examinations to study Western medicine for five years (Cai et al. 1999, 87; K. Taylor 1999; Wang and Cai 1999, 86–87).

The intended unification of Chinese and Western medicine had clear political functions, too, inasmuch as Western medicine was perceived to be a tool with which to remedy the ideological shortcomings of traditional physicians. Mao Zedong, for instance, stated during a meeting of the CCP Central Committee in 1953 that, in the course of uniting the two medicines, "Western medicine definitely must smash the sectarianism [of Chinese medicine]" (Cui 1997, 155).

Economically, too, the state began to undermine the independence of the Chinese medicine sector and to assimilate its physicians into state-controlled institutions. Chinese medicine was initially excluded from the country's new national insurance scheme, although the government established a number of clinics for party cadres. Physicians were encouraged to donate their families' herbal formulae for the public good. The government also encouraged these doctors to join larger cooperative clinics *(lianhe zhensuo)*. While private practice was fully abolished only in 1966, the number of physicians in private practice in Shanghai, for instance, had already declined from 3,308 in 1948 to about 1,000 in 1965 (Wang 1998, 68–70; Zhang and Shao 1998, 140).

Physicians adjusted to these new realities in quite different ways. Those who had entertained close relationships with the Nationalist Party elite emigrated to Hong Kong, Taiwan, and, later, the United States. For some this led to a considerable decline in social status, while others were able to exploit the new opportunities that relocation offered them. Too, it was from within this community of exiles that some of the most important early teachers of Chinese medicine in the West emerged.

On the mainland, Shanghai initially continued to be the center of reform in the Chinese medical arena. The first Chinese medicine improvement school, for instance, was established in Shanghai in 1951, followed in October 1952 by the opening of the first Chinese medicine clinic for party cadres. Both institutions were directed by Lu Yuanlei, who was eventually also appointed chairman of the committee that edited the first Chinese medicine teaching materials commissioned by the Maoist state. In other cities as well, prominent advocates of scientization—such as Shi Jinmo (1881–1969) in Beijing and Ren Yingqiu (1914–1984) in Chongqing—rose to leading administrative and advisory positions. Furthermore, the emphasis the CCP placed on the development of acumoxa therapy allowed acupuncture physicians such as Lu Shouyan (1909–1969) in Shanghai and Wang Leting (1905–1984) in Beijing to move from the margins to the very center of the field of Chinese medicine (Chen 1990; Lu et al. 1999, 54–76, 195–196; Sun 2000; Wang 2003).

In the main, however, the daily practice of Chinese medicine continued much as before. Texts such as the *Gazetteer of Famous Shanghai Physicians (Shanghai mingyi zhi)*, published in 1950, demonstrate that even in metropolitan centers such as Shanghai, a physician's native place and his family background mattered more to patients than his knowledge of biomedical science (Qian 1950). For physicians themselves, establishing personal connections with the new elite involved difficult choices not only on the level of ideology but also on that of personal habits and the organization of one's life. Should one give up a successful practice in order to join a cooperative? To what degree should one get involved in reeducation? Was it worth giving up smoking opium, the tried and tested way of coping with a busy life? These were still individual decisions at the time, as no framework had yet been put in place by which the state could actively intervene at the microlevel of individual teaching and practice. Only during subsequent periods did the new realities of Maoist health care began to touch upon every aspect of daily and professional life, to effect a more profound transformation of Chinese medical practice.

1954–1965

Contemporary Chinese histories of the period claim that the CCP has always taken a principled stance to protect and promote the development of Chinese medicine. More accurately, this position emerged in the years between 1954 and 1956. Furthermore, it did not reflect a conscious policy shift. Rather, it was the outcome of a series of events that led to, and fed off, each other in ways that eventually provided Chinese medicine with an institutional infrastructure and framework of clinical practice that endures to this date. The origins of these developments can be traced to shifts in the balance of power between "reds" and "experts" within the health care sector. In these political struggles, attitudes favoring Chinese medicine initially appear to have been nothing more than a convenient stick with which to beat the biomedical professionals dominating the Ministry of Health, including the minister, He Cheng. However, as mistakes in the ministry's governance of the Chinese medical sector were identified, they obviously had to be corrected. Hence, Mao Zedong, although by no means convinced of its clinical utility, demanded to "take Chinese medicine seriously, to do research to rectify it, and to go further in developing Chinese medicine." By September 1954 Liu Shaoqi pronounced that "despising Chinese medicine is servile and subservient bourgeoisie thinking" (Cai et al. 1999).

As a consequence, Chinese medicine was increasingly accorded value in its own right. It was accepted into the national insurance scheme, and in October 1954 the Culture Department of the CCP Central Committee made recommendations regarding the improvement and strengthening of Chinese medicine. These included the establishment of the China Academy of Chinese Medicine *(Zhongguo zhongyi yanjiuyuan)* and the integration of Chinese medicine into the larger hospitals, as well as a general expansion of the scope of Chinese medical work.

Overall, however, the larger goal of creating a new society and a new medicine still guided this reevaluation of Chinese medicine. Mao Zedong noted that the experience of the preceding years revealed the mistaken assumptions underlying related policies. He therefore changed track, setting a new priority: Western medicine physicians would now study Chinese medicine. Through their studies and commitment to serving the people, these physicians would "abolish the boundaries between Chinese and Western medicine," thereby forming the spearhead of the new medicine (Cui 1997, 155). Mao Zedong's goal at this stage most definitely was not to ensure the survival of Chinese medicine as an independent tradition. Rather, he hoped to subordinate Western medicine to Chinese medicine in an attempt to break existing patterns of behavior within certain institutions. The purpose was "to force doctors from the two traditions to work together in order to create, eventually, a medicine of China capable of serving as a world medicine" (Taylor 2000, 112).

At Mao's specific behest, young doctors of Western medicine from all over the country were summoned to Beijing in 1955 to be reeducated in the first experimental class of Western medicine doctors studying Chinese medicine *(diyijie xiyi xuexi zhongyi yanjiu ban)*. Many of these young physicians, who shared with other intellectuals a perception of Chinese medicine as old and backward, were none too pleased about this invitation (Ma 1993, 583–584). Later, however, the considerable status associated with this class allowed many of its graduates to advance into influential positions within the Chinese medical sector.

Eminent Chinese medicine physicians from all over China—particularly from Sichuan and Jiangsu—were likewise called to Beijing as teachers and advisors to the Ministry of Health. The resulting concentration of senior practitioners in Beijing not only facilitated the establishment there of the China Academy of Chinese Medicine in 1955 but also located these physicians much closer to China's new political center of power (Zhongguo kexue jishu xiehui 1991). In addition, it fed into the quiet resurgence of a tradition of studying with teachers and masters.

This centralization had several important consequences. For the previous fifty years, Shanghai had been the undisputed center of Chinese medicine. It had been the place where most of the influential physicians had lived, studied, practiced, and taught; where the most important schools and colleges of the Republican era had operated; and where all of the key debates of that period had been fought. Now, however, its influence declined in direct relation to Beijing's rise. Facilitated by new personal networks as much as by ideological commitment, politics infiltrated medicine in ways that have not yet been well researched and often can only be ascertained indirectly. The anti-rightist campaigns of the mid-1950s, for instance, coincided with a marked decline in the influence of more radical modernizers such as Zhang Cigong. One of the many results of this realignment was that Five Phases doctrine, long perceived as the most emblematic exemplar of mystical thinking in Chinese medicine, was firmly reintegrated into Chinese medical teaching (He 1997, 59–67; Zhao 2006).

Following Beijing's lead, classes of various duration and quality were soon established throughout the whole of China for Western medicine doctors studying Chinese medicine. These classes were integrated into the curriculum of Western medicine universities, colleges, and schools. By 1960, thirty-seven full-time courses had trained more than 2,300 physicians, while an additional 36,000 Western medicine doctors had received training in Chinese medicine even as they continued to carry out their medical duties (Cai 1999, 14). Physicians of Chinese medicine were also admitted to existing Western medicine hospitals and clinics, and new hospitals of Chinese medicine were established. This strengthening of Chinese medicine's role within the health care sector expressed itself in a new alignment between Western and Chinese medicine, articulated in the slogan "Chinese medicine must become scientific, Western medicine must become Chinese" *(zhongyi yao kexuehua, xiyi yao zhongguohua)* (Ma 1993, 575).

The "integration of Chinese and Western medicine" *(zhongxiyi jiehe)*—a concept initially developed by Mao Zedong in 1956 to describe the second attempt at creating a new medicine in China—thus guided CCP policy from the mid-1950s onward. Unification of both medicines remained the ultimate goal, but it was accepted that this would take longer than previously estimated. Chinese medicine physicians and their supporters, sensing that the political mood had changed, seized the moment to lobby for the establishment of an independent Chinese medicine sector. Their campaign received a major boost in 1956 with the founding of four Chinese medicine colleges (zhongyi xueyuan) in Chengdu, Beijing, Guangzhou, and Shanghai. Resources were made available for developing an administrative infrastructure charged with supervising the research, education, and practice of Chinese medicine at both national and provincial levels. By 1961, tertiary colleges, research institutes, and teaching hospitals could be found throughout the country (Liu and Cui 1998; Zhu and Zhang 1990).

This sudden and vigorous expansion of the Chinese medicine sector caused new problems for policy makers. The most urgent involved manpower. Relying only on physicians graduated from the new colleges would have meant scaling back the ambitious scope of the program. The government therefore decided to revitalize the traditional apprenticeship system, despite its associations with feudal ideology and society. Beginning in 1957, selected students were assigned to established physicians of Chinese medicine, and special classes were set up to supplement such apprenticeship training with lessons in theory, Western medicine, and politics. As a result, the number of physicians of Chinese medicine increased rapidly in both rural and urban areas. In Shanghai, for instance, it almost doubled in the course of less than ten years, although still lagging behind the even more rapid growth of the Western medicine sector (Wang and Cai 1999, 86–95).

If it was the state that had engineered this expansion, it was also the state that decided the direction it would take. Through a series of loosely connected initiatives that have continued to define the identity of Chinese medicine up to the present, the development of Chinese medicine was thereby integrated into the CCP's more comprehensive project of nation building and socialist modernization. Though different in their aim and scope, the common denominator of these initiatives was the simplification, regularization, and systematization of traditional modes of practice. New national textbooks and teaching materials compiled under direct supervision of the Ministry of Health attempted to condense the often contradictory information contained in classical texts into a more coherent system, while translating their content into modern Chinese. The goal was to detach learning from the idiosyncratic interpretations, experiences, and habits of individual teachers and provide all students with equal access to the resources of tradition. As a consequence, even as they claimed to represent the accumulated knowledge of the past, these textbooks delineated Chinese medicine in an entirely new fashion.

Some commentators view this reorganization as so radical that they speak of a paradigm shift separating today's "traditional Chinese medicine" (TCM) from the scholarly medical tradition of old. Others, including Chinese medicine physicians themselves, emphasize continuity and view modern reorganizations of learning and practice as merely another stage in the ongoing development of the tradition. Both sides agree, however, that the model that organizes and, by implication, epitomizes contemporary Chinese medical practice is *bianzheng lunzhi,* or "pattern differentiation and treatment determination."

Bianzheng lunzhi describes an idealized clinical encounter as constituted by two separate yet tightly integrated processes of translation. In the first step— pattern differentiation—the four examinations enable the practitioner to elicit the pertinent symptoms and signs, organizing them into distinctive clinical patterns, descriptions of which can be found in the classical literature. These patterns are similar to syndromes in biomedicine. However, their primary purpose is not to define disease but rather to grasp the moment-by-moment unfolding of pathological processes. In the language of Chinese medicine, patterns of this kind describe pathologies of *qi* transformation *(qi hua).*

In a second step, one responds to these disorders with appropriate treatment strategies designed to balance or control the disordered process. The physician uses him- or herself as an instrument, when making the diagnosis, by looking, listening, smelling and tasting, and feeling, drawing on his or her own embodied experience and subjective understanding of the patient's body. The doctor then distills the result of this interaction with the patient into the formulation of a clinical pattern, or a diagnosis—the differentiation of a pattern and determination of a treatment. This subjective understanding then undergoes a reverse process, as the physician translates it into a set of treatment strategies that include herbal medicines, acupuncture point prescriptions, or other related modes of treatment (Farquhar 1994b).

Although physicians had practiced medicine in just this manner for centuries, the definition of *bianzheng lunzhi* as representing Chinese medical practice per se is the definitive product of its institutionalization in Maoist China. *Bianzheng lunzhi* initially occupied this position because it provided the most effective way of reconciling the multiple forces involved in this process of institutionalization. It continued to hold the position because it has proved itself sufficiently sturdy and flexible to accommodate to the changing contexts of practice since then. It played on ideological, linguistic, and conceptual similarities between older notions of pattern diagnosis in Chinese medicine and modern Marxist dialectics. It also brought together the Maoist emphasis on practice and the definition of Chinese medicine as constituted by "experience" that had been worked out in the 1930s.

Physicians during the 1950s reconceptualized pattern diagnosis as being concerned with recognizing and overcoming the contradictions thrown up by the encounter between human beings and their environment. Focusing on patterns rather than disease, furthermore, provided a useful boundary marker that differentiated Chinese from Western medicine. At the same time, it allowed Chinese medicine physicians to integrate their practices into a biomedically dominated health care system and thereby fulfill their obligation to modernize (Karchmer 2010).

Such integration proceeded at two different levels at once, permitting maximum flexibility in accommodating traditional practices to new contexts of use. In what might best be described as a bottom-up approach, physicians subsumed biomedical techniques and information into Chinese medicine's practices of pattern differentiation and treatment determination. This could mean adding an herb known to reduce hypertension to a Chinese medicine formula prescribed on the basis of more traditional pattern determination. Or it could mean translating the hormonal rhythms of the female menstrual cycle into Chinese medicine patterns and then prescribing ancient formulas with reference to basal temperature charts rather than pulse or tongue. This integration has largely been piecemeal, tied to individual preferences and habits, and transmitted via small networks (from teacher to student, within specific institutions, or via journal articles).

In contrast, the top-down approach that characterized the writing of textbooks attempted to define Chinese medicine *as* Chinese medicine and was aimed at universal applicability. Given the very real power differentials in China's health care system, the continued viability of Chinese medicine within that system depended on finding a way to include its practice within the dominant understanding of the body as defined by biomedicine. The second edition of national textbooks published in 1964 achieved this objective. In their presentation of pathology, diagnosis, and treatment, these textbooks employed biomedical diseases as overarching rubrics, each of which could then be further analyzed in terms of Chinese medicine patterns (Karchmer 2004).

The long-term consequences of this accommodation are still being played out, and it is therefore too early to judge their ultimate effects. On one level, it has allowed Chinese medicine to attach itself successfully to the sociotechnical networks of biomedicine and thereby vastly extend its range of influence—not only in China but also throughout the world. Over time, however, the balance between bottom-up and top-down integration and between the relative priority accorded to biomedical disease and Chinese medical pattern differentiation has gradually shifted. What started out as a flexible process in which diagnosing a biomedical disease was, in practice, an option rather than a necessity is changing into a method where diagnosing the biomedical disease is now both institutionally and practically the primary task on which all later action hinges. Only after a disease is known are Chinese medical patterns—now rendered as "types" (*xing*)—brought into play. The process downgrades traditional methods of diagnosis and their emphasis on local process in favor of diseases as defined by universal biology. Increasingly, the argument is being made that the institutionalization of Chinese medicine predicated on *bianzheng lunzhi* is the beginning of the end of Chinese medicine as an independent and effective medical tradition (Liu 2006). Others, however, believe it has not gone far enough, and that the scientization of tradition remains, as yet, an unfinished project (Zhao 2006).

As in all previous periods of dynastic change, central to government-directed efforts at modernization was a rewriting of history. This rewriting took in all aspects of the Chinese medical tradition, but it has become visible with exemplary clarity in the changing definition of "tradition" itself. In late imperial China, Chinese medicine was commonly imagined as resembling a network of waterways, made up of different currents but descended from a common origin. Any serious scholar had to start his education by traveling upstream to the sources of tradition, because they contained the basic models of all legitimate practice. Thus, when in 1757 the eminent scholar-physician Xu Dachun published a critique of medicine that sought to impress upon its readers the importance of classical learning, he naturally drew on the image of the "source and course" of a river when selecting the title for his book: *On the Origin and Development of Medicine (Yixue yuanliu lun)*.

Almost two hundred years later in 1935, another scholar-physician, Xie Guan (1880–1950), used the same image in a medical history entitled *On the Origin and Further Development of China's Medicine (Zhongguo yixue yuanliu lun)*, a work that redefined Xu Dachun's scholarly medicine as a "national medicine" (*guoyi*). This medicine could not be based on individual insight but had to represent the achievements of a nation (defined in racial terms) throughout the course of its history. Rather than looking backward toward origins, Xie's history was linear, progressive, and modeled on the European West: a golden age (from the Spring and Autumn period to the Tang) during which the nation constructed its own culture was followed by a period of decline (from the Song to the Republic) characterized by foreign occupation, leading to a period of rejuvenation, rationality, and progress (May Fourth and onward) that ultimately would resolve itself in the future, when all differences between nations disappear and history ends.

Xie Guan argued that, throughout the course of its history, the unity of tradition that had characterized Chinese medicine at the start had gradually been swept away by a multitude of competing currents. Hence the apparent crisis of

Chinese medicine in the late imperial era and what needed to be done to overcome it. Western methods of scholarship were to be used to address and correct problems within the Chinese tradition and thereby increase its international competitiveness. But, because this process could also be configured as a link in the unceasing process of change that, according to ancient Chinese philosophy, was the most fundamental pattern of the universe, it did not pose any threat to the validity of the Chinese tradition itself.

Twenty years later, dialectical materialism and Mao Zedong Thought became the guiding lights for scholar-physicians such as Ren Yingqiu, who supplied Chinese medicine in early Communist China with a revised modern history. In *Doctrines of Schools and Physicians of Chinese Medicine (Zhongyi gejia xueshuo)*, Ren celebrated the achievements of previous generations of physicians as aspects of a wider human struggle against disease. He defined the various currents of Chinese medicine not as antagonistic to each other but as tributaries to a single river of knowledge. Holding on to the ancient image of the river, he linked it with Mao's utopian humanism, arriving at a vision in which all the currents of tradition converge in the new socialist medicine of the future. This would be China's unique contribution to the world (Ren 1980, 1981).

To facilitate this process, the Ministry of Health launched a campaign for the exchange of scholarship and learning *(xueshu jiaoliu huodong)*. Ideologically linked to the One Hundred Flowers campaign of 1956–1957, its purpose was to collect all available sources of medical knowledge, distill from them their strengths, and discard their shortcomings. Family medical traditions were encouraged to bring their private medical knowledge into the public domain. Those who refused became politically suspect and risked falling victim to one of the many rectification campaigns that now enforced submission to party policy.

The Ministry of Health issued another directive in 1960, aimed at extracting personal knowledge in an even more immediate manner. It instructed local administrative units to arrange discipleships for young doctors with all the famous physicians of their area. In the course of their studies these doctors would systematically analyze the clinical experience of their teachers and collect their case records (Wang 1998, 83–84; Zhang and Shao 1998, 149–150).

Meanwhile, Cheng Menxue, president of the Shanghai College of TCM, initiated a project to analyze the clinical experience of the city's most important medical currents of the twentieth century. Collaborating directly with these physicians, their disciples, and family members, the college compiled a series of essays that were published one year later, in 1962, in an important collection entitled *Selected Experiences of Chinese Medicine Currents in the Modern Era (Jindai zhongyi liupai jingyan xuanji)*. In its foreword, Cheng Menxue described its purpose as letting the distinct characteristics of each [individual] current and each [individual] scholar-physician become fully apparent [so that] after allowing for ample consultation, they might be assimilated and dissolved [into each other] leading to their [eventual] synthesis. Generalizing and regularizing them in this manner we can greatly raise the level of Chinese medical scholarship. Through sorting out and carrying forward the inheritance of national medicine, we can thus make ever greater and better contributions [to it]. (Shanghai zhongyi xueyuan 1962, 1–2)

In its overall purpose, Cheng Menxue's book project thus fit squarely into a larger political program directed at national unification and individual sacrifice to the socialist collective cause. Physicians had already surrendered their economic autonomy by ceasing to be independent practitioners and becoming salaried workers within the state health care system. They now collaborated in an equally important transformation of social agency, whereby the Maoist state attempted to engineer a break with traditional cultural definitions of individual and group identities. Mutual help *(huxiang bangzhu)* was advocated as a principle of social relations among all members of the new nation, rather than just between members of smaller social groups such as families, lineages, or particularistic associations.

That even cultural conservatives such as Cheng Menxue were by then wholeheartedly committed to this endeavor shows the deeply felt debt that most practitioners and teachers of Chinese medicine experience in relation to the CCP and its leaders. The language of the foreword—replete with references to the "sorting out . . . of national medicine" that were taken directly from the debates of the 1930s—also shows, however, that these physicians did not experience a break between what they were committing themselves to now and what they had been aiming for all their lives. Hence, even as they claimed to let go of adhering to the idiosyncrasies of particular groups in favor of the homogeneity of an emerging national orthodoxy, the writers of the essays in Cheng Menxue's book also reaffirmed their personal attachment to diverse lineages of descent. In this way, they maintained—at least in theory—the tools for an alternative history of their tradition.

In an important sense, therefore, Chinese medicine on the eve of the Cultural Revolution continued to be defined by the same tensions that had troubled it since the Song period. The Maoist state had attempted to create a new kind of Chinese medicine characterized by shared truths and devoted to the health care of the people. To this end, it had devised strategies for smashing sectarianism, modifying the values and beliefs of physicians, and restructuring their daily lives and patterns of medical practice. By and large, members of the Chinese medicine community were grateful for the value accorded to them and their tradition by the state. But they were also reluctant to cut themselves loose from the particularistic social relations that tied them to distinctive lines of descent. And however much they might desire to be part of the new China, they still had not succeeded in constructing a medicine that resolved, once and for all, the contradiction between the authority of tradition (which was, of necessity, tied to models of the past) and the ever-changing problems of the present that constantly required a search for different solutions. The next period in the history of Chinese medicine proposed a revolutionary response to this dilemma, although one that ultimately failed, precisely because of its one-sided radicalism.

1966–1977

Mao Zedong's Great Proletarian Cultural Revolution, which destabilized Chinese society throughout the "lost decade" from 1966 to 1976, can be understood at least in part as a radical attempt to solve contradictions that by then had become visible, and not only in the domain of medicine. Frustrated with the manner in which old social practices and habits continued to undermine China's movement toward socialism, Mao unleashed the power of youth in a struggle against the "four olds": old ideas, old culture, old customs, and old habits. Meanwhile, individuals and groups at all levels of society exploited these campaigns for their own selfish purposes and as simple acts of revenge, to settle private scores against coworkers, neighbors, family members, and others (Thurston 1987).

A short-lived frenzy of violence destroyed much of Chinese medicine's infrastructure, including ancient texts as well as modern institutions. For ideological reasons, medical doctrine was simplified to the greatest possible extent, and practice rather than book study became the proper guide of action. The integration of Chinese and Western medicine became the only legitimate way to practice, and the Chinese medicine sector rapidly contracted below its pre-1949 levels. A survey commissioned by the Ministry of Health in 1978 established that between 1959 and 1977 the number of people employed in the Chinese medical sector declined by a third, from 361,000 to 240,000, while in the Western medical sector it almost quadrupled, from 234,000 in 1959 to 738,000 in 1977 (Meng 1999, 744).

The repercussions of the Cultural Revolution on individual lives were frequently devastating. Renowned physicians who only recently had guided the development of the new Chinese medical orthodoxy under the direct supervision of the party were now branded "forces of evil," subjected to torture and abuse, and prevented from carrying out scholarly work or engaging in medical practice. Some were killed; others committed suicide or died as a result of physical and emotional trauma. Most others were sent down to the country-side or employed in factories in order to attend to the health care needs of peasants and workers rather than those of the party elite.

Equally significant were efforts to break up what remained of the traditional structures of Chinese society. Private medical practice was now completely dis-allowed. Hierarchical teacher-student relationships, "polluted" by Confucian patriarchy, were replaced by a program of mutual study *(xuexi huzhu)* and mu-tual help *(huzhu hezuo)*, in which the teacher had as much to learn as the stu-dent. Even family relationships were to be surrendered to an attitude of serving the people *(wei renmin fuwu)*. The establishment of rural and urban collectives was accelerated in an effort to destroy the vestiges of lineage-based society in rural areas. Family grave sites were ransacked, lineage halls destroyed, and gene-alogies burned. Inasmuch as these institutions had been crucial to the manner in which Chinese medicine had traditionally been taught and remembered, an important link to the past was cut that has never entirely been rebuilt since.

FOLK NUTRITIONAL THERAPY IN MODERN CHINA

Eugene N. Anderson

Chinese folk nutrition in recent centuries drew on the idea that foods could be heating, cooling, wetting, drying, strengthening, or cleansing. The most impor-tant dimensions were heating *(re)* and cooling *(liang;* a few foods were cold, *han)*. These concepts developed from a medieval fusion of Chinese ideas of Yang and Yin with Hippocratic-Galenic humoral medicine introduced from the Near East ("Galenos" is referenced in one fourteenth-century text). Experience of famine also reinforced the realities of food energy and its importance in maintaining body heat. More recent fieldwork in southeast China shows that managing diet remains the first recourse when responding to illness (Anderson 1988, 1996).

Heating foods included those that were high-calorie, subjected to high heat in cooking, spicy or bitter, or "hot" in color (red, orange). Cooling foods were low-calorie, watery, soothing or sour in taste, or "cool" in color (whitish, green). Cooked grain was considered perfectly balanced, serving as a reference point. In contrast, cool foods treated hot illnesses, which involved sores, reddening, rashes, dry skin, and sore throat—symptoms similar to those of a burn (and ill-nesses often recognized by biomedicine as involving vitamin C deficiency). Green vegetables were among the most commonly used.

Typical cool conditions involved low body temperature, chills, pallor, weakness, watery eliminations, and symptoms resembling those of hypothermia. Anemia most commonly fit these criteria, as did tuberculosis and recovery from childbirth. Treatment involved easily digested red and organ meats, ginger, Chinese liquor, wolfthorn berries *(gou qi zi, Lycium chinense)*, and similar foods rich in vitamins and minerals. Such interventions addressed the anemia and alleviated conditions related to conditions of excess coolness. Heating foods were often eaten simply to maintain body heat. Everyone knew, for example, that eating baked goods or fatty meat on a winter day would keep one warmer than would a diet of vegetables.

Strengthening *(bupin,* literally "supplementing" or "patching things") foods were usually easily digested, nutrient-rich protein foods, such as the dark meat of poultry, organ meats, mushrooms, and several herbal foods (Hu 2005). Some specifically strengthened particular organs; these foods usually derived from organs themselves. For example, pork lungs helped human lungs, liver helped liver, and penises of harem-keeping animals such as seals or deer supplemented human male genitalia. Sometimes resemblance was enough: walnut meats strengthened the brain, for example. Red liquids, especially port wine, strengthened the blood. Sometimes a red fruit, such as red jujubes, did the same. Black items (from the meat from a black dog to stout beer) often strengthened the body. Foods with a gelatinous texture possessed a special *qi* and were valued for replenishing Yang. When high in protein and minerals, such gelatinous foods were particularly valued: birds' nests, rare fungi, sea cucumbers, and less common game animals, from tigers to vultures.

Bland to slightly sharp herbs were cleansing *(jing),* clearing away undesirable moisture, phlegm, impurities, and contamination in the body. Some contained chemicals later recognized in biomedicine as antibiotic, astringent, or diuretic. Other foods were "poisonous" *(du),* in the sense that they potentiated poisons in the body. For example, although live male poultry kept away demons and had other ritual functions, when dead they were thought to exacerbate cancer.

In short, practical experience led Chinese villagers and townsfolk to recognize the value of what only later would be reinterpreted as heat energy, protein and nutrients, and antibiotic "contamination-dispelling" action. Indeed, studies of Chinese medicine that talk only of high theory and neglect practice are getting things backward. Chinese medicine in action privileged practice and empiricism. Theory was useful to explain and interpret, to classify, and to extend logically the procedures used, but common experience was always the first consideration.

The search for new treatment methods facilitated by revolutionary zeal, and by a genuine ethos of mutual assistance and help, led to a general opening up, in the long term, of the borders that had hitherto defined Chinese medicine. Folk remedies were included in the *materia medica*; new acupuncture points and treatment techniques were discovered. Some of these achievements, such as the publication of the *Encyclopedic Dictionary of Chinese Pharmacology (Zhongyao dacidian)* in 1977, have had a lasting impact on the practice of Chinese medicine (Jiangsu xinyi xueyuan 1979). However, just as many widely proclaimed medical breakthroughs were quickly discarded again. Thus, on one hand, the widespread repopularization of Chinese medicine—albeit in simplified form—may ultimately have contributed to saving it from becoming a treasured but practically redundant academic museum piece. On the other, the dissociation of medical practice from classical learning only accelerated the disintegration of older styles of therapeutic practice that the reforms of the previous decade had set in motion.

Finally, if the 1950s had witnessed a concentration of resources in the cities—exemplified by Chinese medical hospitals and colleges, and most particularly in Beijing—the period of the Cultural Revolution shifted at least some of these resources to the countryside. Due to the relatively small number of Western medicine physicians, the rural population still relied on a mixture of self-help, Chinese medicine, shamanism, religious healing, and folk practitioners for most of their health care needs. The establishment of the Three-Tiered Health Care Network *(Sanji weisheng baojian wang)*, with its emphasis on the delivery of basic health care needs at the village level through "barefoot doctors" *(chijiao yisheng)*, dramatically changed this balance.

Sometimes condescendingly referred to as "half peasants, half physicians" *(bannong banyi)* by their college-trained peers, barefoot doctors received basic training in both Western and Chinese medicine and then worked under or together with college-trained senior doctors. When not engaged in health care, they would continue to participate in agricultural tasks. Their therapeutic repertoire included the use of biomedical pharmaceuticals where available, acupuncture for toothache and other painful conditions, and Chinese herbal formulas prescribed symptomatically rather than on the basis of the more complex pattern differentiation. Barefoot doctors were responsible for immunization, disease prevention, family planning services, midwifery, and other basic medical care, as well as health education. Problems that exceeded their skill were referred up the network to county- or provincial-level clinics or hospitals, where more specialized care was available (C. C. Chen 1989; Jia 1997; White 1998).

Barefoot doctors and the Three-Tiered Health Care Network into which they were integrated constituted an efficient use of resources much admired by

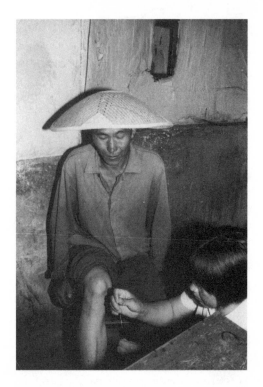

Figure 8.2. A Chinese "barefoot doctor" uses her needles to treat a production brigade worker. Photograph by D. Henrioud. Courtesy of World Health Organization.

foreign experts at the time. The barefoot doctors fundamentally changed patterns of morbidity by greatly reducing the impact of infectious and parasitic diseases, still the main causes of death in rural areas prior to the 1960s. Hence, while images of barefoot doctors administering acupuncture helped to popularize Chinese medicine in the West (Fogarty 1990), their impact on patient behavior in China itself was rather different. They provided access to effective biomedical care on a large scale to a population that had never before been able to afford such luxury. Injections, drips, and those who delivered them became the first port of call for anyone seeking help outside of the home or family (Lora-Wainwright 2006).

If everyone in China today knows that "Western medicine is good for acute disorders, Chinese medicine is good for chronic disorders," few are aware of how recently this truth was established (see Karchmer 2004, 2010). Indeed, in 1936, Zhang Taiyan—a leading proponent of national medicine—could still argue that the strength of Chinese medicine lay in the treatment of seasonal (i.e., infectious) disease. Interviews conducted by the author in Shanghai and rural Jiangsu confirm that until the 1960s, such diseases still constituted the mainstay of Chinese medical practice. Few physicians prior to that time could become famous unless they were perceived as successful in treating these seasonal disorders.

The most violent phase of the Cultural Revolution lasted only until 1968, but it was not until Mao Zedong's death on September 9, 1976, that the revolution's force was finally spent. Two years later, the CCP officially acknowledged its failures. It embarked on an ambitious program of reform and development under the slogan of the "four modernizations" in agriculture, industry, science and technology, and national defense. Creating "socialism with Chinese characteristics" implied that Chinese classical culture could once more be valorized—though this time in the service of a transition modeled on Western market economics (Baum 1982, 1170; Ong 1995). The contours of post-1978 reforms in the health sector reflect these ideological reevaluations and tensions. They can be summarized by four new maxims: (1) to emphasize hospital-based services rather than primary or community care, reversing the priorities of previous policies; (2) to move toward reprofessionalizing medicine (implying that specialist knowledge was to be valued above that of political cadres); (3) to depend on technology, including the transfer of technologies such as tools and personnel from developed countries; and (4) to establish a plural health care system (Henderson 1989).

The contours of this plural health care system emerged incrementally through a series of Ministry of Health meetings and conferences during the late 1970s and early 1980s. In 1976, Chinese medicine colleges resumed teaching degree courses, while the new chairman of the CCP, Deng Xiaoping, personally initiated a program aimed at revitalizing the Chinese medicine sector. In 1980, the Ministry of Health committed itself to the "three paths" policy, which stated: "Chinese medicine, Western medicine, and integrated Chinese and Western medicine constitute three great powers that all need to be developed and which will coexist for a long time." Two years later, in 1982, the phrase "to develop modern medicine and our nation's traditional medicines" (i.e., not only Chinese medicine but also the medicine of China's non-Han minorities) was formally written into the new constitution of the People's Republic of China. The number of Chinese medicine physicians reached a historic high in 1985, while in conjunction with its policy of reform and opening up, the Chinese government began to take more fervent steps toward promoting the globalization of Chinese medicine (Wang and Cai 1999, 17–21).

In the long run, therefore, the Cultural Revolution merely interrupted the process of expansion and modernization that had been set in motion during the previous decade. And yet, inasmuch as it also constituted the endpoint of the Maoist project, it marked a break whose long-term consequences for the field of Chinese medicine are only gradually becoming apparent. As the predominance of the center was shattered, regionalism and particularistic social relations once more became potent forces in Chinese political and social life. Integrated Chinese and Western medicine—so powerfully promoted during the Cultural Revolution—emerged as a potent third force within China's health care system that continuously threatens to disrupt the stability of its parents. As China marches toward a neoliberal market economy that is socialist only in name, Chinese medicine, too, is subject to reconstruction by economic forces that appear to be far more powerful and corrosive than those unleashed by successive waves of Maoist revolution.

During the 1980s—a period that may yet come to be seen as the final flowering of Chinese medicine as an independent medical tradition—such developments were as yet only barely visible on the horizon. It was a decade of ferment and, at least initially, fervent optimism. Economic reforms promised undreamed-of prosperity, and China's intellectuals were dizzy with the new modernity opening up before them. A range of "fevers" swept the country: "new methodology fever" explored the possibilities of rational science, "root searching fever" tried to understand the present through the possibilities of the past, and "*qigong* fever" tried to cure everything by getting in touch with specifically Chinese energies. Meanwhile, "Chinese medicine fever" (*zhongyi re*) had erupted in the West and offered physicians in China new forms of legitimization, new students, and new possibilities of escape (Chen 2003; Wang 1996).

Inventing Qigong

David Ownby

Qigong ("the discipline of the vital breath") is a modern term for physical and mental disciplines based on traditional Chinese regimes of meditation, visualization, and *taiji*-like exercises. Much like the "Traditional Chinese Medicine" formulated by the People's Republic of China, *qigong* was invented and popularized in the 1950s as part of a nationalistic reaction to the perceived threat of Western medicine to traditional medical practices and practitioners. Older traditions were "scientized," their "superstitious" language replaced with new, modern terminology to be employed by newly trained technicians who administered *qigong* to ailing patients in clinical settings. Yet despite some state support through the mid-1960s, the Cultural Revolution (1966–1976) denounced *qigong* as "feudal superstition," and it largely disappeared from official view.

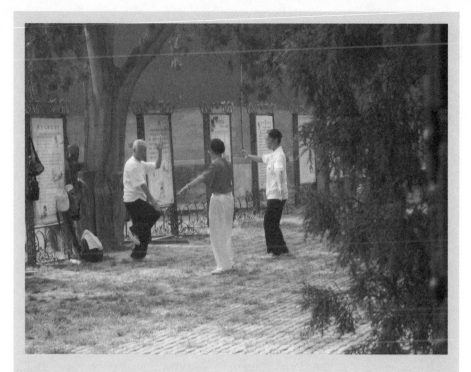

Figure 8.3. Group engaged in public *qigong* practice in Tian Tai Park, Beijing. Courtesy of Linda L. Barnes.

During the mid-1970s, however, individual *qigong* masters began appearing in urban parks. Not part of the medical establishment, they had developed their own healing methods, which—lacking a better term—they called *qigong*. By the late 1970s, laboratory experiments by respected Chinese scientists claiming to prove the material existence of *qi* restored the practice to official favor, expediting its incorporation into China's quest for modernization and the party's for legitimacy.

Advocates included scientists who continued to conduct experiments, journalists who publicized *qigong*'s power and benefits to the Chinese public, charismatic masters whose numbers increased along with burgeoning public interest, and, most important, party and government officials who saw in *qigong* a powerful "Chinese science" as well as a practical, economical means to achieve a healthier population (at a time when China was dismantling its free urban health care system). The China Qigong Scientific Research Association was established in April 1986 as a state organization mandated to oversee *qigong* activities.

The 1980s witnessed a massive *qigong* boom (*qigong re*) involving as many as 200 million practitioners, who elevated some charismatic *qigong* masters to the equivalent of rock star status. The first "grandmaster" was Yan Xin, a previously unknown Chinese medical practitioner. Scores, if not hundreds, followed, including Zhang Hongbao, Zhang Xiangyu, and Li Hongzhi, founder of Falun Gong (literally, "practice of the revolving dharma wheel"). The most popular built nation-wide organizations and carried out national lecture tours. Thousands of enthusiasts bought tickets. Such events, held in local arenas or stadiums, lasted for hours. In addition to *qigong* techniques, masters often preached traditional morality and spirituality, suggestive of new religious or cultural revitalization movements.

Some claimed to "emit *qi*" during their "lectures," a telling difference between the *qigong* of the 1950s and that of the 1980s. Whereas 1950s *qigong* had been a therapeutic practice administered by a trained professional in a clinical setting, post-Mao *qigong* involved the magical power of a charismatic hero. "Therapy" consisted of diffusing his personal *qi* toward a mass of followers. Many taught the cultivation of supernormal powers—of interest to China's military-industrial complex, which dreamed of using *qigong* to speed China's return to great-power status. Many masters took advantage of the newly market-oriented Chinese economy to produce *qigong* books and paraphernalia for an eager public.

By the 1990s, some authorities began to question at least the excesses and abuses of certain masters. Debates arose concerning *qigong's* scientific value. Beginning in April 1999, the boom ended, following a confrontation between Falun Gong and the Chinese government. Although grounded in *qigong*, Li Hongzhi had taken Falun Gong in a more clearly religious direction, failing to respect tacit rules of political prudence by encouraging his practitioners to engage in open—if always peaceful—protests against government and media criticism. Beginning in 2000, *qigong* disappeared from China for several years, but it is currently resurfacing under the title "medical *qigong*," to distinguish itself clearly from Falun Gong.

Although the Chinese medicine sector also became infected, its inherent traditionalism—and perhaps its constant engagement with the materiality of the body—ensured that the fever never reached the levels it did in other cultural arenas. Yet, for a while at least, the strategies and tactics by which Chinese medicine should be inherited and developed (*jicheng fazhan*) appeared to be up for genuine discussion. Some physicians turned with renewed vigor toward the integration of Chinese and Western medicine, hoping to move forward more easily now that they were no longer constrained by Maoist ideology and the material deprivations of revolution. Others went beyond reductionist biomedicine in an effort to align their ancient tradition with the dynamic sciences of the late twentieth century: systems theory, cybernetics, and quantum mechanics (Dong et al. 1990).

On the other end of the spectrum, a renewed interest in China's past allowed physicians to emphasize once more their own genealogies and lines of descent. Just as in the villages of rural China, where lineage institutions experienced a widespread revival, family medical traditions and medical lineages were celebrated once more, while the promotion of individual identity asserted itself as a renewed virtue (Brandstätter 2000). With a center that, for the moment at least, was content to devolve more power to the regions, authorities in the provinces, counties, and cities throughout the country promoted local medical traditions. Doing so represented an effort to project their cultural pedigree onto the national and international stage without challenging the overall dominant power of the state (Hu 1990; Liu and Zhou 1999; Wuzhong yiji bianxiezu 1993).

The 1980s thus witnessed the (re)emergence of diverse genres of writing that juxtaposed the state-promoted orthodoxy of a unified national medical tradition, on one hand, with perspectives emphasizing individuality and plurality, on the other. This literature included the personal experience of individual physicians transmitted in case records (yi'an) and medical essays (yihua), as well as officially sponsored research into local medical traditions and scholarly currents. The authors and publishers of this literature and their motivations for writing it were as diverse as the spirits of the time. They included individual physicians and their families interested in promoting or enhancing a particular image or reputation, publishing houses on the lookout for new market niches in a newly competitive market, and historians in state institutions working under the direction of national, regional, and provincial political bodies.

Leading this search were the laozhongyi, the "senior physicians" of Chinese medicine, for whom the politics of "inheriting and developing" opened up a space in which they could regain some of the pride and status stripped from them a decade earlier. Their need was matched by an equally strong yearning among younger physicians for idols untainted by revolutionary excess and for genealogies of descent through which they could reconnect as individuals to Chinese medicine as a living tradition. Judith Farquhar has shown how this convergence of interests expressed itself in a series of widely acclaimed and often intimately personal biographies entitled Paths of Famous Senior Physicians (Ming laozhongyi zhi lu). Written by China's most famous laozhongyi and their students and published during the mid-1980s in the journal New Chinese Medicine (Xin zhongyi), these biographies depict Chinese medicine not as an

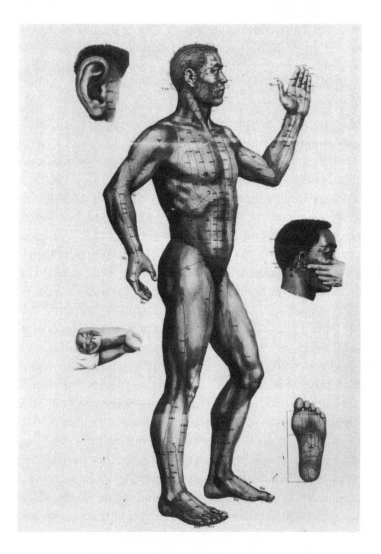

Figure 8.4. A modern anatomy chart for Chinese medical students shows the acupuncture points and meridians. Courtesy of World Health Organization.

abstract medical system but as a personal achievement realized through a life of ongoing struggle (Farquhar 1994a, 1995; Zhou et al. 1981–1985).

These *laozhongyi* were the same physicians, of course, who twenty years earlier had labored to create a space for their own teachers within Mao Zedong's treasure house. If, at the time, they legitimized their efforts by linking them to the Maoist project of systematization, synthesis, and nation building, they now added a rhetoric of self-cultivation that harked back to the moral codes they had learned in their youth. Those *laozhongyi* who regained their previous positions within the medical bureaucracy and institutions, furthermore, devoted whatever time and energy they had left in their lives toward translating these personal memories into social facts. If ultimately they failed in diverting Chinese medicine away from the attractions of science and technology and back toward a tradition based on personal self-cultivation, they succeeded, at least, in creating some of the narratives through which Chinese medicine continues to remember itself in the present.

1989–Present

In 1989 the Chinese state once more used brutal force to reassert its hegemony in the cultural and political domain. Neither Chinese medicine students nor their professors were known for their radical politics, however, and the events in Tiananmen Square did not cause visible ruptures within the field of Chinese medicine. Their aftereffects, rippling across its apparently tranquil surface, continue to be felt today as the development of Chinese medicine mirrors that of the nation at large. The policy of paying equal attention to Chinese and Western medicine remained in place throughout the 1990s, as did the official rhetoric of "developing and carrying forward" the heritage of the Chinese medical tradition. From this point on, however, that project was joined to the establishment of a neoliberal economy that favored a more unregulated market with less government involvement. This orientation places the onus of providing for health care needs back onto the individual and has as its goal the integration of China (and Chinese medicine) into the networks of the emergent global economy.

For the politically orchestrated expansion of Chinese medicine onto the world stage, this meant that regularization and standardization—necessary for any practice seeking to escape the attachment to specific local contexts—acquired a new urgency. Beginning in the late 1980s, multiple directives were passed that sought to define standards in everything from diagnosis and treatment to technologies and management. As of January 2010, 305 standards have been issued and five professional technical national committees established. Increasingly, China is pushing to impose these standards internationally, culminating in 2009 in the submission of a proposal by the Standardization Administration of China (SAC) to the International Organization for Standardization (ISO) to establish a technical committee for the development of standards in Chinese medicine (Zaslawski and Lee 2010). Imposing its own standards globally is not merely a tool in globalizing Chinese medicine but also in maintaining control of that process, and in warding off the competing interests of other East Asian medical traditions.

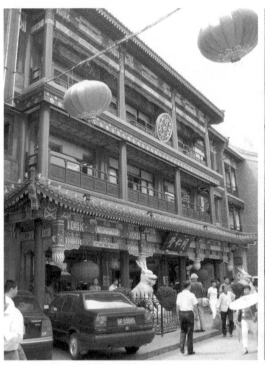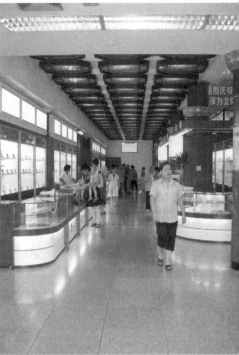

Figure 8.5. *Left:* Exterior of Tongrentang Pharmacy in Beijing. *Right:* Interior of Tongrentang Pharmacy. Tongrentang is one of the oldest pharmacies in the city. Courtesy of Linda L. Barnes.

Research mirrored on biomedical paradigms has become the only acceptable way to carry tradition forward. Universities of Chinese medicine now collaborate with international pharmaceutical companies in the development of new drugs to be placed on world markets. For half a century, scientization had always been the stated goal but Maoist dialectics and the importance of practice left sufficient room for self-cultivation and the development of personal styles of practice. Now, younger physicians openly suggest that the only logical conclusion of this development is for Chinese medicine to be gradually assimilated into a single and universal biomedicine. A good example would be the debate on the future of Chinese medicine conducted in the *Shanghai Journal of Chinese Medicine and Pharmacology (Shanghai zhongyiyao zazhi)* in articles published in 1999 and 2000.

This vision strikes fear in the hearts of older physicians. As animal experiments, molecular genetics, randomized controlled trials, and the language of evidence-based medicine rather than the understanding of medical classics become the foundation of medical practice and the management of individual careers, many of the older generation feel bitter and left behind. They complain

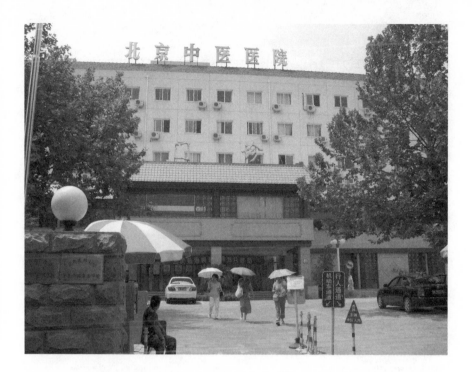

Figure 8.6. The Traditional Medicine Hospital of Beijing. Courtesy of Linda L. Barnes.

that their students can speak English but are unable to read the *Inner Canon*, that in the search for "knowing why" *(zhi qi suoyiran)* they have lost sight of the fact that what matters most in medicine is "knowing how" *(zhi qi ran),* and that their tradition is undergoing a dramatic decline (Wang 2003).

Objective facts support these claims. Following the expansion of the Chinese medicine sector in the 1980s, it has dramatically contracted since then. At the end of 2002, for instance, only 66 percent of all counties still had a Chinese medicine hospital, while the average number of Western medicine hospitals stood at 4.45 per county. Of 85,705 medical institutions in the country, only 3,801, or less than 5 percent, belonged to the Chinese medical sector. By the end of 2006, this number had fallen by yet another 20 percent, to a mere 3,009. The number of consultations in the Chinese medicine sector, too, is falling dramatically. In 2001, this number stood at roughly 900 million, or about 20 percent of all consultations in the official health care sector. By 2006, this number had fallen to just 300 million. As hospitals have been forced to generate revenue for themselves, Chinese medicine—in particular, labor-intensive practices such as acupuncture—are increasingly considered uneconomical. Physicians are actively encouraged to use revenue-generating biomedical tests, insidiously enhancing the importance of biomedical data in Chinese medical practice (Köster 2009, 67).

Chinese Medicine as Popular Knowledge in Urban China

Judith Farquhar

By the turn of the millennium the barefoot doctor and her hybrid version of Chinese-Western medicine were long gone. However, new fusions of Chinese and Western medicine constantly appear in the booming health information market. Increasing state efforts in the early 2000s to fund health insurance for rural and urban residents privilege biomedical services, but these new programs remain inadequate to meet the needs of the seriously ill. Those at risk for expensive illnesses, especially aging people on limited retirement stipends, often turn to preventive health care. For this they use home resources to craft wholesome daily regimes, especially drawing on the literature of classical Chinese medicine. Many of these swimmers, joggers, taiji practitioners, kite flyers, meditators, and ballroom dancers refer to their healthful activity as *yangsheng,* "nurturing life."

A plethora of medical information is available to Chinese urbanites. Radio programs on managing diabetes through diet, lectures in community halls on keeping one's memory sharp, television features demonstrating the benefits of acupressure massage, and advertising in every medium for dietary supplements (calcium is favored, as is ginseng)—these are just a few examples of a vast public health discourse. We recognize throughout these media the global proliferation of medical information, ever changing and often self-contradictory, that has Americans eating hormone-free beef and Japanese office workers running on treadmills. But in China, traditional Chinese medicine forms a significant part of the popular literature.

Consider the many books available in the large "life nurturance and health maintenance" *(yangsheng baojian)* sections of Beijing's neighborhood bookstores. One impressive example is the *Complete Life Nurturance Writings from the Inner Canon of the Yellow Emperor,* ten paperback volumes that reorganize advice from the classic for easy reference and practical use. The *Life Nurturance Canon,* by contrast, is pocket-sized but just as useful: it organizes inspiring quotes from classical works into short thematic chapters about everyday health. Other titles announce their topics: *Chinese Medical Methods for Building Brainpower, Ancient Chinese Maxims on Life Nurturance, Famous Senior Chinese Doctors Discuss the Dao of Life Nurturance*—the list of such works goes on, even when we focus only on those with significant classical medicine content. Such works reveal the persistent hybridity characteristic of "traditional" medicine in the twentieth century: disease names (diabetes, high blood pressure) are often biomedical, while therapies are often separated from whole regimes of treatment or health maintenance. What is declared to be "Chinese medicine" or "ancient maxims" has been retooled for modern use.

Popular literature maintains little distinction between Chinese and Western medicines or medical knowledge. Deep logical contradictions between the two would seem to require consumers to make some choices about which "system" they most "believe" in. Certainly in today's Beijing, one meets people who proclaim their adherence to traditional medicine and their distrust of biomedicine. But the historical affiliation of information is less important than its practical use. When asked how they find reliable information, most people privilege personal experience. If a product or procedure has worked once for someone whose joys and ills are well known, it is worth trying, whatever its cultural character.

Classical Chinese medicine, moreover, can be used without requiring doctors, laboratory tests, or expensive drugs. *Yangsheng* practices are more easily incorporated into one's life than biomedical care. Thus, a persistent category for organizing health information is the classical concept of *qiju*, or

Figure 8.7. Popular books, including business, biography, and health-related self-help works, being sold on the street in Beijing, 2007. Courtesy of Judith Farquhar.

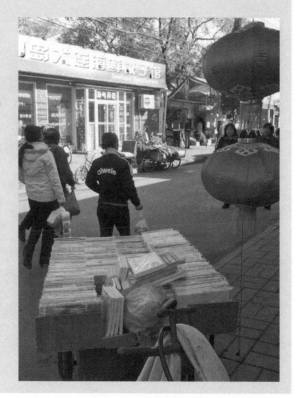

"rising and resting." The term is often translated, appropriately, as "daily life." It includes common sense about dressing warmly, sleeping enough, eating regularly, and getting outdoors. Some of these tidbits are classical. All are practical. Yet even through this mundane category, the unmistakable voices of the medical classics can still be heard in the modern cacophony of advice about health.

Within China, with the introduction of market reforms in the 1980s, the Three-Tiered Health Care Network has been dismantled. Its comprehensive insurance scheme, based on a concept of shared social responsibility, has been replaced by a cash-for-service system that denies access to even the most basic health care to those who cannot afford it—especially peasants in rural areas. In this system, patients shop for health care much as they would for other goods on the market. This approach has further been encouraged by the state, which has relaxed rules for the sale of over-the-counter remedies.

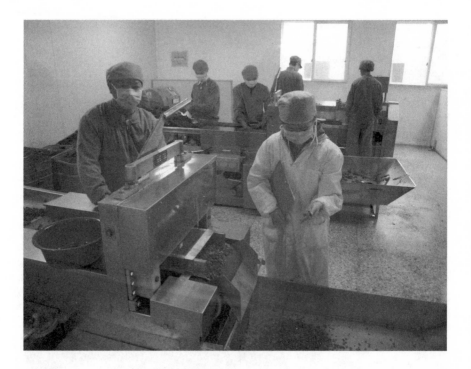

Figure 8.8. Herb production. Courtesy of Erich Stoeger.

Seal Penis, Viagra, and Sexual Potency in Post-Mao China

Everett Zhang

Heightened anxieties about male sexuality have attended post-Mao consumer culture and capitalist competition, accompanied by a flourishing "medicine for males" *(nanke)* to address the problem of male impotence, as well as changes in related medicines. For example, earlier prescriptions for impotence in Chinese medicine and other nonbiomedical traditions contained animal parts such as cock liver, carp gallbladder, crow eggs, seal penis *(wanaqi;* also called *haigoushen,* literally "sea dog kidney"), and reindeer velvet *(lurong).*

Some of these animals are endangered. When Viagra, an anti-impotence drug, entered the Chinese market, one researcher predicted it might help protect some endangered species. He speculated that impotence patients would choose Viagra over Chinese medicine, decreasing the demand for seal penises and reindeer velvet (von Hippel 1998). Yet this prediction was not borne out. Researchers have looked for related trade statistics (von Hippel and von Hippel 2002) but have not established causal links between consumption of animal parts (e.g., seal penis) and fluctuations in the animal trade (e.g., seal meat) (Hoover 2003). The researchers even sought clinical evidence that patients were leaving traditional practices in favor of Viagra (von Hippel et al. 2005). Yet although many men in China did use Viagra, and some did leave older practices, these changes did not necessarily contribute as much as had been hoped to protecting endangered species.

Historically, impotence has often been seen as resulting from deficient kidney Yang, an etiology dating from the Ming period. Because *haigoushen* and *lurong* are on the Yang side, both have been used to nourish the liver and the kidney meridians. However, as clinical experience and an epidemiological study from the late 1990s show, this etiology has changed over the past two decades, challenging this earlier dominant model. One prominent example emphasizes Liver Stasis and related emotional problems, requiring smoothing of the Liver or nourishing Kidney Yin, instead of strengthening Kidney Yang. This shift may trace to changes in male bodies and the potency of the general male population, related to significant changes in nutrition over the past two decades in China or to greater caution with strong minerals, herbs, and animal parts (reindeer velvet, for example, is now considered too powerful). Most contemporary prescriptions contain neither *haigoushen* nor *lurong* but, rather, herbs.

Moreover, although Viagra induces erections, many patients still value recovering or strengthening potency, defined not just as the ability to get an erection but also as overall vitality. The latter requires nourishing the whole body (e.g., seminal essence) to restore the general balance of *qi*. Those who use Viagra may take Chinese medicine concurrently, alternating between the two medicines and related ethical regimes—the new focus on satisfying desire and the historical emphasis on cultivating a combination of sexual potency and vitality. To a large degree, this "switching between Chinese medicine and Viagra," or the "blending" of two medicines (von Hippel et al. 2005, 237), accounts for the low sales of Viagra during its early years in the Chinese market.

Indeed, China is one of the places in the world where Viagra sales have not matched manufacturer expectations. Early optimism derived from the establishment of men's medicine following the 1980s and the Maoist period. Men now felt encouraged to pursue their own gratification—a marked change from the collectively oriented Maoist regime, which had been hostile to individual desire and self-cultivation. It is thus possible that although biomedical anti-impotence technology may have a growing impact on people's sex lives, it may not be as dramatic as expected. Rather, medicine in China continues to epitomize the value of difference, whether in the body, medicine, or ethics.

In the countryside in particular, much of Chinese medicine was thus pushed into the private sector, with many former barefoot doctors opening their own practices. In the cities, where hospital physicians on the whole are still not allowed to run their own practices, dosages of Chinese medicine formulas are steadily creeping up, because physicians earn a percentage of what they prescribe. Tied in various ways to older practices of life cultivation, Chinese medicine is also discovering and moving into new markets: beauty therapy, weight loss, psychology, and the treatment of male and female infertility. Shamanism and other forms of non-state-controlled healing also reemerged, filling a gap in the market for those to whom access to Western or Chinese medicine is being denied, or whom it has been unable to help (Farquhar 1996a, 1996b; Jia 1997).

Religious Healing in the People's Republic of China

Thomas DuBois

Today, religious healing continues to coexist with both Chinese and Western medicine, especially in rural areas. Although the People's Republic has managed to bring at least basic medical care to even the remotest villages, many continue to seek the services of such healers. The reason is not a disdain for medicine but the recognition of different types of sickness. Using terms borrowed from Chinese medical theory, religious healers will often divide sickness into Substantial *(shi)* and Insubstantial *(xu)* types. The first are identifiable medical conditions, such as infection or cancer, which should be treated by a doctor of either Chinese or Western medicine. The second are those caused by supernatural forces and can manifest as general weakness, erratic behavior, or unexplained physical symptoms. These conditions are beyond the power of doctors to cure and should be referred to religious healers. Such healers continue to practice in large numbers, and in many areas every village will have at least one, usually an older woman.

In southern Hebei, these practitioners are known as Incense Masters *(xiang-tou)* and heal through the power of fox spirits. When a patient is brought before them, an Incense Master will determine whether the sickness is Substantial or Insubstantial by burning three sticks of incense, the Ghost Incense *(guixiang)*, Life Incense *(mingxiang)*, and Transcendent Incense *(xianxiang)*. If the center stick burns brightest, the patient has a Substantial sickness and should be referred to the village doctor. If the left or right stick burns brightest, the patient is being afflicted by a disaffected human ancestor or mischievous animal spirit, respectively. The patient must then determine whether he has somehow offended these spirits.

In one case, a villager was made ill for by neglecting to sacrifice to the spirit of his dead mother; in another it was because he had beaten a stray dog to death. In both instances, the first act of the healing regimen was to make restitution to these spirits. Occasionally spirits will make children sickly in order to shorten their life span and hasten their return to the spiritual realm. Such cases are treated by "switching children" *(huan tongzi)*, a ritual that involves burning a doll to ascend to heaven and act as a proxy. In other cases, the cause might be a spirit who is simply evil. Such spirits must be exorcised, either

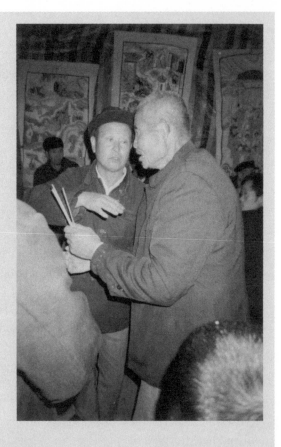

Figure 8.9. A *xiangtou* (the man on the left) instructing a patient to burn incense as appeasement for a past misdeed. Courtesy of Thomas DuBois.

through a scripture-chanting ritual or by giving the patient tea leaves or ashes that have been blessed by the fox spirit. Either way, the Incense Masters themselves do not have power to diagnose or heal, but rather serve as conduits for outside spiritual forces who work through them. (DuBois 2005, 65–85)

It is only quite recently that this trend is beginning to change as the state is rediscovering Chinese medicine as a tool to make health care available once more to a rural population that had simply been priced out of the market. In a movement harking back to Mao's creation of barefoot doctors, the recently passed Twelfth Five-Year Plan for Chinese medicine envisages the training of 15,000 Chinese medicine clinicians for hospitals at county level by 2015, and of 30,000 Chinese medicine general practitioners for grassroots medical facilities. By the same year, every Chinese city at prefecture level is to have a TCM hospital, while 95 percent of community health care centers and 90 percent of township health clinics will also provide Chinese medicine services (Xinhua News Agency 2012).

In the cities meanwhile, with an increasingly affluent middle class able to spend money on health care, famous Chinese medicine doctors are becoming, once again, sought after providers of highly valued personal skills that can earn them fortunes. Riding on the back of the recent root-searching *(xungen)* movement, Chinese medicine professors like Qu Limei from Beijing or Liu Lihong from Guangxi have turned themselves into national media stars, writing best-selling books on how to employ the *Inner Canon of the Yellow Emperor* for purposes of personal self-cultivation, or speaking for an authentic tradition that lies beyond urban state-controlled institutions (Qu 2008; Liu 2006). Hence, classical texts are more readily available than ever before in bookshops as well as on CDs and the Internet.

In recent years, a movement has sprung up that vociferously criticizes the modernization of Chinese medicine over the past few decades, arguing for a return to more classical medicine or claiming that truly effective Chinese medicine can now only be found in the countryside. Local and regional medical currents are making a revival supported as in earlier eras by local money and local pride. Some of these local traditions have even become internationally recognized brands. One example is the "Fire Spirit Current" *(huoshen pai)*, a style of Chinese medicine that originated in Sichuan in the late nineteenth century and emphasizes the use of high dosages of warming medicinals such as aconite *(fuzi)*, ginger *(ganjiang)*, or evodia *(wuzhuyu)*. It now has vociferous proponents throughout the world who hail it as one of the most effective forms of Chinese medicine (Lu 2006).

The global expansion of Chinese medicine feeds such yearnings for ancient traditions unpolluted by the dark sides of modernization even as it increasingly becomes commercialized along biomedical lines. On June 4, 1997, the State Council decided to implement a national research program during the period from 1998 to 2010. Research into Chinese medicine formulas was listed as one of forty-two projects in the program and was allocated funding of approximately U.S. $7 million, the largest grant for Chinese medicine research ever awarded at the national level. This research program has, as its main objectives, enhancing the understanding of formula composition and efficacy and advancing technologies of production for traditional pharmaceutical products in order to introduce them into the mainstream of international pharmaceutical markets (Li and Liang 2007). A decade later, this policy is beginning to reap its first rewards. Early in 2012 *Di'ao xin xue kang*, produced by the Chengdu-based Di'ao Group, received marketing authorization from the Medicines Evaluation Board of the Netherlands, making it the first Chinese traditional drug to be identified as a therapeutic medicine in the European Union (Cheng 2012). Tasly Pharmaceutical Co. Ltd., based in Tianjin, is currently involved in

Phase III trials to license a similar Chinese medical product with the FDA (Icon 2012). Many Chinese medicine physicians, therefore, self-consciously envision the twenty-first century to be the century of Chinese medicine (Wang 1995)—leaving us to wonder whether the laments of their elders regarding the loss of tradition from "traditional Chinese medicine" express instead mourning about the loss of their own power in a country that increasingly values youth over age.

In the future, therefore, historians may once again need to change their perspective in order to understand and describe medicine in China. The analysis may require moving away from an emphasis on Western and Chinese medicine and their confrontation, interaction, and interpenetration, turning instead toward a more fractured field of medical practice. This field is at once increasingly open to global influences that include not only the global techno-cultural networks and markets to which it has sought access over recent decades but also global disease vectors rapidly transmitted across borders. It is also open to these influences precisely because it is constituting itself as a market to the needs and choices of local consumers.

SARS, Bird Flu, and Media Transparency in China

Hepeng Jia

Severe acute respiratory syndrome (SARS), which killed 774 people worldwide before abating in July 2003, affected not only China's struggling public health system but also its media practices. After first holding back information about the outbreak, the Chinese government responded to pressure from the public, other governments, and international organizations such as the World Health Organization by setting up a daily reporting system in April 2003, and maintained it until the epidemic subsided. It restored this system during two small-scale outbreaks in late 2003 and April 2004, as well as during the spread of H5N1 bird flu in 2004 and 2005. Government departments provided experts to address media questions, and the Ministry of Health released epidemic-related information through a spokesperson.

Official channels such as Xinhua News Service, *People's Daily,* and China's central TV station covered the outbreaks, making other media reports redundant. This apparently self-regulated reporting provided background, discussed research, featured people's reactions, and examined the spread of the diseases

TABLE 5

Number of SARS articles published by four sampled newspapers through June 2003

	February and before	March	April 1 to April 20	April 21 to June 30 (to July 2 for Southern Weekend due to its weekly publication)
People's Daily	5	3	45	648
Health News	10	1	96	430
Southern Metropolis News	86	11	114	936
Southern Weekend (Weekly)	7	0	2	55

(Source: Author's statistics)

abroad. A sampling of such media shows no negative reporting related to the government's prevention and treatment measures. (See Table 5.) Sensitive information was often delayed or contradicted, and domestic media reports were blocked internally.

The government refuted reports about the initial human H5N1 infections. It denied research findings that isolated the virus from a poultry market in Fujian province, which the government had declared a virus-free zone, and would not acknowledge the detection of a new viral strain of H5N1 (Smith et al. 2006). Rather, the government argued that the virus had spread from other countries into China, whereas Hong Kong virologist Guan Yi's discovery of the genomic structure of the wild-type virus indicated that it had actually originated in China itself, in a poultry market in Fujian province, which the government had declared a virus-free zone.

No evidence suggests that these gaps in reporting derived from direct censorship. Indeed, a ban would have been impossible because much of the information not yet reported in China had already circulated through the international media, reaching some Chinese through the Internet. It may be, however, that media leaders and editors, after years of following the "right" propaganda direction (and witnessing measures taken against those who strayed from it), had learned to self-censor. For example, on December 27, 2003, the Guangzhou-based *Southern Metropolis News (Nanfang dushibao)* reported without authorization that a suspected SARS patient had been found in a Guangzhou hospital. The Ministry of Health confirmed the story that same day, but the deputy editor in chief responsible for allowing the report was sacked. The imprisonment of the paper's general manager for alleged corruption followed.

Although no Chinese media overtly challenged the government's control over information, some provided key details through oblique descriptions of real situations. For example, China did not acknowledge the cases of human H5N1 infection and death that had occurred in a Hunan village in late October 2005 until mid-November. Prior to this acknowledgment, the financial review *Caijing* had reported on village rumors surrounding deaths that followed a family's eating sick chicken. In other cases, rather than addressing the government's denial of unfavorable claims, Chinese media have reported those claims, as with Guan's findings on a wild type of H5N1 virus. Chinese media thereby avoided directly criticizing the government while also providing the public with information about serious public health issues. Still, the blocking of unfavorable messages, sporadic punitive measures against "disobedient" media, and media leaders' self-censorship have contributed to a style of medical reporting in China constrained by what is deemed orderly and politically safe.

Conclusion

Chinese medicine's history in contemporary China has been a history, above all, of having to adapt to the changing realities of a plural health care system created and directed from above by a powerful state. Yet if the state demanded change in order to fit into the system(s) it laid out, it also provided Chinese medicine, in return, with a degree of autonomy and a safe environment in which it was able to experiment with various forms of modernization. Yet now, as the power of the state itself is threatened by the demands of the global socio-technical networks to which it has opened itself up, and a new accommodation between local identities and universal process is called for, it is perhaps not surprising that a new wave of attacks on the very right of Chinese medicine to exist has been launched.

On October 7, 2006, Zhang Gongxi, a professor at the Research Institute for Science, Technology, and Social Development of Zhongnan University, published a petition on the World Wide Web that called for "Chinese medicine to be abolished." Although government institutions quickly assured Chinese medicine physicians and the public that they had no plans to act on Zhang's petition, a lively debate about the place of traditional medicine in a modern society has erupted in the media and Internet chat rooms throughout the country. In March 2007, the influential *China Newsweek* (*Zhongguo xinwen zhoukan*) led with a cover story on the state of Chinese medicine that painted a picture of a tradition in severe crisis (Li and Liang 2007). That same month, China Union Medical University Press published a four-volume series of books entitled *The Great Debate About Chinese Medicine in the New Century (Zhongyi xin shiji dalun zhan)*, which allowed both sides in the debate to square off against each other in the public domain.

Whatever else divides the participants in these polemics, they agree that Zhang Gongxi's proposals constitute but the "third wave" of an attack first launched by Yu Yunxiu's draft law to the National Assembly in 1929 and followed by the Proposals for the Reform of Chinese Medicine of the early 1950s, both having been conceived with a similar purpose in mind. On each occasion, the supporters of Chinese medicine were able not only to deflect these attacks but also to use them as a springboard from which to consolidate their position within society. These victories carried a heavy cost, however—the surrendering of Chinese medicine's autonomy to powerful outside influences, most important among them the state and biomedical science. If this forced opening up corroded Chinese medicine's authenticity as a self-defining medical tradition, the 1920s and '30s, and then the 1950s and '60s, also proved to be periods of intense creativity. Precisely because their very survival was at stake, Chinese medicine physicians were forced to (re)define their relation to past, present, and future. In the eyes of some, it is precisely this ongoing questioning of what is at stake in one's practice that is the hallmark of any living tradition. In that sense, current debates about Chinese medicine's value to China and the world in the twenty-first century attest that, even as it struggles to survive, it remains very much alive.

NINE

A WORLD OF CHINESE MEDICINE AND HEALING: PART ONE

Linda L. Barnes

IN LATE 2006, the World Federation of Chinese Medicine Societies sponsored the first issue of the *Journal of World Chinese Medicine*. The editorial committee and senior consultant group included "more than 100 famous physicians and leading scholars." The journal proposed to reflect "the present level of the development of Chinese medicine all over the world, so as to promote international communication and cooperation in R&D, medical service, education, information exchange of medical and pharmaceutical products, and scientific management of Chinese medicine among countries" (WFCMS 2009).

When, in 2002, the World Health Organization (WHO) published its strategy related to traditional medicine, it repeatedly cited "Traditional Chinese Medicine" (TCM) as an example (WHO 2002). The study recognized not only that traditional medicines were widely used in their countries of origin but also that many such medicines had migrated into Western countries, first as "unconventional medicine," next as "alternative medicine," and then as "complementary/alternative medicine," moving toward the category of "integrative medicine." Issues of policy, safety, assessment, and quality took on new importance in connection with global health.

Yet the very word "traditional" would prove unexpectedly complicated. Something could be defined as traditional only in contrast with something else—whatever was considered "modern," for example. As Volker Scheid has pointed out, "Many so-called traditional medicines are revealed as inventions of distinctly modern regimes of knowledge and institutional practice, while the political needs of healers and the epistemological desires of researchers converge in the construction of distinctive medical practices for description, classification, and comparison" (Scheid 2002b, 136; see also Jennings 2005).

The formal identification of Chinese medicine and related healing practices as a world tradition by such highly placed organizations highlighted a reality that had been part of Chinese Diaspora experience in East Asia, Oceania, South Asia, Africa, the Middle East, Europe, and the Americas for as long as outside voyagers and overland travelers had journeyed to China, learned about its healing practices, and returned with knowledge about what they had observed (Barnes 2005b). Over the past centuries, some immigrant practitioners have also left behind letters, prescriptions, and, in a few cases, their actual herbal collections.

Yet relatively little systematic study has focused on the dissemination and flourishing of Chinese healing traditions throughout the world over time. Scholars such as those represented in this chapter have directed their attention to particular local settings; this is an essential step toward developing a more comprehensive picture, but much work remains to be done. It calls for sifting through archived newspapers and magazines—both immigrant Chinese and non-Chinese—including their advertisements; family letters and photographs; museum collections and family artifacts; and histories of the Chinese in different locations, because in those histories one often finds references to practitioners and practices.

However, as the chill of the Cold War lifted, the People's Republic of China (PRC) sought to promote not only its revolutionary model in general but also that model's application to medicine in the renaissance of acupuncture and the creation of the "barefoot doctor." It also dispatched doctors of its own "Traditional Chinese Medicine" to different parts of the world as part of larger diplomatic and commercial initiatives. Some Western imaginations were stirred, and small numbers of pilgrims went to the margins of China, or to other parts of the Chinese Diaspora, to study acupuncture and related healing arts, meditation practices, and alternative approaches to religious and spiritual life.

For others, teachers proved to be closer at hand—longtime practitioners in Chinese immigrant communities or, as immigration policies changed in different parts of the world, newer émigrés from the PRC (sometimes brought out of China by prospective students in Europe and the United States). Texts generated in the PRC provided new sources for thinking about Chinese medicine and healing, as did the genre of martial arts films coming out of Hong Kong, along with teachers of Buddhism and Daoism sought by a generation of spiritual seekers, particularly in some of the Western countries. Earnest students and followers produced their own books, recordings, and sometimes films to transmit what they were being taught—both to promote the work of their teachers and, increasingly, to spread the hybrid understandings of those teachings that were taking shape outside China.

Yet the paradox of this burgeoning phenomenon lies in its inversion of previous relationships and balances between the various branches of Chinese medicine as a whole, and in particular its positioning of acupuncture as the face of Chinese medicine. As previous chapters have richly demonstrated, until the twentieth century acupuncture had never played a central role in Chinese medicine. Yet now it is the one branch of the tradition that routinely comes to mind, at least for non-Chinese. There is a history to this change, which this chapter will address. It is important to add that although the chapter reviews developments in different parts of the world—an undertaking greatly enhanced by the discussions provided by the other authors in this volume—many of its examples and illustrations will be drawn from the United States, as that is the country within which the author has conducted her research. This is in no way to suggest that the United States stands as an exemplar for Chinese healing arts as world practice; rather, as a large country, with a rich Chinese American legacy, it provides useful case material with which to compare and contrast the lay of the land in other parts of the world.

Waves of Migration

Chinese medicine and healing arts have entered parts of the world outside of China through multiple pathways and trajectories. This phenomenon first occurred in the countries surrounding China, leading to the varieties of schools and strains of practice that took root in Taiwan, Hong Kong, Korea, Japan, Vietnam, and other countries in the region. This historical process dates back centuries.

Chinese have also migrated to other parts of the globe for various reasons: economic pressures; an increase in the number of avenues for leaving the country, whether legally or illegally; changing immigration regulations; and emergent social options for educated and professional groups, businesspeople, and the poor. Such factors have generated waves of immigration characterized by variations in these factors. Each wave has also varied in the degrees and ways that women were included.

Much of the early traffic occurred through trade, whether conducted by Chinese merchants taking up residence in surrounding countries or by foreigners trading with China. Many foreigners involved in the China trade employed Chinese sailors, carpenters, and other workers at various times, as the Spanish did in the 1600s when they hired Chinese labor through the galleon trade that rounded Africa and India and which from China went on to the west coast of the Americas. By the eighteenth century, Chinese sailors were settling in American cities such as New York, where some married Irish women and set up boardinghouses, restaurants, and other services for their countrymen (Barnes 2005a). Many were from China's southeast and spoke Cantonese, Chaozhou, Hakka, and Min Nan dialects.

Earlier groups often clustered in communities where Chinese businesses and services had concentrated. In part, this provided a more familiar and welcoming setting; in part, exclusionary policies, combined with local violence, often made it safer to live among other Chinese immigrants. These "Chinatowns" took root around the world. Some existing Chinatowns have expanded with migration from different parts of China, as in the new Fujianese section of New York's Chinatown; elsewhere, new ones have sprung up, as in Flushing, a neighborhood in the borough of Queens in New York City. Some of the most recent arrivals have entered the United States, Canada, various countries in Western Europe, Australia, New Zealand, and other Pacific island nations with undocumented status, aided by gangs of smugglers known as "snakeheads" (shetou), and consequently have been forced to live under the radar.

Groups with greater resources were likely to eschew these Chinese neighborhoods to the extent that local practice or policy didn't restrict where they could live. They were then more likely to go to the local Chinatown on weekends for groceries, supplies, restaurants, medicines, and practitioners. More recently, different Asian groups in cities such as Houston, Texas, have joined together to build malls with a concentration of Asian businesses. These business centers are called Chinatowns, too, and serve not only Asian customers but also non-Asians. Yet regardless of how they came into the country, each group brought its healing traditions—often interwoven with its religious worldviews, and nuanced by factors related to the group's departure from China and its reception in its adopted country.

For some Chinese immigrants settling among other groups, it was the first time they had been forced to experience themselves as "Chinese" in ways defined by others. This included finding themselves inserted into categories of race, ethnicity, and class over which they often had little control. For example, during the nineteenth century in the United States, Chinese immigrants in some of the western states were legally assigned to the same racialized category as Native Americans and prohibited from testifying in court. In the state of Mississippi, however, the Supreme Court ruled in 1927 that the Chinese belonged to the same category as African Americans, making them a "colored race" subject to segregation law. More recently, the census category of "Asian" has overridden differences between disparate "Asian" ethnicities and cultures.

Chinese workers arrived in early twentieth-century South Africa to work in the mines. Although most returned to China by 1910, the eventual institution-alizing of apartheid classified them as "colored," excluding them from voting, denying them equal opportunities in business and education, and preventing them from living in white communities. Then, following the establishment of an economic alliance between Taiwan and South Africa in 1970, Taiwanese im-migrants were granted the status of "honorary whites"—which had the indirect effect of reducing some of the stigma imposed on more-established Chinese South Africans and decreasing some of their vulnerability to segregation. Although not considered "honorary whites," the latter group still began to be accorded more of the privileges enjoyed by white South Africans. However, since 1994, additional waves of immigration have resulted in some 300,000 Chinese in South Africa. In a somewhat surprising turn, the Chinese Associa-tion of South Africa sued the government in 2006, arguing that being treated as white now excluded them from benefits being extended to victims of apart-heid. The high court ruled in their favor, reclassifying them as "black" and

TABLE 6

Timeline 1: 16th century through the 1930s—events cited

16th–19th c.	Mexico: First known Chinese immigrants to Mexico
	United States: Chinese immigrants entering North America; following 1785, entering through China trade
1897	United States: Foo and Wing Herb Company publish *The Science of Oriental Medicine*
1927	France: Soulié de Morant begins translating Chinese works and training French doctors
1930s	China: John Shen *(Shen Hefeng)* founds Shanghai Medical College
1938	China: John Shen founds Shanghai Medical Clinic
1939	France: Soulié de Morant's *L'Acuponcture Chinoise* (1939–1941)
	Japan: Kodo Fukushima becomes acupuncturist, develops theory and techniques for blind practitioners

thereby rendering them eligible for affirmative action programs. The court ruling, however, benefits only those ethnic Chinese whose families were in South Africa prior to 1994 (Canaves 2008).

Whether externally imposed or sought out, such classifications have filtered into how Chinese medicines and healing arts have been viewed and represented not only by surrounding groups but also by Chinese practitioners themselves, marketing to other groups. Non-Chinese who adopt Chinese practices may reconfigure their own identities depending on choices provided by their era and surroundings (and sometimes in reaction to those choices). Such factors further complicate the meanings assigned to "Chinese" healing around the world.

Acupuncture and Moxibustion

The modalities of acupuncture and moxibustion have spread throughout the world via multiple channels. The following sections sketch some of these trajectories, with the recognition that in a work of this scope, any such review is inevitably incomplete. The objective is to illustrate that what is frequently represented as a single channel of transmission is, more accurately, a set of diverse streams generated by multiple stakeholders. Some have played a minor role internationally while being significant locally; others have reached national and even international prominence. As the PRC's version of TCM assumed global dominance, the other currents faced the challenge of differentiating themselves and, in some cases, defending their place in the larger field. Yet with time, they have resurfaced or resumed their earlier influence in different quarters, suggesting the fluid configuration of relationships between them.

Transmission through Immigration

By the nineteenth century, the first immigrants to leave China came from the circles of merchants, diplomats, scholars, and businesspeople, many of whom intended to return to China eventually. Most met with a generally welcoming response in the receiving countries. However, as economic crises in southern China led growing numbers of unskilled workers to emigrate and traffickers to profit from transporting them, the welcome often dwindled, forcing immigrants into contained enclaves.

Such communities relied on self-care and other therapeutic interventions, as well as seeking reassurance that spiritual forces were acting on their behalf. Some individuals trained in Chinese medicine journeyed to these locations and set up practice; sometimes the practitioners were self-taught individuals who had read a variety of books and then learned in the field. Gradually, many of them began treating patients from the receiving culture.

Yet their introduction of acupuncture into different parts of the world did not necessarily occur in a vacuum. In France, England, Scotland, Germany, Italy, the British colonies in North America, and eventually the United States, surgeons in particular were already familiar with reports brought back from China by missionaries, traders, and diplomats; in some cases they themselves had written about and experimented with both acupuncture and moxibustion, beginning at least as early as the seventeenth century (Barnes 2005b; Bivins 2000). However, this did not lead them to seek out Chinese immigrant practitioners. On one hand, they accepted acupuncture and moxibustion as variations on their own practices of bloodletting, cauterization, and electrical stimulation. At the same time, as their articles and reports attest well into the nineteenth century, they rejected theoretical frameworks grounded in such concepts as the Dao, *qi,* Yin and Yang, and the Five Phases (Barnes 2005b). This dynamic would, to varying degrees, characterize acupuncture circles and eventually organizations in these countries. Constituted largely along ethnic lines, such groups often saw only partial intersections. Only since the 1980s have these organizational intersections increased.

Transmission through France and Vietnam

French interpretations of acupuncture predated developments in the PRC. In addition to the information about acupuncture that entered France through Jesuit reports beginning in the seventeenth century (Barnes 2005b), in the early twentieth century Georges Soulié de Morant (1878–1955) played a pivotal role in this transmission process. Having learned Chinese in childhood, he initially considered going into medicine, but entered banking instead, and then eventually joined the French diplomatic corps. As a French consul in China, he observed acupuncture during the cholera epidemic in Beijing, leading him to seek training from teachers in cities where he served. One of those cities, Yunnan, was close to the Indochinese border of the time. Thus, some of the styles influencing his understanding of the modality originated in what would later become Vietnam.

Following his return to France in 1918, Soulié de Morant took his daughter in 1927 to see physician Paul Ferreyrolles (1880–1955), an advocate of alternative therapies. Ferreyrolles, who participated in a study group interested in such therapies, learned of Soulié de Morant's experience with acupuncture. The group persuaded Soulié de Morant to translate related Chinese works and train French doctors in its use. His writing drew on texts such as the *Great Compendium of Acupuncture and Moxibustion (Zhenjiu dacheng)* and *Introduction to the Study of Medicine (Yixue Rumen)* and the teachings of Japanese acupuncturist Takeshi Sawada. He also built on his own experience from testing needling on himself (Deshpande 2001).

In addition to numerous articles, Soulié de Morant published *Précis de la vrai acuponcture chinoise* (1934)—which contributed to his being nominated for a Nobel Prize in 1950—and then the first part of *L'Acuponcture chinoise* between 1939 and 1941. He completed the whole work before his death in 1955. The full text appeared in 1957, with an English translation in 1994. Yet, despite its role in the acculturation of acupuncture in Europe, the text was slow to gain traction in the United States. In 1981, acupuncturist Paul Zmiewski found in a Sri Aurobindo ashram in Pondicherry, India, an English translation prepared by a French-American team (Felt 2006c). This discovery occurred during what were still the relatively early days of Chinese-to-English translations of Chinese medicine texts. Translators such as Nigel Wiseman had begun to develop lists of terms in what would become a longer-term project to develop a standardized nomenclature. Both he and Zmiewski were connected with Paradigm Publications, under the direction of Bob Felt, who decided to sponsor a full translation. The project finally came to fruition in 1999 and involved collaboration with the heirs of Soulié de Morant, who provided the actual index cards he had used while writing the book (Felt 2006c).

A second intellectual tributary representing French understandings of acupuncture came through Dr. Roger de La Fuÿe, whose father had served as a general in the French army in Vietnam (then Indochina)—a period that saw exchanges between French and Vietnamese doctors in Hanoi and Saigon and with doctors in France. As a result, a number of French military hospitals established acupuncture consultations. De La Fuÿe founded both the French Acupuncture Society (Société française d'acupuncture) in 1943 and the International Acupuncture Society (Société internationale d'acupuncture) in 1946. His work influenced developments not only in France but also in Austria and England, especially through physician Felix Mann.

A third French tributary involved Dr. Paul Nogier (1908–1996), who decades earlier had helped organize the Ligue Homéopathie Internationale (International Homeopathy League). In the early 1950s, Nogier observed small burn scars in the ears of some of his Algerian patients. They told him about Madame Barrin, a lay practitioner who had treated them for sciatica by cauterizing particular points in the ear. Nogier went to North Africa to learn more (Borsarello 2005). After much experimentation, he determined that if certain points in the ear were tender when palpated, they corresponded to specific dysfunctions in other parts of the body. He argued that problems with different organs manifested in different zones of the ear, a connection predicated in part on the premise that the external ear bears a resemblance to an inverted fetus.

In 1956, Nogier was encouraged by Jacques Niboyet (1913–1986) to present his work to the Mediterranean Society of Acupuncture, a group founded the year before by Niboyet, who himself had studied acupuncture with a Chinese man (Borsarello 2005). In turn, German doctor Gérard Bachmann heard about the work, translated it, and published it in a German acupuncture journal in 1957 (see Nogier 1956, 1957). Japanese practitioners picked up Nogier's system, which then entered China, where it encountered the resurgence of interest in acupuncture and underwent extensive testing. Alongside acupuncture analgesia and scalp acupuncture, the PRC adopted it, eventually folding it into the training of the barefoot doctors (see Hsu 1992, 1996). In 1958, the PRC published a Chinese version of the Ear Chart, later recognizing Nogier's influence by giving him the sobriquet "father of modern auricular therapy."

A fourth line of transmission arose through Dr. Albert Chamfrault, a student of Soulié de Morant, who went to Vietnam as a naval officer. Eventually Chamfrault wrote *Traité de médecine chinoise* (Treatise on Chinese Medicine), the six volumes of which were published from 1954 to 1969. The coauthor of the final volume was Dr. Nguyên Van Nghi (1909–1999), originally from Hanoi.

Both Van Nghi and Felix Mann (see below) had studied *Introduction to Chinese Medicine (Zhongyixue gailun)*, a foundational text on Chinese medicine commissioned by the PRC for the new TCM colleges (Nanjing Zhongyi xueyuan, 1958). The Vietnamese Communist government in Hanoi had the book translated as *Trung Y Hoc* in 1959, which Van Nghi's *Pathogénie et pathologie énergétiques en médecine traditionnelle chinoise* regularly cited. Ironically, the PRC government did not go on to privilege this pre-TCM version of Chinese medicine, deciding instead in favor of other constructions.

Yet another French transmitter was Jacques Lavier, who developed an interest in Chinese calligraphy as a child, eventually combining the practice of medicine with an interest in sinology (Wu 1962) and going on to study, practice, and write about acupuncture (see Lavier 1966, 1974, 1977). Some of his students—J. R. Worsley, Oscar Wexu, Richard van Buren (see below), and Mary Austin—played key roles in disseminating the practice internationally. Such interpretations provided foundations for acupuncture in Italy; only later would the Italians turn more directly to developments in the PRC (see Candelise 2008). For decades, the Chinese and Vietnamese traditions that had informed French styles remained largely unrecognized outside of Europe, except by the students of the

Table 7

Timeline 2: 1940s–1950s—events cited

1940s–1960s	China: Ding family's College of Chinese Medicine in Shanghai teaches more than 70 percent of leading traditional physicians
1943	France: Dr. Roger de La Fuÿe founds Société française d'acupuncture in 1943 and Société internationale d'acupuncture in 1946
1949	England: Ilza Veith translates first thirty-four chapters of *Huangdi neijing*
1950s (early)	England: J. R. Worsley pursues acupuncture training in Taiwan, Singapore, and Korea
	Japan: Dr. Yoshio Manaka invents ion-pumping cords
1952	England: Johannes Diedericus van Buren begins learning acupuncture in 1952, eventually studying in France under Jacques Lavier
1954	England: Joseph Needham publishes vol. 1 of *Science and Civilization in China*
	France: 1954–1969 Dr. Albert Chamfrault, *Traité de médecine chinoise*, 6 vols.
1956	England: Worsley founds College of Traditional Acupuncture in Leamington Spa, England
	France: Dr. Paul Nogier presents his work, which is published in a German acupuncture journal in 1957
1958	China: *Nanjing Zhong yi xue yuan*, a foundational text on Chinese medicine commissioned by the PRC for the new TCM colleges; PRC publishes a Chinese version of Nogier's Ear Chart
1959	Vietnam: Vietnamese translation *Trung Y Hoc*

different writer-practitioners and the individuals they in turn had trained (see "Transmission through Québec," below).

It should be noted, too, that between 1990 and 2000, a Vietnamese professor named Nguyên Tai Thu—founder of the Tan Cham (new acupuncture) school and known for his use of *mang cham* (snake needle) practice, which employs needles of up to eighty centimeters in length—trained thousands of Mexican physicians in acupuncture. Some Mexican medical schools have started acupuncture courses, and four centers have been established to provide treatments. The Vietnam Central Acupuncture Hospital graduated twenty Mexican practitioners in 2007 from a three-year training program ("Vietnamese Acupuncturists" 2007, "World Famous Acupuncturist" 2007).

ACUPUNCTURE IN ARGENTINA

Betina Freidin

Acupuncture has had a long-standing presence in Argentina and is currently practiced there by East Asian immigrants, biomedical doctors and other health professionals, and by Argentinean practitioners. It is thought that Japanese and Chinese immigrants informally introduced acupuncture into the country in the early twentieth century (Remorini 2005). However, the greater numbers of immigrants arriving from Taiwan during the 1980s and from mainland China during the 1990s contributed to its popularizing (Bogado Bordazar 2003; Sui Lee 1999; Zhu 2002). During the 1980s, these immigrants initiated a process of formal organization by opening schools of acupuncture and other modalities of Chinese medicine and creating professional associations (Zhu 2002; Remorini 2005). At the same time, Argentinean acupuncturists, trained either in Argentina or abroad, opened other training centers.

In 1997, hoping to raise their members' professional status, the Association of Chinese Acupuncturists in Argentina invited the Committee of International Examination of the World Federation of Acupuncture-Moxibustion Societies (WFAS) (Zhu 2002). This strategy did not pay off, however, since WFAS credentials lack official recognition in Argentina. In 2000, the Association of Acupuncturists and Naturopaths (CAN) was founded to certify non-MD acupuncturists. Since 2001, CAN has brought bills before the National Congress to pass certification and licensing laws; these efforts have also been unsuccessful.

Although acupuncturists who are not medically qualified had always risked prosecution for practicing medicine illegally, the National Ministry of Health's passage of physician-supported Resolution 997 in 2001 worsened matters by restricting the practice to MDs. In 2008, the ministry also authorized physical therapists to practice acupuncture. Neither measure improved the situation of practitioners who did not have a degree in biomedicine or physical therapy. Moreover, Argentinean physicians' long-term interest in acupuncture and the strategies they employ to monopolize the practice have been key factors in deterring the advancement of non-MD practitioners.

Attracted by the spread of medical acupuncture in France, a small group of Argentinian physicians began practicing it in the late 1940s, organizing the Argentinean Society of Acupuncture (Sociedad Argentina de Acupuntura, SAA) in 1955 as a branch of the International Society of Acupuncture. Since 1959, the SAA and the Medical Institute of Acupuncture (founded in 1960) have offered courses for MDs. Yet medical acupuncture, despite its promising beginnings, has lagged in Argentina in comparison with other Latin American countries, remaining largely marginal within the biomedical profession. Only recently have a few medical schools offered courses in acupuncture.

Outside of a few states, no health policies integrate medical acupuncture into Argentina's health system. Social insurance programs and private insurers do not cover treatments (World Health Organization 2005). The passing of Resolution 997/01, however, has favored expansion of medical acupuncture in the public sector. MD acupuncturists have resorted to extensive international biomedical research into the efficacy and physiology of acupuncture. They have lobbied the National Congress to pass legislation recognizing acupuncture as a medical act and limiting its practice to MDs. To date, this legislative battle has not succeeded.

With the collapse of the national economy in 2001, many immigrant acupuncturists either returned to their homelands or emigrated to the United States or other Latin American countries. Those who stayed in Argentina counted on transnational political and academic capital to try to create a niche for educational programs in Traditional Chinese Medicine and acupuncture, as officially taught in mainland China and promoted by global professional associations such as the WFAS and the World Federation of Chinese Medicine Societies. Institutes run by Argentinean non-MD acupuncturists have also resorted to foreign academic sponsorship in order to stay in the market. They promise training and credentials based on international standards, to prepare trainees for the eventuality of the CAN-supported bills getting passed (Freidin 2008). Such efforts notwithstanding, these groups remain at the margins of the health system in the midst of loose governmental controls.

Transmission through Québec

Oscar Wexu was a Romanian physiotherapist who had moved to Paris to flee the Nazi invasion. There he had studied acupuncture, and cofounded the International Society of Acupuncture (ISA) with Van Nghi and Jean Schatz. Eventually Wexu relocated to Montreal with what he had learned from Lavier and Soulié de Morant. In 1972, he established the Institut d'acupuncture du Québec (Quebec Institute of Acupuncture), as a section of the ISA (Reid 2008). As Van Nghi became more involved with the style of TCM found in the PRC, his influence led Wexu to change the program's name to the Institut de médecine traditionnelle chinoise du Montréal (Institute of Traditional Chinese Medicine of Montreal) in the early 1980s.

The legacy of the Quebec program has continued. Although Wexu's school itself did not survive, his students exercised considerable influence, contributing to official recognition of acupuncture as a profession in Quebec with the adoption of the *Loi sur l'acupuncture* in 1994. Collège Rosemont in Montreal, a junior college, is the now only institution in Québec to offer certified acupuncture training; funded by the province, tuition for the intensive three-year acupuncture program (taught in French) is virtually free (Reid 2008). In the United States, the program's influence has carried down through its American students, as the following section details. Additionally, the Tri-State Institute of Traditional Chinese Acupuncture, founded in 1982 in Stamford, Connecticut (and now the Tri-State College of Acupuncture in New York City), started by Mark Seem and Walter Bosque, was originally founded as an affiliate of the Institute of Traditional Chinese Medicine of Montreal.

Transmission through Harlem

Over time, students from the United States began to attend the Wexu's school in Montreal. For example, in 1970, Lincoln Hospital in the South Bronx in New York hired Mutulu Shakur (b. 1950, also stepfather of revolutionary rapper Tupac Shakur [1971–1996]) as a political education instructor for their drug detoxification program for victims of heroin addiction, who were being given methadone. He, along with community activists in New York City from groups such as the Black Panthers, the Young Lords, the Health Revolutionary Unity Movement (a Bronx-based group of health workers), and White Lightening (a group of former victims of addiction) led the initiative, for what became known as the Lincoln Hospital Detoxification Program, or simply the People's Program (Burton-Rose 1997).

At around this time, two of Shakur's children were injured in a car accident. Through activists from the I Wor Kuen (named after the original Boxer Movement), a revolutionary Chinese American organization in New York that ran a health service for the older Chinese community, Shakur learned about traditional Chinese medicine. The group connected him with an Asian woman acupuncturist, who treated and cured his children, leading him to take an interest in China's historic struggle with opium addiction (Friends and Family N.d.).

Counselors at the clinic learned about the work of Dr. Hsiang-Lai Wen (1923–) in Hong Kong. Wen, who had heard of the PRC's application of acupuncture with anaesthesia, applied needles to the ear of an opium addict undergoing surgery. The patient noted not only that the needles reduced his pain but also that his withdrawal symptoms diminished. After that, Wen began testing acupuncture and electroacupuncture to treat addiction, publishing his findings (Wen and Cheung 1973a, 1974; Wen, Cheung, and Mehal 1973).

In 1974, the Lincoln clinic introduced acupuncture to help with heroin and methadone detoxification. Staffers came across a book on ear acupuncture by Oscar Wexu's son Mario. Some of the counselors—Shakur, Urayoana Trinidad, Walter Bosque, Richard Delaney, and Wafiya among others—went to Montreal to study with Oscar Wexu at the Quebec Acupuncture Association, where Shakur and others obtained a Doctorate in Acupuncture in 1976. He was licensed to practice acupuncture in the State of California that same year, later became Director of the Lincoln Detox Acupuncture Research Unit, and went on to visit the People's Republic of China, and to speak in wide circles about his work at Lincoln hospital.

One of the Lincoln clinic's open houses for potential volunteers attracted Mark Seem, to whom Shakur gave the task of translating Van Nghi's *Pathogénie et pathologie énergétiques en médecine traditionnelle chinoise* and other instructional materials in French, to enable English-speaking students to access the course more easily. Some of these American students also earned diplomas in acupuncture over the next few years. Wexu's son Mario even moved to New York City for a year to help establish the Lincoln Detox School of Acupuncture and to supervise the final phase of the students' clinical acupuncture training. (Other prominent American acupuncturists, like Misha Cohen, first studied at the Bronx school.)

In 1977, Lincoln Hospital closed its clinic to the acupuncture school and volunteers; the police confiscated the records of the clinic and school (Federal agents claimed that Shakur was using both as a front for resistance activities). Psychiatrist Michael Smith, who had trained in acupuncture and served as one of the physicians required by law to supervise nonphysician practitioners, was put in charge of the acupuncture detox program, which was renamed the Lincoln Acupuncture Clinic. He was subsequently credited with having initiated and developed it. Shakur and others went on to establish the Harlem Institute of Acupuncture, a separate branch of the Quebec institute. In August of 1980, Shakur also began the Black Acupuncture Advisory Association of North America (BAAANA) while continuing his involvement in Black liberation movements.

The FBI's counterintelligence program accused Shakur of participating in a clandestine paramilitary group and of taking part in robbing armored trucks between 1976 and 1981 to fund the acupuncture clinic and other Black liberation initiatives. He was indicted in 1981, leading him to go underground. At the same time, the FBI raided the acupuncture school, depleting its resources and eventually forcing its closing (Barbanel 1981a, 1981b; McFadden 1981a, 1981b). Shakur himself was arrested in 1986. He was convicted and sentenced to sixty years' imprisonment (Announcer 1992; "MutuluShakur.com" 2009). Shakur is now held in prison in the United States Penitentiary, Victorville, in Adelanto, California, with a projected release in 2016.

The Menghe-Ding Transmission

During the late nineteenth century, the town of Menghe, which lies about halfway between Shanghai and Nanjing in southern China, emerged as a medical hub, its literati doctors exercising national influence. One family, the Dings, became particularly well known, eventually producing Ding Ganren (see Chapter 7). This elite medical network continued to shape medical developments in China throughout the twentieth century. According to Ding Yige, great-grandson of the founder, from the 1940s into the 1960s the Ding family's College of Chinese Medicine in Shanghai taught more than 70 percent of the leading traditional physicians ("Producing New Disciples" 2008); this group would shape the early directions of the PRC's version of TCM and thereby influence international understandings of Chinese medicine. In New York, therapeutic relationships between members of the Ting (Ding) family—particularly Dr. Ching Yuen Ting (Ding Jingyuan)—and family members of key political figures in the state opened doors to legislative support for legalization (Brody 1971; Scheid 2007).

During the 1930s, John Shen (Shen Hefeng, 1914–2001), from a wealthy Shanghai family, went to the Shanghai Medical College both as a student and then as an apprentice, and studied pulse and facial diagnosis as well as herbal medicine. In 1938, he founded the Shanghai Medical Clinic. Ten years later, with the

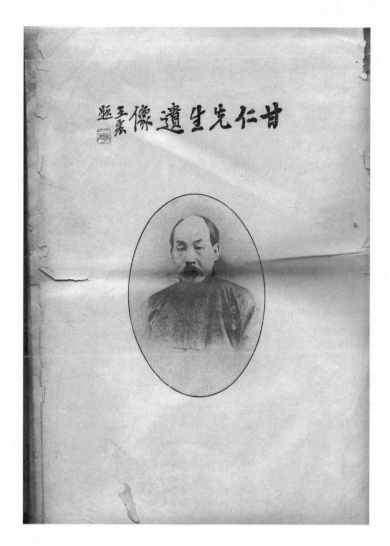

Figure 9.1. Ding Ganren. Courtesy of the Ding family and Volker Scheid.

outbreak of the revolution on the mainland, he relocated to Taiwan, where he practiced for seventeen years. He also continued to practice and learn in other settings, including Vietnam. There he may have encountered a local family tradition of pulse diagnosis. From 1965 to 1971, at the invitation of the National Medical Association of Malaysia, he traveled throughout Southeast Asia, working as a consultant and seeing more than fifty thousand patients (Scheid 2001; Rosen and Stickley 2007).

In 1971, Shen moved to New York. Eventually he set up clinics in New York and Boston, his reputation growing not only among patients (including the socially elite) but also among practitioners, many of whom hoped to study with him. He became famous in particular for his expertise in pulse diagnosis and his ability to resolve complex cases, and he taught key figures in the United States, including Leon Hammer, Mark Seem, Giovanni Maciocia, Jane Lyttleton, and Lonny Jarret.

Hammer became one of Shen's best-known students. A successful psychiatrist, Hammer changed course midcareer to study acupuncture with Dr. Johannes Diedericus van Buren (1921–2003) in England between 1971 and 1974. Beginning in 1974, Hammer apprenticed with Shen for eight years, and he worked closely with his teacher over the course of more than two decades. In 1990, Hammer began to offer pulse workshops, and in 2001 he helped to found the Dragon Rises School of Oriental Medicine in Gainesville, Florida—a program known particularly for its emphasis on pulse diagnosis. Hammer, in turn, influenced the next generation of practitioners, including Will Morris, Heiner Fruehauf, Ray Rubio, and Brandt Stickley, who would go on to found their own schools or contribute to key developments in Chinese medicine in the United States. Shen returned to Shanghai for the final years of his life, dying there in 2001 (Scheid 2007).

Transmission from the People's Republic of China

As Volker Scheid has observed, one the Maoist government's objectives was to reorganize and revise Chinese medicine in ways that would modernize *(xiandaihua)*, regularize *(guifanhua)*, scientize *(kexuehua)*, and sort out *(zhengli)* its theoretical underpinnings. Nor was this initiative entirely new, as we have seen in Chapter 7 and Chapter 8. Rather, the adoption of a Maoist, Marxist framework, with its focus on social transformation, reoriented earlier emphases. Elite literati physicians largely directed the project, except during the Cultural Revolution, when many of these same individuals were marginalized (Scheid 2002).

Occasional stories about these initiatives filtered into media overseas, with reports of large-scale public health campaigns, the application of acupuncture and, in some cases, herbal medicines. During the late 1960s, the image of the barefoot doctors *(chijiao yisheng)* inspired a small number of leftward-leaning Americans. Some, such as Ted Kaptchuk, Dan Bensky, and others, went to East Asia during the 1970s to study acupuncture and herbs. Upon returning to the United States, they became some of the earliest non-Chinese promoters of Chinese medicine. Others found teachers locally in cities like New York and San Francisco and became apprentices.

These examples notwithstanding, the classic account about the introduction of acupuncture into the United States points to a story filed in 1971 with the *New York Times* by reporter James "Scotty" Reston following the removal of his appendix, using standard surgery, at the Anti-Imperialist Hospital in Beijing. Subsequently Reston suffered severe postoperative pain, which Dr. Li Chang-yuan treated with acupuncture (Reston 1971). The story somehow reached an American audience in new ways, giving rise to what some Chinese-American practitioners would later call the "acupuncture heat."

This phenomenon generated new levels of national and even international interest in acupuncture in particular. Some Chinese medicine doctors who had learned in pre-PRC schools or from family lineages had previously focused on herbalism. Those who left mainland China following the revolution found public interest directed primarily to their acupuncture training, whether or not they had used the modality extensively prior to their arrival. Medical missions also went to the PRC, while researchers attempted to align Chinese and biomedical concepts and to figure out how acupuncture worked. Master practitioners were recruited to teach in other countries. For example, Dr. Ju Gim Shek (known as Dr. Kim), who had taught a small group of non-Chinese students in San Francisco, took one of them, Steve Rosenblatt, to Hong Kong to meet his own teacher, Dr. James Tin Yau So. Dr. So accepted Rosenblatt's invitation to come to Los Angeles, and in 1975 he founded the New England School of Acupuncture just outside of Boston, Massachusetts, with some of his students.

The advent of the Cultural Revolution imposed considerable hardship on older doctors of traditional medicine in the PRC, as well as on any TCM doctor viewed as politically suspect. The explosion of interest abroad resulted in some joining the faculties of foreign schools of Chinese medicine. Their influence, coupled with growing international exchanges between schools and practitioners, gradually resulted in the TCM of the PRC becoming a dominant international influence on conceptual frameworks, curricula, standards, and ways of thinking about the integration of Chinese and biomedicine. This widespread outcome often generated the impression that Chinese medicine was and is synonymous with TCM.

Transmission through England

Johannes Diedericus (Dick) van Buren was born in Jakarta, Indonesia, to Dutch parents who were also Theosophists, and who later moved the family to India. During World War II, van Buren went into the Dutch army; he was taken prisoner in Java by the Japanese and held for four years. Following the war, he trained in England as a naturopath, osteopath, and homeopath. He began learning acupuncture in 1952, eventually studying in France under Jacques Lavier, and later in Taiwan, where he was awarded a doctorate in acupuncture. In 1972, he founded the International College of Oriental Medicine in England and Holland, attended by many European students. He would teach Leon Hammer and Giovanni Maciocia (who also studied with J. R. Worsley). Van Buren died in May 2003.

Jack Reginald Worsley (1923–2003) came from a working-class background in Coventry, England. While in the British army as an education officer, he also studied physiotherapy, and eventually osteopathy and naturopathy. At the time, although word of acupuncture was filtering into England through developments in France, there were no British training programs. During the early 1950s, building on his engagement with nonbiomedical modalities, Worsley pursued acupuncture training in Taiwan, Singapore, and Korea, where he encountered styles of practice independent of the version of TCM emerging in the PRC. More particularly, he was exposed to orientations based on the Five Phases or Elements.

In 1956, he founded the College of Traditional Acupuncture in Leamington Spa, England, where he practiced, developed his own understanding of the Five Elements, and taught. Fifteen years later, in 1971, a group of Americans visited him for treatments. Impressed with the treatments' efficacy, the Americans brought him over to the United States in 1972 to give public talks at Big Sur, California, and other sites. Some thirty American and Canadian students subsequently went to Kenilworth, England, to study with him. That first group included individuals who would go on to become key figures in the lineage he was transmitting: Bob Duggan, Dianne Connelly, Fritz Smith, Harriet Beinfield, Efrem Korngold, and Jim McCormick, who described themselves as "latter-day hippies and New Age idealists" (though Worsley wore his customary three-piece tweed suit). For four weeks, ten hours a day, the group attended daily lectures, after which Worsley sent them out to practice.

They quickly decided that they needed further clinical training, which Worsley provided the next year. During the years that followed, these students recruited others. They also returned to the United States and Canada to start their own clinics and, in some cases, to found schools. Bob Duggan and Dianne Connelly, for example, incorporated the College of Chinese Acupuncture in Maryland in 1974 as an outgrowth of Worsley's program. The school changed its name to the Traditional Acupuncture Institute (TAI) four years later, and in 1985 it became the first program accredited by the National Accreditation Commission for Schools and Colleges of Acupuncture and Oriental Medicine (NACSCAOM, now ACAOM). TAI added the School of Philosophy and Healing in Action (SOPHIA) in 1987. For years, American practitioners recognized TAI SOPHIA as the first of the Worsley schools in America, although Worsley himself went on to establish other schools. The SOPHIA program has continued into the present.

One of Worsley's students, Judy Becker from Florida, originally trained as a lawyer, received her license in 1974 and went on to get her bachelor's, master's, and doctoral degrees in the field. By the early 1980s, she was traveling with Worsley to assist in teaching and consulting with patients. They married in 1991 and remained devoted colleagues and partners throughout the rest of his life. As one of Worsley's students recalls:

> He spoke of the elements and suddenly we saw them as never before, vibrant or dying, creative or useless. . . . He spoke of the desolation of a barren field, of rivers drying up and terrifying droughts. Over and over again he would bring alive the consequences to the body/mind/spirit of fire that burns instead of warming, of earth that smothers instead of nourishing. He spoke of the twelve officials in such a way that they became as familiar to us as our friends. You could see the Official of the Small Intestine failing in his task and confusing pure with impure, or could watch a sick Gall-Bladder Official making sick decisions. . . . He aroused a deep pity for the distress of illness and gave us a way of understanding even the most disagreeable of people. (Darby 2003)

A critical part of Worsley's teaching occurred through what he called consultations. Student-practitioners would bring their own patients, observe his treatments, and then discuss the cases together.

Worsley gave master of acupuncture academic certificates to the students he trained. In 1996, one of his students, Sandra Lillie, incorporated the Institute of Taoist Education and Acupuncture (ITEA) in Louisville, Colorado. Currently ITEA is the only degree-granting school in the United States that is recognized within the lineage as transmitting the tradition directly: Judy Worsley continues to teach there, and J. R. Worsley's daughter, Hilary Skellon, is the institute's director. In 1997, J. R. and Judy Worsley established the Master Apprentice Program to train selected senior students dedicated to transmitting the tradition as passed on by Worsley himself; the program continues to award the designations of Master Apprentice and Apprentice. Worsley died in June 2003, having designated his wife as his successor (Gumenick 2003; Darby 2003).

Born in Germany, Felix Mann (1931–) first became a biomedical physician in England and then worked in other countries to explore other therapeutic theories. In France, he observed the effective application of a needle below the knee of a patient with appendicitis. This experience inspired him to study Chinese and train with European, Vietnamese, and Chinese teachers, going to

China several times. Eventually he founded and served as the president of the British Medical Acupuncture Society in England.

Like Nguyên Van Nghi, Mann's own early work focused on acupuncture with an emphasis on Channel (*jingluo*) pattern identification and treatment as these were understood and practiced prior to the PRC series of reformulations and standardizations (Mann 1962, 1973a, 1973b). Writings by both Van Nghi and Mann included *tuina* and *qigong* external practices, but not material related to herbology. Ironically, the sway of the PRC reformulations over a period of twenty years resulted in prevailing assumptions that Van Nghi and others had invented their own versions of practice deriving from Vietnamese or French tradition. In fact, they were transmitting a pre-PRC version of Chinese medicine (Seem 2010).

Mann went on to practice, teach, and write the first widely used English-language textbook on the modality, *Acupuncture: The Ancient Chinese Art of Healing* (Mann 1962). (Van Nghi himself cited Mann's early texts.) For many English-speaking practitioners, Mann's works were a formative influence during the 1960s and 1970s, as were mimeographed sheets of acupuncture points from Worsley's early classes, Mark Seem's translations of Van Nghi's works, lecture notes from teachers who had studied with Oscar and Mario Wexu of the Quebec Institute of Acupuncture and, later, Dianne Connelly's *Traditional Acupuncture* (1979).

Ironically, over time Mann redefined his understanding of acupuncture, eventually rejecting theories of acupuncture points and Channels altogether and arguing that neither existed. His books reflect this reversal, particularly *Reinventing Acupuncture* (1992). Over time, both he and Van Nghi allowed their earlier works to go out of print, removing their previous theoretical emphases from circulation.

Transmission through Japan

Japan's acupuncture world is complex and pluralistic and involves both licensed acupuncturists and biomedical physicians. The following are only several examples of a larger world of practice.

One of these involves the practice of acupuncture by blind practitioners—an approach attributed to Waichi Sugiyama (1610–1694), who lost his sight while young. Among other innovations, Sugiyama introduced the use of a guide tube to govern the depth to which the needle can be inserted. He went on to establish forty-five acupuncture schools to train blind practitioners, although lack of financial support following his death resulted in their all closing. Blind

TABLE 8

Timeline 3: 1960s–1970s—events cited

1960s	China: Barefoot doctors
1962	England: Felix Mann, *Acupuncture: The Ancient Chinese Art of Healing*
1969	US/California: Homer Cheng, MD, founds SAMRA (Sino-American Medical Rehabilitation Association), Los Angeles
1970s	US/California: Ted Kaptchuk, Dan Bensky, and others go to East Asia to study acupuncture and herbs
1970	England: Group of Americans visits Worsley for treatments
	US/New York: John Shen moves to New York, sets up clinic; community activists establish Lincoln Detox Community Program
1971	US/New York: James Reston publishes *New York Times* story on acupuncture in China
1972	England: Van Buren founds International College of Oriental Medicine in England and Holland
	Québec: Oscar Wexu establishes Institut d'acupuncture du Québec
	US/California: Worsley talks at Big Sur, California
	US/Maryland: Dianne Connelly's *Traditional Acupuncture*
1973	US/California: Dr. Effie Poy Yew Chow founds East West Academy, San Francisco
	US/Nevada: First state to designate traditional Chinese medicine a "learned profession"
1974	Sri Lanka: Dr. Sir Anton Jayasuriya goes to PRC to study acupuncture
	US/California: Miriam Lee arrested for practicing medicine without a license; Gov. Ronald Reagan declares acupuncture an experimental procedure

(continued)

TABLE 8 *(continued)*

US/Maryland: Bob Duggan and Dianne Connelly incorporate College of Chinese Acupuncture

US/New York: Leon Hammer apprentices with John Shen; Lincoln Detox introduces acupuncture for detoxification

1975   China: *The Outline of Chinese Acupuncture*

England: Mary Austin's *Textbook of Acupuncture Therapy*

Québec: Mario Wexu publishes *The Ear: Gateway to Balancing the Body*

US/California: Steve Rosenblatt recruits Dr. James Tin Yau So from Hong Kong; So goes to Massachusetts to found the New England School of Acupuncture

1976   US/California: Governor Jerry Brown legalizes acupuncture

US/New York: First round of Lincoln Detox students receive Wexu diplomas

1977   US/New York: Lincoln hospital closes detox clinic to school and volunteers; Michael Smith put in charge

1978   Soviet Union: WHO and UNICEF declaration of Alma Alta

US/California: Dr. Joseph Helms develops Medical Acupuncture Program

US/New York: Mutulu Shakur cofounds Black Acupuncture Advisory Association of North America

---

acupuncture persisted for almost a century, but as a minority tradition, until a new private school for the blind was established in 1878. Gradually, more schools came into existence, reviving Sugiyama's tradition. There are now some sixty-nine schools, all government funded.

A second style—Toyohari—was developed by Kodo Fukushima, who lost his sight in 1932 during the war between China and Japan but went on to become an acupuncturist in 1939. He refined the theory and techniques for blind practitioners, who are taught to heighten their sensitivity to the point where they not only diagnose using pulse and abdominal palpation but also do not practice actual insertion of needles into the skin; rather, they hold a needle over a point and insert it into the *qi* system slightly above the skin. It is said that in the practice of this style, sighted practitioners are generally at a disadvantage.

A third orientation traces to Dr. Yoshio Manaka (1911–1989), who first trained as a biomedical physician and then studied the Japanese herbal medicine tradition *(kampō)* and, later, acupuncture with leading acupuncturists in Japan. During the 1950s, he invented "ion-pumping cords" that attached to needles, allowing flow of the patient's electrons between the clips. His own methods drew on international developments, introducing multiple innovations into Japanese acupuncture. For example, he applied color stimulation to specific points and experimented with polarized objects—not only the ion-pumping cords but also north-south magnets and gold and silver needles—to demonstrate the flow of *qi* (see Manaka 1980, 1995).

Three of Manaka's students—Stephen Birch, Kiiko Matsumoto, and Miki Shima—further spread his influence through their own work. Matsumoto, for example, taught first at the New England School of Acupuncture and then at the Tri-State College of Acupuncture (TSCA), and has developed her own style.

As a whole, Japanese approaches to acupuncture differ from some other systems in their emphasis on diagnosis using abdominal palpation, their application of a guide tube, the use of small grains of moxa rather than larger cones, and what to TCM-trained practitioners may appear to be extremely superficial insertion. Instead of inserting needles and leaving them for an extended period of time, practitioners insert needles and then check the patient's pulse, abdomen, joint mobility and pain, and pressure and pain responses in order to gauge the impact of the insertions. The practitioner continues to apply treatment in small increments, then examines these indicators to get feedback from the patient's system before inserting further needles (Fratkin 1999; Fixler and Kivity 2002; Kobayashi, Uefuji, and Yasumo 2007; Ishizaki, Yano, and Kawakita 2010). It should be noted that the Classical Five Element acupuncture transmitted by J. R. Worsley resembles Japanese styles in this last respect.

Transmission through Sri Lanka

In the movement toward a global vision for public health, the World Health Organization and UNICEF held a meeting in 1962 at the University of Kazakhstan at Alma Ata, in the Soviet Union. A formal conference convened in 1978 at Alma Ata produced a declaration calling for health for all by 2000 and supporting both biomedical and traditional modalities.

Biomedical physician Dr. Sir Anton Jayasuriya (1930–2005) of Sri Lanka, who had attended the 1962 meeting to learn more about the use of traditional medicines in different parts of the world, was charged with exploring ways to study, teach, and apply these methods. In 1974, through a scholarship from his government and the WHO, Jayasuriya went to the PRC to study acupuncture. He subsequently collaborated in the establishment of a teaching center at the University of Utrecht, in Holland, and Medicina Alternativa Institute, an international organization at the University of Kazakhstan. However, the costs of studying in Western Europe created enough of a barrier to potential students from developing countries that, in 1987, Jayasuriya established an affiliated program in Sri Lanka, at the Colombo South General Hospital in Kalubowila (Mendis 2005).

In addition to training students in acupuncture practice, Jayasuriya's free government acupuncture clinic allowed physicians and students to spend an intensive month in a paid internship under his supervision. As one student described it: "Hundreds of people were sitting on benches under the shade of huge Temple Flower (Aralia) trees. Many more were moving on paths leading in and out of the clinic, so packed that you could only shuffle slowly along" (Josephs n.d.).

The program represents a minority influence in the larger world of acupuncture. In small pockets of that world, however, it is well known. For example, practitioners such as the Rev. Dr. Richard Browne, founder of the Acupuncture and Massage College in Miami, Florida, trained there, and recalls the program's intensity. Philippe Manicom, founder of Acupuncture at Sea (see below), remembers that before going to France to study, he first learned with a practitioner in Guadeloupe who had studied acupuncture in Sri Lanka.

Transmission through Returns to Old Sources

Each of the branches discussed above views itself as rooted in some authentic branch of Chinese medicine, often characterized as "ancient," and legitimized using a variety of criteria: it was developed within the PRC; it was *not* developed within the PRC; it derived from an old family or temple line, representing previously secret teachings now revealed to outsiders; it carried on traditions that would otherwise be lost; it adapted the tradition to meet the needs of a receiving culture; and the like. Some early immigrant practitioners claimed to have been physicians to the emperor of China.

It is too simple to state that texts serve to transmit traditions. Such a statement leads to further questions: Which texts? Which versions or revised editions? Whose commentaries? In which environment were the texts being used? Some early immigrant practitioners had their own collections of medical books. Doc Ing Hay (see Chapter 10), for example, built up a personal library of Chinese sources on a wide range of topics, even though he lived in the easternmost end of Oregon. Other practitioners—particularly those who were largely self-taught—also relied on Chinese medical books. Occasionally these practitioners wrote their own books in other languages, to garner support and understanding for their medicine. Such was the case with the Foo and Wing Herb Company's 1897 publication *The Science of Oriental Medicine,* out of Los Angeles.

As non-Chinese groups and individuals sought to learn various traditions, it was natural that they resorted to texts written or recommended by their own teachers, or about which they had read in other sources—a process that invariably and necessarily resulted in partial exposure to that tradition. What confounded the process was the disproportionate influence of redacted sources coming out of the PRC. Moreover, as China underwent its own internal transitions, emphases within the medicine shifted as well. Therefore, what was presented as TCM was itself a somewhat fluid body of material.

One early and influential translation was *An Outline of Chinese Acupuncture,* compiled by the Academy of Traditional Chinese Medicine and published in 1975 in Beijing. The compilers positioned the book as a support to Chairman Mao's characterization of Chinese medicine and pharmacology as "a great treasure-house." Readers were encouraged to accept "the guidance of the revolutionary medical line of Chairman Mao" and the "correct path of combining Chinese and Western medicine," which the chairman is quoted as having advocated as early as 1928. Qing period rulers were characterized as having despised acupuncture and moxibustion; it was "the broad masses of the labouring people" whose acceptance and belief in the therapy sustained it (Academy of Traditional Chinese Medicine 1975).

The *Outline* alluded to the *Inner Canon of the Yellow Emperor, Basic Questions* and a number of other texts. However, at the time, few translations were available, outside of a relatively small number in English, French, or German. Ilza Veith (b. 1915), a German historian of medicine who relocated to the United States in 1937, had translated the first thirty-four chapters of the *Inner Canon of the Yellow Emperor.* The massive *Science and Civilization in China,* edited by British historian of science and sinologist Joseph Needham (1900–1995) and his longtime collaborator and eventual wife Lu Gwei-Djen (1904–1991), and particularly their book *Celestial Lancets* (1980), provided a history of acupuncture and moxibustion, along with the other branches of Chinese medicine. However, such scholarship—along with the work of historians Nathan Sivin (b. 1931) and Paul

Unschuld (b. 1943)—made it clear that the story was far more complex than the one told in PRC texts. It became glaringly apparent that the access most researchers and practitioners had to older sources was painfully inadequate.

The project of generating translations would not only result in a voluminous and growing body of sources but also unleash intense and sometimes acrimonious debates over what translation actually means, as well as how such translation and interpretation should be done. In each case, the core question involved what it meant to remain faithful to the terms, concepts, and historical meanings of the texts, as well as the cultural translation.

One approach argues for as precise and standardized an English rendering of each Chinese term as possible, an orientation advocated by leading translator Nigel Wiseman and publishers Bob Flaws of Blue Poppy Publishers and Bob Felt of Paradigm Publications—two of the leading presses relaying Chinese medicine resources to English-speaking practitioners. In contrast, practitioners Harriet Beinfield and Efrem Korngold—authors of the widely read *Between Heaven and Earth: A Guide to Chinese Medicine* (1991)—argue in favor of a more fluid approach that reflects the transplanting of a tradition into new soil (Emad 2006). A differing approach appears in the translations and arguments of scholar-practitioner Dan Bensky, who advocates linking multiple English terms to given Chinese medical vocabulary, to introduce a context-linked flexibility. Bensky's work largely has been published by, and in these debates identified with, Eastland Press in Seattle, Washington.

All agree that Chinese terms are polysemous, with multiple dimensions and meanings. All support the importance of flexibility and sensitivity to context. At the same time, they differ in how they think about actual implementation. What one contingent calls "rigid," the other may view as necessary "rigor." The differences in approach also complicate being able to link discussions about one set of translations with another. As researcher-practitioner Marie Ergil observes, "The terminological choices made by both Chinese and non-Chinese authors and translators of traditional Chinese medicine have greatly affected what students and practitioners learn and understand about traditional Chinese medicine" (Ergil n.d.; see also American Association of Oriental Medicine 2006; Felt 2006a, 2006b).

The debate has also raised the question of whether practitioners should be required to learn Chinese medical language, in order to read sources for themselves. Some schools outside of Chinese-speaking countries have opted to include and, in some cases, require courses in the Chinese language as part of their curricula. Some teach an introductory familiarity with Chinese medical terms; some foster the cultivation of full written and spoken fluency. The Seattle Institute of Oriental Medicine, for example, has its students study Chinese medical language throughout one of its programs, to the point where they can translate case studies and articles.

For some programs, these initiatives coincide with a conceptual commitment to bypass or at least supplement the PRC's version of TCM and to formulate an understanding of the classical roots of Chinese healing traditions. As defined by Dr. Heiner Fruehauf, for example, this has meant integrating Daoist medicine, Jinjing qigong, *Treatise on Cold-Damage Disorders (Shanghan lun)* pulse diagnosis, Sichuan Daoism, and traditional Sichuan folk art and music—"long lost and rediscovered"—into the curriculum of the School of Classical Chinese Medicine at the National College of Natural Medicine in Portland, Oregon. Analogous initiatives have taken shape at the Tri-State College of Acupuncture in New York, among others, with a return to pre-PRC texts and the Confucian and Daoist traditions. The Chinese Medicine Database (2006), an international project dedicated to translating classical Chinese medicine texts and disseminating those translations, has furthered access to previously unavailable works. It is still too early to tell what long-term outcomes this return to older sources will have.

Institutionalization

Schools and programs that had developed around the world prior to the founding of the PRC would, in many cases, continue their work after the establishment of the PRC regime. After publication of the Reston article in 1971 these groups gradually began taking steps to legalize the practice of acupuncture. In the United States, for example, the process has varied from state to state; a few states still have no practice law at all or are still in the process of developing one. Some have not removed the requirement that an acupuncturist work under the supervision of a biomedical physician, and others allow only MDs to practice. And only in 1996 did the Food and Drug Administration reclassify acupuncture needles from the category of experimental device to accepted medical instrument.

The first state to designate traditional Chinese medicine as a "learned profession" was Nevada. As would often prove to be the case in other states, the decision came about largely because of the direct experience of treatment. A New York attorney and real estate developer, Arthur Steinberg, had been deeply impressed by his wife's experience with leading Hong Kong acupuncturist Dr. Lok Yee-kung while they were in Hong Kong seeking help for her headaches.

When the Steinbergs relocated to Nevada, Arthur Steinberg invited Lok to come and introduce the medicine. He then took steps to persuade the Nevada state legislature to issue Lok a temporary license as an emergency bill. Lok set up a clinic in a room above a casino and for three weeks provided free treatments to sixty members of the legislature. So many of them experienced benefits that, as one staff member put it, "it looked like a little Lourdes around here." Shortly thereafter, the governor signed a law allowing the practice of Chinese medicine, including acupuncture, by practitioners who did not have to be biomedical physicians ("The Nation: Acupuncture in Nevada" 1973; Spiro 1973; Edwards 1974).

Sometimes, however, it took court challenges. Miriam Lee (1926–2009), a nurse-midwife, left mainland China in 1949 for Singapore, where she lived for seventeen years. She then went to California and worked in a factory while treating patients, first out of her home and then in an office she shared with an MD. In 1974, after her arrest for practicing medicine without a license, her patients came to her defense at her trial, and then Governor Ronald Reagan established the modality as an experimental procedure. Two years later, Governor Jerry Brown legalized it. Lee herself went on to train many of northern California's acupuncturists. In addition to playing a pivotal leadership role in the state, she was particularly known for transmitting the work of one of her teachers, Dr. Tung Ching Chang (1916–1975), who represented the eleventh generation of a long-standing and closely guarded family acupuncture tradition. Tung himself had left mainland China in 1949, going instead to Taiwan.

Even as practitioners worked for legalization and licensing regulation, they also took steps to transform classes with individual teachers into full-fledged schools, and then these into accredited institutions. In turn, the faculty, graduates, and allies of these institutions lobbied for state-based licensing laws. Over time, with the founding of national associations, an accreditation commission, a council of colleges, and development as a discipline, the field has emphasized growing as a profession within the larger therapeutic world of the country (Barnes 2003b).

In the United States during the 1970s and 1980s, almost three times as many schools opened on the West Coast as on the East Coast. Additional schools grew up during the 1990s. Not all survived. As of the writing of this chapter, in August 2012, the number of accredited and candidate programs varies slightly, depending on the source. The most reliable number, however, comes from the Accreditation Commission for Acupuncture and Oriental Medicine (ACAOM), according to which there are now fifty-three accredited masters programs and one candidate program under review (Accreditation Commission for Acupuncture and Oriental Medicine 2012; see Furth 2011). These programs prepare students to take state licensure and national certification exams. There are now also nine doctoral programs.

Acupuncture in Germany

Gunnar Stollberg

The early history of acupuncture in Germany remains to be written. Although two propagators of knowledge about acupuncture were native Germans, they represent European colonial history. Engelbert Kaempfer (1651–1716) worked as a physician on Dutch East India Company ships and for two years in the company's Nagasaki branch. Kaempfer published *Amoenitates exoticae* (1712); his reports on moxa and acupuncture, like those of the Dutch doctor Willem ten Rhyne (1647–1700), were quoted repeatedly into the nineteenth century. The second, Andreas Cleyer (1634–1697/98), also worked as a Dutch East India Company physician. Some European authors quoted from his *Specimen medicinae Sinicae* (*Examples of Chinese medicine*, 1682) and *Clavis medica ad Chinarum doctrinam de pulsibus* (1686).

During the first half of the nineteenth century, multiple testimonials reflected the use of acupuncture in France, England, and Italy. In 1832, German physician Theodor Kerber quoted from some sixty English, French, Italian, and German authors on acupuncture. He contrasted European and East Asian practices, insofar as Europeans inserted needles at the locus of pain, not according to the channels (Kerber 1832, 29).

Acupuncture's more recent presence in the West started before World War II with Georges Soulié de Morant (1878–1955) in France. During the 1950s, it spread to western Germany (Gleditsch 2001). For example, Dr. Gérhard Bachmann (1895–1967), founding father of the Deutsche Ärztegesellschaft für Akupunktur (German Medical Acupuncturist Association, DÄGfA), adopted the ideas of Dr. Roger de La Fuÿe (1890–1961). The latter served as a military physician in Indochina and published textbooks on acupuncture and "homoeosiniatry," a combination of homoeopathy and acupuncture (Arnold 1976). Dr. Heribert Schmidt, DÄGfA's chair from 1967 to 1970, had learned *kampō*, the Japanese version of Chinese medicine, in Japan. Thus, non-Chinese forms of acupuncture were prevalent prior to the 1970s, when American journalists showcased the acupuncture formulated by the People's Republic of China. Today, German professional organizations mostly teach forms of acupuncture related to this PRC version.

The actual number of acupuncturists and the extent of acupuncture use in Germany are unknown. Many German physicians and some nonbiomedical practitioners belong to acupuncture organizations (see Table 9). Many medical

TABLE 9

Membership of Acupuncturist Associations in Germany, 2003

German Academy for Acupuncture and Auriculomedicine (Deutsche Akademie für Akupunktur und Aurikulomedizin, DAAAM), established 1974	13,600
German Acupuncture Society for Physicians (Deutsche Ärztegesellschaft für Akupunktur, DÄGfA), established 1951	11,000
German Society for Acupuncture and Neural Therapy (Deutsche Gesellschaft für Akupunktur und Neuraltherapie, DGfAN), established 1971 in the former GDR	3,200
German Acupuncture Society Duesseldorf (Deutsche Akupunktur Gesellschaft Düsseldorf, DAGD), 2002	1,600
Association for Classical Acupuncture and TCM (Arbeitsgemeinschaft für klassische Akupunktur und traditionelle Chinesische Medizin; AGTCM), non–medically qualified Heilpraktiker, established 1954	1,050

acupuncturists practice a biomedically dominated integration of biomedicine and acupuncture, using the latter as a complementary rather than alternative modality (Frank and Stollberg 2004a).

Initially skeptical of acupuncture, biomedical organizations turned to trials and regulatory models. As recently as 2001, the Federal Joint Committee (FJC, Gemeinsamer Bundesausschuss), which authorizes new diagnostic and therapeutic methods, published a critical report. Physicians on the committee are funded by public insurance companies, the *Gesetzliche Krankenkassen*—highly regulated statutory sickness funds that cover some 90 percent of the German population. (Private companies cover the other 10 percent) (see www .g-ba.de). The report situated acupuncture among therapies not tested using randomized controlled trials (RCTs).

In 1999, however, a group of these companies initiated acupuncture RCTs as part of a debate over whether they would continue to cover selected physician-administered treatments. Based on the results of these trials, in April 2006 the FJC added acupuncture to "acknowledged methods of diagnosis and treatment" for chronic low back pain and arthritis of the knee (Baecker, Tao, and Dobos 2007; Stollberg 2006). Coverage, however, did not include treatment for headache or migraine. Pointing to good results from the placebo group, researchers refused to acknowledge a placebo treatment as efficient. Given reductions in coverage, some experts anticipate that acupuncture could die out. This remains to be seen.

In 2003, the German Medical Association (Bundesärztekammer) published rules for further education in acupuncture, which are now becoming a model for some German states. These regulations establish an additional title, *Zusatzbezeichnung,* or "medical acupuncturist." In Germany, mostly physicians offer acupuncture treatment, unlike some other European states where more non-biomedical practitioners do so. Thus, acupuncture has become integrated into normal medical practice, while other forms of TCM (herbal teas, *tuina* massage, etc.) are situated in the wellness area.

In some other countries, such as Germany, France, Italy, Argentina, and Iraq, only biomedical physicians can legally practice acupuncture. In contrast, physicians in the United States who wish to practice acupuncture are not required to fulfill the curriculum requirements of the accredited acupuncture programs, because their medical license already permits them to insert needles. Those who incorporate acupuncture into their therapeutic repertoire are more likely to take the continuing-education medical acupuncture program for physicians developed by Dr. Joseph Helms.

First developed in 1978, Helms's program eventually became a three-hundred-hour Continuing Medical Education course for biomedical physicians. Helms drew on what he has referred to as "French energetic acupuncture," delineating it as a further offshoot in that stream of transmissions growing out of China and Vietnam. His objective has been to train physicians to incorporate acupuncture into their own medical specialty. Physicians can also attend a course offered at Harvard Medical School, or registered programs in New York leading to certification in acupuncture for physicians and dentists. Such programs have generated considerable controversy in the United States, because they require only three hundred hours of training, as compared with the three-year curricula of the acupuncture schools, and do not require the usual requirements for licensure that a practicing acupuncturist must fulfill. They do, however, meet or exceed the WHO's guidelines for abbreviated training of physicians in acupuncture, which established two hundred hours as the minimum standard.

Over time, each state formulated its own scope-of-practice laws, which resulted in disparate definitions of what it meant to practice as a licensed acupuncturist. Nonetheless, by 1982 acupuncture had coalesced as a recognized profession in the United States, with founders and educators from schools across the country agreeing to refer to it as "acupuncture and Oriental medicine" (AOM). This designation acknowledged the prominence of acupuncture in the public imagination. The term "Oriental" acknowledged the role of the many East Asian traditions alongside that of TCM. (The implications of Edward Said's *Orientalism* [1978] had not yet entered discussions in the field.)

In addition to coming to consensus around an encompassing frame of reference, a second challenge involved the many different legacies that had shaped orientations to practice, including those discussed above. The East Coast schools, for example, had been strongly influenced by European currents of transmission, whereas the West Coast schools privileged a TCM model that required training in acupuncture and herbal medicine for licensure. These differences made the task of determining national standards for training and national board examinations a difficult one. The challenge was taken up by the newly formed National Council of Acupuncture Schools and Colleges (now the Council of Colleges of Acupuncture and Oriental Medicine), with Mark Seem as its first president.

TABLE 10

Timeline 4: 1980s—events cited

1980	China: Publication of *Essentials of Chinese Acupuncture*
	England: Joseph Needham and Lu Gwei-Djen's *Celestial Lancets*
	United States: Acupuncture school founders and educators agree on "acupuncture and Oriental medicine" (AOM)
	US/California: American College of Traditional Chinese Medicine founded
1981	United States: Centers for Disease Control and Prevention recognize "acquired immunodeficiency syndrome" (AIDS)
	US/New York: Mutulu Shakur indicted
1983	US/California: Emperor's College starts (Santa Monica)
	US/Massachusetts: Ted Kaptchuk's *The Web That Has No Weaver*
	US/Oregon: Oregon College of Oriental Medicine founded
1984	England: Royston Low's *Secondary Vessels of Acupuncture*
	US/California: San Jose Five Branches University founded

1985	US/New York: Michael Smith and others found National Acupuncture Detoxification Association
1986	US/California: American College of Traditional Chinese Medicine becomes first college in US to award a M. Sc. degree
	US/New York: Shakur arrested; sentenced to sixty years in prison
1987	Sri Lanka: Jayasuriya establishes program in Sri Lanka
	United States: National Council of Acupuncture Schools and Colleges established; core curricula in TCM, but diversity also preserved
1988	US/Massachusetts: AIDS Care Project, nonprofit public clinic
1989	US/California: Brothers Daoshing and Maoshing Ni found Yo San University in memory of their grandfather Yo San Ni

The three leading schools in the East—the New England School of Acupuncture, Tri-State College of Acupuncture, and the Traditional Acupuncture Institute—were founding members. The organization was joined by the Midwest Center of Oriental Medicine, founded by Brian Manuele and Paul Zmiewski in Chicago, which also taught pre-TCM Chinese and French acupuncture styles, and the Northwest Institute of Oriental Medicine in Seattle. The East Coast and midwestern schools supported protecting such diversity in acupuncture education. Seem and Bob Duggan in particular voiced this position (Seem 2010). In contrast, the Chinese practitioners who played a key role in the California schools advocated for making the PRC's version of TCM the national standard. The latter included the American College of Traditional Chinese Medicine, Emperor's College, and the East West Academy, among others.

Because of the growing availability of texts from the PRC, by 1987 a compromise had been reached. TCM would provide the common foundation for curricula, school accreditation, and national examinations. At the same time, any school could also teach diverse traditions and styles, elect to focus on acupuncture, and not include herbal medicine in its curriculum. Provided graduates could pass TCM-based examinations for licensure, they could then go on to practice any style they chose.

These different orientations resulted, for a time, in different schools emphasizing different texts, limited by what was available in English. Such works included Felix Mann's earlier works, Royston Low's *Secondary Vessels of Acupuncture,* Mary Austin's works emphasizing Five Elements theory, and Ted Kaptchuk's *The Web That Has No Weaver,* which introduced TCM as taught in the PRC. Students circulated lecture notes and copies of class mimeographs from teachers such as James Tin Yau So and J. R. Worsley, some of these becoming the basis for later textbooks. For those who read French, there were the works of Chamfrault and Van Nghi; students who had gone through the Wexus' program had access to the Seem translations. The PRC also disseminated its own translated texts—*The Outline of Chinese Acupuncture, Essentials of Chinese Acupuncture,* and *Chinese Acupuncture and Moxibustion* (Seem 2010). By the 1990s, however, the revisiting of older texts and non-PRC approaches to practice had gained traction outside of mainland China. At the same time, dissenting scholars and administrator in the PRC have began to question and even criticize the TCM model and its intensified biomedicalization, and to bring elder Chinese medicine physicians back into the discussion (Fruehauf 2010).

Textuality and Truth in U.S. Chinese Medicine Education

Sonya Pritzker

The transmission of a therapeutic tradition from one culture and language to another invariably poses challenges of translation and interpretation, whether in relation to actual practices or texts or to the interplay between the two. The theories and practices known today as "Chinese medicine" (CM) can thus be understood as a process whereby living, breathing practice engages with the written record. In the United States, for example, CM students face the challenge of discerning how to interact with this written material in a way that leads to some degree of clinical aptitude. Factors mediating this process include the English-language publishers who supply textbooks for American acupuncture schools and the curricula of the different schools, as well as the hopes and desires of individual students, their past experiences with Chinese medicine and biomedicine, and their particular views on the way language and texts relate to daily practice.

American students quickly find that their reliance on textbooks and guides, most of which are translations, further complicates the process, particularly insofar as the authors of many of these works support conflicting approaches to the interpretation, translation, and nomenclature of CM texts. Moreover, as in China, specific teachers and institutional contexts significantly mediate the relationship that students form with the written archive of CM, and thus the type of clinical practice they later develop (Hsu 1999). Students must then navigate divergences between all of the above.

Schools of CM generally characterize their required texts as authoritative. Students are directed to interact with these works as expressions of the relevant truths of CM, memorizing the knowledge contained therein and reproducing it in class, on tests, and in the clinic. Yet individual teachers may offer different perspectives on the validity of this knowledge. In a first-year class at one school, for example, a teacher may tell students, "The [CM] nomenclature in [state-board-required] textbooks is misleading and not clinically relevant." Therefore, she says, "you've got to *learn* things the wrong way, and then you've got to *apply* them clinically in a completely different way." She goes on to differentiate between what she feels students must memorize to pass licensing exams and what they really need to understand in order to treat patients, often explaining the latter in terms of embodied, experiential knowledge. She encourages students to explore their own experience in relation to pulse taking and other CM diagnostic methods—an experience that eventually becomes the primary "truth" for their clinical practice.

A different teacher at the school may also tell these same students that the information in their required texts is "wrong." He admonishes them instead to try to read classical texts that, according to him, contain knowledge that is more legitimate. However, because students' training rarely includes instruction in the Chinese language, most of these classics remain inaccessible to them. Both instructors thus reinforce an argument that textbook knowledge is suspect. Yet although the first offers some hope through the acquisition of experience, the second counters with the frustrating perspective that truly valid knowledge remains beyond the students' reach, distant and locked in the secrets of a language they learn only indirectly, through translation.

This case illustrates ways in which students may receive conflicting information about how best to engage with the texts available to them, contributing to ambiguity about what constitutes authentic knowledge. In such cases, American students may be left feeling ambivalent about the relationship between textuality and practice. Although the effects for each student may differ substantially, the process can still leave them challenged by the sense not only that they are learning a medicine in translation but also that these very translations may distance them more from the medicine than take them into it.

Public Health Applications

Although the founding activists at the Lincoln Hospital program were, for the most part, no longer present, work there continued. In 1985, Smith and others founded the National Acupuncture Detoxification Association, or NADA (the acronym means "nothing" in Spanish, referring to a drug-free approach to addiction treatment). As an organization, NADA provides advice on starting similar treatment programs, trains and certifies practitioners to use its five-point auricular treatment protocol (known as "acudetox"), and cross-trains chemical dependency specialists and acupuncturists to work together more effectively (Serrano n.d.; NADA 2008).

The use of a group setting became standard practice, to which was added an herbal detox tea to help with relaxation and sleep. The formula draws on both Western and Chinese sources and includes chamomile, peppermint, yarrow, hops, skullcap, and catnip, each for a specific purpose, and is given to patients to take home after each acupuncture treatment. Group therapy is also commonly used (NADA 2008).

The protocol is now used not only in programs for addiction treatment but also in mental health facilities, harm reduction and similar outreach projects, homeless shelters, jails, prisons, and halfway houses. During the aftermath of the attack on the Twin Towers on September 11, 2001, not only did biomedical personnel go to Ground Zero to care for first responders from the police and fire departments, but groups of acupuncturists and other complementary/alternative care providers donated time as well. In particular, they treated for stress, anxiety, difficulties with sleep, and cravings for alcohol and drugs, symptoms later more widely recognized as indicative of post-traumatic stress disorder (PTSD).

Inspired by that example, the group Acupuncturists Without Borders (AWB) coalesced under the direction of Diana Fried in response to the impact of Hurricane Katrina, wildfires in southern California, floods in the Midwest, and the earthquake in Haiti (Acupuncturists Without Borders 2009a). Over time, volunteers have been invited to provide treatments inside Red Cross shelters as well as in local malls and other relief sites. In Ohio, they worked alongside the Tzu Chi (Zi Ji) Buddhist Charitable Organization, which offered relief at Ground

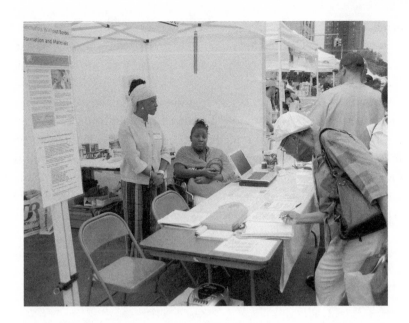

Figure 9.2. Acupuncturists Without Borders fund-raiser in 2007 in Harlem, New York: (standing) Julia Bennett, L.Ac., (seated) Saleema Render. Courtesy of Dr. RoBert J. Woodbine.

Zero and numerous other disaster-relief initiatives. Other practitioners have taken the NADA approach to countries around the world (Porter and Sommers 2008; Mandell 2002; Editorial Staff 2005).

Military Applications

Military conflicts in Iraq and Afghanistan involving American military personnel have resulted in grave injuries and extensive post-traumatic stress disorder. AWB responded with what was originally called the Veterans Project and is now known as the Military Stress Recovery Project; the renaming was intended to make it clear that clinics were open not only to veterans but also to servicepeople on active duty, reservists, and their family members. As with its other initiatives, AWB volunteers use the NADA protocol as a point of departure. Groups such as Black Veterans for Social Justice, in Brooklyn, New York, have provided space for this initiative, as have other groups throughout the United States. This response represents a significant cultural shift from the Vietnam era, when acupuncturists identifying with the counterculture often came out of groups protesting military actions.

The U.S. military itself has also now adopted acupuncture in multiple ways. Faced with 300,000 Iraq and Afghanistan war veterans who suffer from PTSD or major depression, and roughly 320,000 who have suffered mild concussions or combat-related brain injury, as well as the rising incidence of suicide, the Pentagon has been searching to find innovative ways to treat troops. By 2008, it had spent some $5 million to study acupuncture, yoga, and other complementary modalities (Zoroya 2008).

Colonel Richard C. Niemtzow, a radiation oncologist and flight surgeon, had received his medical education in France before returning to the United States. He later would take the Medical Acupuncture for Physicians course with Dr. Joe Helms. Beginning in 1999, Niemtzow became the first full-time medical acupuncturist in the armed forces, and in 2001 he coined the term "battlefield acupuncture" to characterize the application of acupuncture to treat pain in combat situations (World Center for EFT 2010).

ACUPUNCTURE IN IRAQ

Lazgeen Ahmad, MD (Interview by Douglas Newton)

Dr. Lazgeen Ahmad, MD, now lives in Kurdistan and is working to open a TCM clinic there—the only one of its kind in the region. His interview illustrates the entry of acupuncture into a politically challenging context, in contrast with the other illustrations presented in this chapter.

DN: When did acupuncture use in Iraq begin?

LA: To my knowledge, it started in 1978 when one Iraqi doctor, a gynecologist, was invited to visit China to see how acupuncture is used during caesarean sections. After 1980, two anesthesiologists had been sent to China to take a course in acupuncture. These doctors came to practice acupuncture for limited pain conditions. In 1991, after the Gulf War [when Iraq attacked Kuwait], economic conditions worsened in Iraq, and physicians experienced a shortage of drugs. This problem was widespread enough that the Ministry of Health [MOH] needed to find an alternative way to treat illness.

In 1996, a pain center was established in Baghdad in the Alwasety Hospital for burn wounds and reconstructive surgery. Of course there was great opposition from doctors, who were against the idea of using TCM. Later, this center was transferred to the neurosurgical hospital. Acupuncture was used by one anesthesiologist and two general practitioners who had limited education in acupuncture. Over time, a guest instructor from Pakistan came annually to give acupuncture lectures and treat patients. During this period, I was senior anesthesiologist in the Teaching Central Hospital for Children, while also practicing acupuncture in my private clinic in the late afternoons. In Iraq, all doctors from the medical college work after graduation in the governmental hospital. After they finish their residency or postgraduate work, they can practice in a private clinic in the afternoon.

I visited the center regularly, particularly when guest TCM lecturers arrived from Pakistan. In 1999, two doctors and I received diplomas in acupuncture from Pakistan, and I became a member of the Pakistan Institute of Acupuncture and Medical Sciences. In 2000, the pain center was renamed the TCM Center and transferred to the Al-Shaheed Adnan Hospital [now called the Specialized Surgical Hospital]. Only four doctors worked at this center. One left for personal reasons. Two left to [go to] China for acupuncture training.

In January 2003, the Ministry of Health transferred my job to the TCM Center. After the war in 2003, I became manager of the center. At that time, three doctors worked there. In 2006 and 2007, the MOH sent me to China for additional TCM training. In 2007, I left Baghdad due to unfavorable conditions and moved to northern Iraq, leaving the center with two doctors and eight assistants [physiotherapists].

DN: How many still practice TCM in Iraq?

LA: Now only two doctors work officially in the TCM Center in Baghdad. In Kurdistan there is only one doctor practicing acupuncture in his private clinic, a doctor trained in China. In 2006, I received the assent of the MOH to open a TCM clinic in one of the bigger hospitals in Baghdad. We trained three doctors for three months to be ready to work in this clinic, under the center's supervision.

DN: Was the beginning of acupuncture use in Iraq a direct result of the war?

LA: Yes. As you know, there were two wars, one beginning in 1991 and the other in 2003. After the first conflict in 1991 there was a drug shortage. After 2003, everything was destroyed.

DN: How is the current practice situation?

LA: After the war, conditions in the MOH were unstable, with continuous changes in officers. This instability affected our planning, and they [the officers] were also busy with many other problems. Political conditions also prevented many patients from continuing their treatment. But I think when conditions stabilize, acupuncture will expand.

In a different but related model, Joe Chang, a second-generation acupuncturist, began working with postdeployment soldiers in a PTSD program based at Fort Bliss Restoration and Resilience Center, William Beaumont Army Medical Center, providing full one-on-one treatments. From there, he joined a pilot initiative, the Warrior Combat Stress Reset Program, at Carl R. Darnall Army Medical Center, at Fort Hood in Texas, where his acupuncture treatments complement other modalities such as tapping, *qigong*, yoga, and pharmaceutical medications. This combination of modalities has enabled many of the veterans to reduce the number and dosage of medications they take.

HIV INITIATIVES

In 1981, the U.S. Centers for Disease Control and Prevention recognized a new disease in the United States: acquired immunodeficiency syndrome (AIDS). Two years later, advanced infection from the human immunodeficiency virus (HIV) was identified as responsible for AIDS. Both conditions have resisted cure. During the 1980s, not only did fatalities accelerate, but secondary symptoms and opportunistic infections compromised patients' quality of life. It was during that same decade that groups of acupuncturists—particularly in larger cities—began to use Chinese medicine paradigms to diagnose and treat people with HIV/AIDS. Rather than starting from a biomedical diagnosis, they used Chinese medicine diagnostics. Acupuncture and Chinese herbs effectively addressed their patients' sleep disturbance, night sweats, chronic diarrhea, pain, and digestive issues, and proved to be effective at managing medication side effects (Moffett et al. 1994; Burack et al. 1996; Beal and Nield-Anderson 2000).

For example, the AIDS Care Project, a nonprofit public clinic begun in Boston, Massachusetts, in 1988, has continued to provide both free and low-cost acupuncture, Chinese herbs, and *shiatsu* (a form of acupressure) treatments to patients with HIV and AIDS. It is the largest such clinic in the United States and provides more than thirteen thousand treatments each year ("About the National Acupuncture Detoxification Association" 2010; Sommers 2010). In California, practitioners like Misha Cohen developed protocols with which to treat people with HIV/AIDS (Cohen et al. 1999) and infectious diseases such as hepatitis C (Cohen, Gish, and Doner 2007). Many acupuncturists have donated time to such clinics, been funded by state or federal programs, or treated patients on a sliding scale of payments.

THE COMMUNITY ACUPUNCTURE NETWORK

In 2002, Lisa Rohleder and her partner Skip Van Meter set up a treatment setting in which reclining chairs ringed the room for communal treatments. The approach was modeled on arrangements used in some hospitals in mainland China and was not unlike that used in the NADA clinics. Their mission was to contribute to social change in American health care by making acupuncture widely available to everyone, regardless of whether they had insurance, while being able to make a living. Their clinic in Portland, Oregon, evolved into Working Class Acupuncture, and the movement into the Community Acupuncture Network. Their work has inspired an international community acupuncture movement, with more than eighty clinics now in the United States, Canada, and Israel (Chang 2007; Crain 2007; Rohleder 2008; Weeks 2008).

Get on Track with Subhealth: Changing Trajectories of "Preventive Medicine"

Mei Zhan

"Get on track with the world" *(yu shijie jiegui)* was one of the most popular government slogans and everyday expressions in China around the turn of the new millennium. In practice, this "world" encompasses mainly the European Union, North America, and affluent regions of East Asia. For traditional Chinese medicine, it means reinventing itself as a novel "preventive medicine" that preserves and enhances holistic health and overall well-being and deals specifically with health conditions associated with urban, middle-class lifestyles.

The seemingly new "global" orientation of traditional Chinese medicine should not obscure the fact that it had already circulated translocally as a preventive medicine—albeit a different kind—in the 1960s and 1970s (Zhan 2009b). Characterized as "a bundle of needles [acupuncture], a handful of herbs [herbal medicine], and a pair of hands [*tuina*]," traditional Chinese medicine then was a low-tech component in China's health care system that aimed at forestalling mass outbreaks of infectious diseases and satisfying basic health care needs, especially in rural areas. This brand of preventive medicine also became a trademark of Chinese medical teams that went to Third World countries in China's effort to forge and champion a proletarian world (Eadie and Grizzell 1979; Hutchison 1975).

In the cultural production of this new preventive medicine, however, places such as California now play a central role. In the 1960s, the counterculture movement in the United States recast Chinese medicine as a naturalistic, holistic alternative to the biomedical establishment. Today, herbal medicine and especially acupuncture are increasingly familiar concepts to many Californians. Having an acupuncturist has come to signal well-being and a good quality of life, with acupuncture and herbal medicine used primarily for conditions associated with urban living, for which biomedicine is less effective or ineffective. Such conditions include, on the one hand, cancers or serious illnesses resistant to conventional biomedical interventions, and, on the other, chronic conditions such as allergies, asthma, insomnia, and various pain syndromes (Eisenberg et al. 1998; National Institutes of Health 1997; Zhan 2001, 2009b). Excepting those who work in ethnic Chinese communities, acupuncturists in California regularly tell me that the overwhelming majority of their patients are young or middle-aged and come from white, middle-class backgrounds.

Acutely aware of this trend, Shanghai's entrepreneurially minded practitioners now promote Chinese medicine as a new preventive medicine with a Californian flair. Since the 1990s, the marketization and privatization of health care have prompted many practitioners in Shanghai to search for a new professional identity and clientele. To this end, some propose a new health concept they call "subhealth" *(yajiankang),* which they insist came from "foreign experts." Although there is no standardized definition of subhealth, proponents think of it as a liminal state between being healthy and being ill (Zhan 2009b).

In practice, subhealth applies to cases where, in the absence of any diagnosed or diagnosable disease, a person suffers from low energy, fatigue, headaches, insomnia, heart palpitations, loss of memory, or a general sense of being unwell. It is estimated that 70 percent of residents in Shanghai are trapped in the state of subhealth (Luo 2006), viewed as potentially leading to more serious health problems and even premature death. As public concern grows, subhealth provides a unique niche for marketing traditional Chinese medicine. The old saying "A doctor of the highest caliber treats an illness before it happens" *(shanggong zhi weibing)* is regaining popularity in both the pedagogy and practice of traditional Chinese medicine, which reemerges as a preventive medicine for the urban middle classes of Shanghai and California (Zhan 2009a).

Therapeutic Massage, Dit Da Jow, and Bone Setting

External forms of treatment had appeared quite early in China, coming to be known as *anmo,* which referred to manual rubbing. For example, oracle bone inscriptions query whether use of early forms of massage would help a particular condition. They also indicate that women were involved in the practice. The

Inner Canon of the Yellow Emperor and the Fifty-Two Medical Formulas from Mawangdui note the use of different forms of pressing, rubbing, compression, gliding, scratching, and other techniques. Various related instruments were also listed.

Different teachers and practitioners of the martial arts, and by extension those involved in military actions, by necessity found that they had distinct therapeutic needs. In response, they developed herbal formulas, baths, and soaks; massage oils, poultices, liniments, and plasters; and dietary changes with which to promote the breaking up of stagnation and to restore the healthy flow of *qi*. Many of their formulas represented closely guarded family knowledge, transmitted from one generation to the next. The actual massage techniques, which drew on Chinese medical theory as a foundation, move the body's protective *qi* by pressing, kneading, pinching, rubbing, tapping, and brushing areas between the joints, using the thumbs, fingertips, and knuckles, with particular attention to the effects of injuries on muscles, tendons, and bones. Some martial arts teachers also created different formulas for Dit Da Jow (literally, "fall hit wine"), an herbal liniment used to treat bruises, sprains, and swelling to prevent the cumulative effect of trauma. Another, San Huang San (Three Yellow Powder Medicine), has remained a commonly used herbal poultice for more acute injuries, such as broken bones.

Under the influence of the PRC, *anmo* came to refer mostly to popular practice, whereas *tuina* referred to the medicalized therapeutic massage that became part of the curriculum in the schools of Chinese medicine—as is the case in many of the schools in the United States. *Tuina* was generally taught through apprenticeship, and some practitioners still learn through direct transmission. Daoist and Buddhist influences on the different schools of martial practice filtered into conceptualizations of injury and healing, and, by extension, into ideas about how to heal injuries. Some martial arts teachers still teach it to their advanced students so that they can treat the bruises, sprains, and other injuries that can result from training. Other teachers offer stand-alone training and certification programs, reaching out not only to acupuncturists, *qigong* practitioners, and *taiji* and martial arts practitioners but also to massage therapists, physical and occupational therapists, yoga teachers, nurses, and Reiki practitioners, among others. The practice is therefore expanding into other fields, finding permeable points of entry. Other programs provide tours to the PRC, where they spend an abbreviated, intensive training period at Chinese massage hospitals.

More recently, throughout some large Chinese communities—such as New York's Chinatown—a plethora of *tuina* salons have sprung up, advertising foot massages and reflexology services. Within a single block, there may be seven or

Table 11

Timeline 5: 1990s–2000s—events cited

1990	Mexico: 1990–2000, Prof. Nguyên Tai Thu trained Mexican physicians in acupuncture
	US/New York: Leon Hammer begins to offer pulse workshops
1992	England: Felix Mann's *Reinventing Acupuncture*
1994	Quebec: Adoption of *Loi sur l'acupuncture*
1996	United States: Food and Drug Administration reclassified acupuncture needles from the category of experimental device to accepted medical instrument
	US/Colorado: Sandra Lillie incorporates Institute of Taoist Education and Acupuncture in Louisville, Colorado
1999	United States: Paul Zmiewski and Nigel Wiseman's full translation of Soulié de Morant's *L'Acuponcture chinoise;* Richard Niemtzow becomes first full-time medical acupuncturist in armed forces
2001	US/Florida: Leon Hammer helps found Dragon Rises School of Oriental Medicine in Gainesville, Florida
	US/Maryland: Richard Niemtzow coins term "battlefield acupuncture" for acupuncture treatment of pain in combat situations
2002	US/Oregon: Lisa Rohleder and Skip Van Meter set up a treatment setting that evolves into Working Class Acupuncture
2005	US/New Mexico: Diana Fried founds Acupuncturists Without Borders
2007	US/New York: Kiiko Matsumoto formalizes her own approach
	Vietnam: Vietnam Central Acupuncture Hospital graduated twenty Mexican practitioners
2008	US/Texas: Fort Bliss Base introduces acupuncture to treat soldiers with PTSD

eight of them, generally in basement store spaces. Some of the practitioners are well trained, representing multiple generations; others have learned the rudiments after being hired and receive only tips for payment. Gradually these businesses have begun to spread into other parts of the city.

Because one must have a medical license to set bones, it is illegal for other kinds of practitioners to do so in the United States. However, prior to the 1970s (and in all likelihood since then), bone setters worked within ethnic Chinese communities, with word getting out to non-Chinese martial arts students and small circles of outsiders. More recently, practitioners with this skill have learned overseas, some through one-on-one training in the lineage tradition. Vince Black, for example, learned not only internal arts and *taijiquan* from martial artist Hsu Hung-Chi (1934–1984) in Taiwan but also bone setting. Black, in turn, trained practitioners such as Tom Bisio when the two met at an instructor training camp for Pekiti-Tirsia Kali martial arts in the Philippines. Bisio, in turn, set up a practice in New York, Zheng Gu Tui Na, which collaborated with the Kamwo herbal pharmacy to manufacture and sell "liniments, *gao* (poultices), soaks, powders, ointments and pills for trauma and orthopedic conditions" (Zheng Gu Tui Na 2010).

Practitioners in the United States who do bone setting tend to do so only with people who are already their patients, those whom they know personally, or those who have been referred by someone else they know. As far as learning the practice, some have studied in formal PRC government-sponsored programs. Moreover, works originally published in China by doctors trained in traditional orthopedics have been translated into English (Zhang 1996) and are available through sources like Amazon.com. More informally, individuals turn to Internet sites to ask questions about where to find practitioners and exchange information under the radar.

PLACEBO-CONTROLLED RANDOMIZED TRIALS AND CHINESE MEDICINE

Ted J. Kaptchuk

By the late twentieth century, Chinese medicine had established itself as a viable health care option throughout the Western world, offering what was construed as natural, holistic, exotic, and nontechnological (Kaptchuk 2002). Within a broader movement toward alternative therapy options, patients have sought relief and health from acupuncture, Chinese herbs, *taiqi,* and *qigong.* A licensed, registered, and organized Chinese medicine profession has successfully established itself to meet this growing demand. But insofar as the field seeks scientific legitimacy and mainstream acceptance, Chinese practices must successfully navigate the mechanisms of the randomized controlled trial (RCT), originally developed to test biomedical pharmaceuticals (Kaptchuk 1998a, 1998b).

Since the 1970s, almost one thousand RCTs in Western scientific centers have examined acupuncture's efficacy for various illnesses. These trials have predominately targeted chronic pain conditions but have also studied conditions such as asthma, irritable bowel syndrome, depression, and anxiety. Hundreds of herbal trials have been conducted, while *taiqi* and *qigong* trials are becoming common.

The results have disappointed the Chinese medicine community. Acupuncture has consistently outperformed a placebo control only in the more than forty RCTs testing its value for nausea and vomiting that occur after chemotherapy and after surgery. Results for pain and other illnesses have been contradictory: for any particular condition, some trials are positive, while others show no difference. Studies of herbal medicines—which contain many known active agents—have been somewhat more positive (e.g., in eczema and asthma studies), but the adverse effects profile of the herbs has also been unexpectedly high. *Taiqi* and *qigong* trials remain in their infancy.

Chinese medicine practitioners blame insufficiently sensitive research methodology for these less than impressive outcomes. They argue that testing acupuncture or herbal combinations is not as simple as testing a pharmaceutical. They may be right. Because acupuncture can only be single-blinded, acupuncturists may have an expectation of a positive treatment outcome, which is likely to introduce significant bias. The quest for a matching placebo control—one that is both inert (has no active properties) and identical in appearance and sensation to the insertion of an acupuncture needle—is ongoing. Two acupuncturists may not select the same points to treat the same condition; a single acupuncturist often varies the treatment protocol from one session to another, raising additional problems of standardization and replicability. How much does a trial represent the quality of the acupuncturist rather than the acupuncture?

Testing herbs poses other difficulties, including inadequate scientific assessment of active chemical components; insufficient information concerning optimal dosages; lack of consistency in chemical composition between manufacturers or between different batches from the same manufacturer; chaotic or commercially determined forms of standardization; contradictory or difficult-to-determine traditional claims; poor monitoring for deterioration of potency; and contamination and adulteration.

Debunkers argue that the evidence already shows that Chinese medicine has failed the RCT's scientific challenge. Yet a more dispassionate reviewer could reasonably say that the RCT biomedical epidemiological and epistemological jury has yet to render clear verdicts. One thing, however, has emerged from acupuncture RCTs, especially from a series of large trials sponsored by German insurance companies: the placebo effects of acupuncture are inordinately high, with a significant impact on illness (Kaptchuk et al. 2006). People get better in trials if they expect to get better, whether the treatment is genuine or placebo. As for the conditions tested, both genuine and placebo acupuncture perform better than, or at least as well as, usual biomedical care (Linde et al. 2007). Thus, although high placebo effect complicates detection of any difference between acupuncture and placebo acupuncture, East Asian medicine definitely seems to be helping patients (Kaptchuk et al. 2008).

The Biomedicalization of Practice

In every setting where Chinese healing traditions have arisen, biomedicine has also tended to be present, generally now as the dominant or official health care system. Practitioners from other traditions have found themselves under direct or indirect pressure to define themselves in relation to it, particularly by trying to look more "scientific" and "professional" (with biomedicine having laid many of the foundations for professional identity) (Barnes 2003b). At the same time, these classifications no longer fully serve, insofar as multiple models of integrated practice have emerged.

Such mixing has led to a number of ambiguities. In the state of New Mexico in the United States, for example, one relatively small group of licensed acupuncturists argues—much to the dismay of other practitioners in the state—that if a practice comes out of China, it must be recognized as a part of Chinese medicine. This argument has been used to buttress such practices as the unregulated injection of human growth hormone. In the state of Florida, the originators of the licensing law for acupuncturists included the use of hypodermic needles, as well as the practice of homeopathy, under the scope of what acupuncturists can legally do. Anyone wishing to practice homeopathy in Florida must therefore secure an acupuncture license, while licensed acupuncturists can use hypodermic needles to inject homeopathic remedies into acupuncture points.

In France and Germany, only biomedical physicians are allowed to practice acupuncture; in contrast, many licensed acupuncturists in the United States

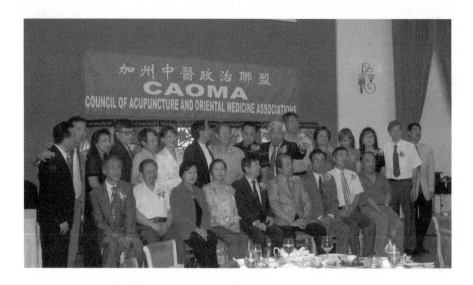

Figure 9.3. Group photograph at a 2008 fund-raiser of the Council of Acupuncture and Oriental Medicine Associations, in Los Angeles, California, as part of an initiative to lobby for enhanced insurance coverage of acupuncture at the state level. Courtesy of Linda L. Barnes.

view physician involvement as suspect unless these doctors have also gone through a full program at one of the acupuncture schools. The boundaries between who can do what, how they learn what they do, and who authorizes them to practice are frequently contested, with each party framing its arguments in relation to its own definition of practice, scope, and legitimacy.

Some of the impetus to designate things as "medical" comes from the PRC. Even when TCM is being practiced in hospital or clinical settings, there is an increasing tendency to foreground biomedical diagnosis. To the extent that developments in the PRC version of practice influence training in other parts of the world, this aspect of cross-fertilization spreads outward from mainland China. Correspondingly, as biomedical schools and institutions in countries like the United States and others emphasize an evidence-based approach to practice, the press is on to demonstrate efficacy of practices such as acupuncture. Researchers, therefore, sought ways to transfer randomized controlled trial methods to different aspects of Chinese medicine, often with ambiguous results at best (Barnes 2005a).

Such outcomes have led to alternative formulations of evidence, featuring authoritative texts, the clinical experience of master practitioners (Barnes 2009), consensus processes that distill the perspectives of leading practitioners, case histories, and practice guidelines that reflect the input of authorities in the field. More recently, researchers working from within the field have incorporated new questions that explore how to study complex systems, connective tissue, and other subtle bodily mechanisms, and to apply strategies such as magnetic resonance imaging (Langevin et al. 2007; Napadow et al. 2009; Wayne et al. 2009). But it is also in response to such developments that we see the call for a return to pre-PRC versions of Chinese medicine—a call that is finding a growing voice as well in mainland China.

TEN

A World of Chinese Medicine and Healing: Part Two

Linda L. Barnes

DESPITE THE WIDESPREAD PROMINENCE of acupuncture, this chapter—like the others before it—aims to present a more complex scenario, in which Chinese medicine also encompasses other branches, many of them arising from common conceptual roots, such as *qi* and the Five Phases *(wuxing)*. They include food therapy *(shiliao)* and herbal medicine; *taijiquan* and other movement traditions, along with related forms of practice (e.g., bone setting); therapeutic massage *(tuina)*; and practices related to inner cultivation and to the healing of others, such as *qigong*.

The last set of practices overlaps with related breathing, visualization, and meditative techniques transmitted by Buddhist and Daoist teachers, as well as from the Confucian self-cultivation disciplines. Additionally, practices discussed in previous chapters of this book that were particularly targeted during the Cultural Revolution and following years are now not only beginning to resurface in mainland China but also, like acupuncture, are spreading worldwide. These include temple practices and systems of divination such as *fengshui*, the *Classic of Changes (Yijing* or *I Ching)*, and face reading *(mianxiang)*.

No practitioner or user of one of these arts necessarily employs the others. Each of the arts may constitute a worldview and lived tradition with which someone has grown up. Or an individual may first be drawn to a particular practice otherwise foreign to him or her and, from there, proceed to learn about some or all of the others. In still other instances, the person may pick up one practice, using it only as long as he or she has an immediate need.

There is, in other words, a spectrum of involvement. Or, as Louis Komjathy characterizes Daoists in the United States, we may find a spectrum of "family resemblances" ranging from "close relations" (such as Daoist priests, lineage holders, acupuncturists and herbalists, or *fengshui* practitioners) to "distant relations" (those drawn to popularized sources such as *The Dao of Pooh* or a Tao Te Ching widget downloaded to their computer). Together, these different dimensions of engagement represent the transmission of Chinese medicine and healing as a whole.

Moreover, some participants may be deeply invested in the scholarly versions of practice—in its texts, and in "philosophical" versions of the tradition that, in some cases, they differentiate from matters "religious." Others may root what they do in the rituals or the religious or lineage hierarchies and dynamics of a particular community, prioritizing the communal dimensions of a tradition. Still others may embrace the personal dimensions of practice, focusing on the pursuit of healing and health, self-cultivation, and/or wisdom (Komjathy 2004; Kohn 2001).

Such an inclusive umbrella reflects differences between how various parties define "Chinese medicine"—an unexpectedly ambiguous term, as Elisabeth Hsu has observed in relation to such practices in Tanzania. There, for example, the term *dawa ya Kichina* can refer to "China's medicine" (that is, "medicine from China"), "medicine of the Chinese" (anything practiced by a Chinese physician, including biomedicine), or "medicines from China" (Chinese medical drugs in some cases, and Chinese-manufactured Western biomedical drugs in others) (Hsu 2002).

CHINESE MEDICINE IN AFRICA

Elisabeth Hsu

East-South medical technology transfers from China to Africa have mostly been studied with regard to Zaire (Bibeau 1985) and Tanzania (Hsu 2008; Langwick forthcoming). Such flows—countervailing the globalization of Western goods and services, yet intricately entangled with it—extend far beyond those two socialist-oriented states and have affected most of sub-Saharan Africa. Three trajectories of transfer prevail, to which a newly emergent fourth can be added.

1. *Medical expert teams.* In the 1960s and 1970s when African states rose to independence, the Chinese project of world socialism dispatched medical

expert teams on two-year missions (Zhan 2002), often to remote district hospitals. These teams, which included a dozen biomedical professionals of various specializations and one acupuncturist who focused on primary care, are today remembered for being as expert in their work as they were modest in their lifestyle. In fact, despite its decline since its heyday in the 1970s, this medical aid program has been hailed as the most successful of the twentieth century (Snow 1989).

2. *The "barefoot doctors."* When the World Health Organization (WHO) issued the declaration "Health for All by the Year 2000" at Alma Ata in 1978, it drew inspiration from the Chinese "barefoot doctors" of the Cultural Revolution (1966–1976). The primary health care programs that the WHO advocated—like the barefoot doctor initiatives—aimed at holistic health care but, again like the barefoot doctor programs, accorded traditional medicines and their holistic care only a marginal role. Ironically, the WHO instituted primary health care programs on African soil in the 1980s, at the very time that barefoot doctor programs were being dismantled in the People's Republic of China (PRC). Moreover, African health bureaucracies have never embraced Mao Zedong's vision of integrating Chinese and Western medicine *(zhongxiyi jiehe),* which was central to the revival of the PRC's construction of Traditional Chinese Medicine (TCM) during the 1950s (see Chapter 8). Some African policy makers argue that any attempt to integrate modern and traditional medicines would breed charlatans, an opinion they justify by their observation that self-professed "modern-traditional" healers are increasingly populating unregulated African medical markets.

3. *Medicine as business.* The acceleration of Deng Xiaoping's economic reforms after the Tiananmen Massacre in 1989 coincided with the global neoliberal turn. This reformulation of the international economic playing field also included "modernized" traditional medicines (Hsu and Høg 2002), and in the last two decades urban African health markets have accommodated numerous Chinese medical clinics. These clinics, which cater to all walks of society, inhabit diverse geographies, from the hustle and bustle of bus stations to quiet residential areas and the shopping centers of the suburban elite. The Chinese medical doctors who staff them range from biomedical or TCM professionals to nurses, lab assistants, and health product merchants. Some health shops thrive under the patronage of powerful bureaucrats and politicians; others are increasingly marginalized, and their staff are on the verge of joining the ranks of local drug sellers.

Chinese medical drugs have been modernized in many ways. New avenues of ethnochemistry have resulted in a rich arsenal of "formula drugs" (also called "proprietary medicines"). Sometimes it is merely their appearance that is new, as is the case with pills that contain ingredients of otherwise unaltered formulas *(fangji)* from the scholarly Chinese medical archive. Some formula drugs derive from age-old folk recipes, while others consist of a mixture of Chinese and Western medical substances. There are also stand-alone extracts from a single plant of the Chinese *materia medica,* such as ginseng.

Still other formulas are entirely new, developed according to Chinese or Western medical rationales. Some more recently developed syntheses contain a combination of Chinese and African herbs. Since these proprietary medicines often can alleviate locally recognized symptoms, they are lucrative products for over-the-counter transactions. Their promoters praise these hybrids as the epitome of TCM biotechnology, but, as instantiations of an "alternative modernity," they have become a nightmare for the dominant biomedical regulative bodies (Hsu 2009). Their business thrives in neoliberal health markets, but it may be short-lived.

4. *The antimalarial* qinghaosu *(Qinghaosu),* also called artemisinin, and its derivatives have made unprecedented inroads into sub-Saharan African health care for at least two reasons. First, the burden of malaria there outrivals that of any other disease, including AIDS. Second, the potency of artemisinin is unparalleled. It clears fevers rapidly, has few side effects, and has been used in Southeast Asia for more than twenty years without giving rise to any significant resistance. The discovery of this unique drug goes back to the days of the Vietnam War, when malaria caused more deaths than combat, prompting governments on both sides of the Pacific to search for antimalarial substances. The Americans focused on artificial substances and developed a synthetic analogue of quinine, mefloquine, which has been on the market for decades despite its serious side effects.

At the same time, Chinese scientists of Maoist legacy sifted through the herbs of the Chinese *materia medica.* They extracted the pure chemical substance artemisinin from the Chinese medical herb *Artemisia annua (qinghao).* The bioscientific reification of *qinghao*'s antimalarial properties depended critically on scientists working in the same institution as historians, for the latter pointed to Ge Hong's (fourth century C.E.) recommendation of soaking the fresh plant in water, wringing it out, and drinking its juice (Hsu 2006), which is the earliest record of *qinghao*'s application against acute intermittent fever episodes. Translated into modern chemistry, Ge Hong's recommendation meant that cold extraction should be applied (Prof. Tu Youyou, personal communication, 2005). Considering, inter alia, the neurotoxicity of other *Artemisia* species (used, for instance, for making absinthe), the WHO was slow to recognize artemisinin as a first-line antimalarial. The WHO began to recommend it only in 2005, and then only against the most dangerous strain, *Plasmodium falciparum.* However, due to the danger of recrudescence (reappearance of the plasmodia in the bloodstream), it soon annulled the recommendation. Consequently, the WHO currently recommends artemisinin only in combination with antimalarials produced by the Western pharmaceutical industry. This regulatory intervention has effectively halted the dispensing of the Chinese brands of artemisinin which, prior to 2005, had constituted more than 50 percent of over-the-counter transactions in Chinese medical clinics. Some Chinese medical businesses have been sorely affected as a result.

In summary, the twentieth century saw diverse medical transfers from China to Africa, some much appreciated by local populations. The motives for these East-South trajectories ranged from Mao Zedong's vision of world socialism to the WHO's development-oriented humanitarianism and, more recently, to opportunistic health business. However, given that neoliberal health markets are not entirely unregulated (Ong 2006), it is possible that some of the current trajectories will diminish, while new ones will emerge. The Chinese medical archive has the potential to be further developed in many different ways.

A receiving culture has its own customs, traditions, and views of newcomers, all of which can be projected onto practitioners and practices coming out of China. The interface between the two parties leads to translations framed in ways the receiving culture can grasp and, to varying degrees, accept while, at the same time, having to expand its frames of reference to accommodate new ways of seeing the world. The matter of family resemblances must therefore be extended to encompass the variations of different Chinese healing arts as these are practiced in new milieus around the world. In the course of the exchange, all parties are changed.

So what holds them together? It has been argued that practitioners at least share conceptual foundations, such as *qi* or, in some cases, the Five Phases *(wuxing)*. Despite their differences, they constitute a loosely connected "speech community"—"a string of people who share a symbolic code of speaking practices and meanings for those practices, although they may be separated by distance as well as race, class, gender, age, and so forth" (Ho 2009; Fitch 1998; Fitch 1999, 46). The more pervasive the practices become, the more such terminology filters into local vernaculars, taking on popular meanings as well. Terms such as "Yin-Yang," *fengshui*, and "acupuncture" have so entered public parlance in different parts of the world, for example, that they appear everywhere from academic journals to tabloids.

Moreover, people combine practices, often in idiosyncratic says. Vasudha Narayanan (2006) observes in connection with Hindu traditions that practitioners and users alike tend to draw on the full repertoire of available approaches to healing, from whatever source, in order to customize their own practices. As has long been noted in the circles of medical anthropology, such choices are further shaped by factors such as the individual's and group's worldviews; the logistically and financially available options; the gravity of the actual problem and its impact on the lives involved; how the origins of the problem are conceptualized in relation to what those parties feel needs to be done; the interventions the person or group has already tried, sometimes with unsatisfying results; and the social and political consequences of specific choices. This customizing of practice occurs as well in connection with Chinese orientations to healing. Much of it involves day-to-day practices related to maintaining and improving one's overall health.

Many practitioners of different kinds, if asked, will attribute the roots of what they do to a Daoist cosmology, understood in different ways. As noted earlier, this frame of reference includes *qi,* Yin and Yang, the Five Phases, and the Dao. For some non-Chinese, the adoption of such concepts may accompany a rejection of inherited religious worldviews and a preference, instead, for what can be construed as "spiritual." It matters little to some of them that such concepts and, sometimes, texts sometimes wove their way into Confucian or Buddhist worldviews and practices as well. Chinese practitioners, in contrast, may view these same concepts as so integral to how they view the world that they can't be considered "religious" or even spiritual; such phenomena would, instead, be found through home altars, temples, or clan halls. The following discussion explores some of the ways in which these conceptual matters play out in these other branches of Chinese medicine and healing.

Food Therapy

One of the most basic ways in which Chinese-based approaches to health have appeared is in food. It was for this reason that immigrant communities not only imported foods from China but also, when possible, grew them for themselves. Such immigrants also sometimes served as ambulatory vendors in states like California, peddling fresh produce among Chinese and non-Chinese by the 1870s. In 1909, a collaborative set up between Chinese, Anglo, and Japanese vegetable growers led to the founding of the City Market Wholesale Produce Terminal in Los Angeles. Wherever Chinese communities grew up, merchants immigrated to establish stores that sold foods otherwise unavailable, as well as remedies for self-care. In the current Chinatown mall complexes in

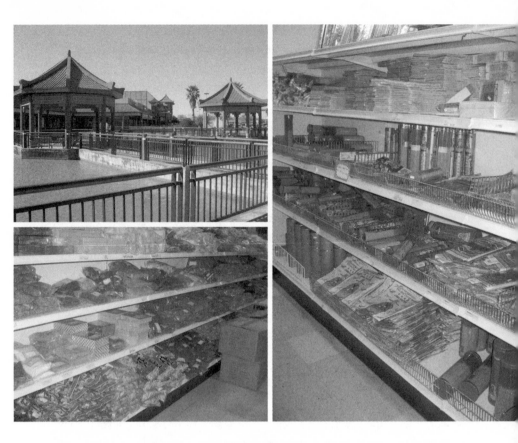

Figure 10.1. Hong Kong Market, at Houston's Chinatown. *Top left:* fountains and moats outside of the Hong Kong Mall, to adjust the site's *fengshui. Bottom Left:* bulk herbs on sale at Hong Kong Market. *Right:* Funeral supplies—spirit money, incense, paper representations of comforts of life—for burning at gravesites. Sold in the Housewares section of the market, together with home altars and related items. Courtesy of Linda L. Barnes.

places such as Texas, there is almost invariably a large supermarket where customers can purchase, for example, patent remedies and prepackaged herbs for tonic soups. There is usually at least one herbal store as well.

Part of family practice in Chinese American homes—depending on how recent the arrival and which generations are involved—may include the use of herbal tonics that combine prepackaged combinations of herbs with meat and vegetables. Parents or grandparents tell the younger generations when to avoid peanuts, spicy foods, or fried foods, and what is best to consume in the summer or in the winter. To different degrees, these instructions translate into a way of life. Yet for those seeking more explicit instruction, cookbooks with recipes for therapeutic soups and stews are available not only in Chinese but also in translation. They include works published in Hong Kong and Taiwan as well as a number published abroad, such as *The Wisdom of the Chinese Kitchen: Classic Family Recipes for Celebration and Healing* (Young 1999; see also Flaws 1995a, 1995b; Zhao and Ellis 1998; Simonds 1999). Even Betty Crocker has gotten in on publishing low-fat Chinese recipes, which sit alongside other low-calorie, fat-free, and heart-healthy Chinese-food cookbooks.

Some of the Chinese medicine schools provide at least basic introductions to Chinese dietary theory and methods, so that practitioners can make recommendations to their patients. But such instruction is most often reserved for those who pursue training in herbal medicine, which not every school requires its students to do, or which may be offered as an optional additional year of training. A teacher such as Daoist priest and chef Nam Singh, in San Francisco, teaches actual courses in Daoist cooking, with direct attention to its health-related properties. Dr. Singh, an Ethiopian American who spent part of his childhood and adolescence in a Daoist monastery in Taiwan, where he also received his medicine training and degrees, practices the full scope of Chinese medicine but has elected to concentrate on the *qi*-based properties of food and on teaching a related medicinal cuisine.

Herbal Medicines

Because the ingredients of food and Chinese *materia medica* overlap, there is little clear boundary between the two. For that reason, in countries such as the United States, Chinese herbs have been represented as "dietary supplements" and have thereby avoided regulation by the Food and Drug Administration (although health food stores have, since the 1980s, periodically circulated flyers flagging impending federal effort to change this policy). Among non-Chinese users, however, who may be unfamiliar with Chinese therapeutic cuisine, the distinctions may appear more clear-cut.

Countries engaged in early trade with China were well aware of the country's herbal resources. Nor did it take long for traders, diplomats, and other foreign observers to become aware of such herbs and drugs as matched their own commercial interests and medical knowledge (Barnes 2005b). For example, wild ginseng from Canada and the American colonies (later the United States) became a stock article in the China trade, transitioning eventually to the actual cultivation of the roots, generally as a form of supplemental income. In the nineteenth century, farming magazines began to sell instructions on ginseng growing and trade, and growers' organizations formed in the early twentieth century (Carlson 1986). Such farming has continued to the present, although there has been a return to the search for wild ginseng, particularly in U.S. states such as Wisconsin and Tennessee. So lucrative has this trade become in recent years that poaching has posed a growing problem for local and state governments (Lienwand 2007).

Anytime a practice migrates from one setting into another, it changes—even when those who practice it insist they are doing as they always did. The very fact of a new location means that the individual or group now lives among others in some measure foreign to them. The circumstances for acquiring the tools of one's art are different: things may not be readily available, and when they are, they may be more expensive or not precisely what one had always used. For example, some nineteenth-century Chinese herbalists in the United States incorporated local plants into their *materia medica,* particularly in the western states. Others, in some of the more remote areas, grew their own.

A widely circulated truism is that until the burst of media attention directed to acupuncture beginning in the early 1970s, Chinese American practitioners had largely cared for patients within their own ethnic communities; only recently, it was routinely claimed, had non-Chinese communities become aware of and begun to use these practices. Nothing could be further from the truth. Although it is certainly true that the early immigrant herbalists served their own communities, in relatively short order they also began to tend to patients from Native American, European American, African American, and Latin American backgrounds. Indeed, the specifics depended primarily on the demographics of particular localities.

One of the best-known examples is Doc Ing Hay (1862–1952), who ran a small pharmacy within an all-purpose store he shared with his business partner Lung An (1863–1940) in John Day, Oregon. Over the years, as work dried up for Chinese workers in eastern Oregon, Doc Hay built a patient base among the local population, most of whom were European American. Hunters brought him animal parts they knew he used in his prescriptions, while patients at a greater distance sent telegrams, letters, and checks requesting refills.

By the 1890s, Chinese herbalists in the United States were advertising not only in San Francisco and Los Angeles but also in Chicago, Boston, New York, and Atlanta—and doing so in English-language newspapers. That these ads often ran week in and week out for years indicates that they proved successful in attracting patients. (During that same period, however, and spilling over into the first decades of the twentieth century, increased regulation of medical practice in the United States led to the arrest of Chinese herbalists in cities throughout the country for practicing medicine without a license.) When possible, some of these practitioners passed their learning and their work on to

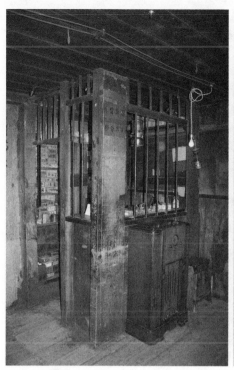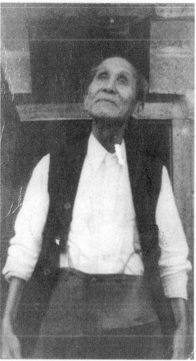

Figure 10.2. Doc Ing Hay in his later years, and his herbal pharmacy, in the Kam Wah Chung building in John Day, Oregon. *Left:* Courtesy of Linda L. Barnes. *Right:* Courtesy of the Kam Wah Chung Museum.

their descendants. This was all the more the case during the years when they couldn't gain entrance to medical or pharmacology schools or, as happened to Willard Jue in Seattle, Washington, they got such a degree but then couldn't get a job in an Anglo-owned business.

"Trialing" Chinese Medicine in Colonial Australia

Rey Tiquia

During the mid-nineteenth century, the British colony of Victoria in Australia became an epicenter of gold fever. Hundreds of thousands of people from all over the continent and around the world flocked there in search of gold, increasing the risk of diseases such as diphtheria, a virulent bacterial infection that produces a leathery membrane on the throat and, sometimes, fatal suffocation. (In Chinese, diphtheria is *baihou,* "white throat.") By midcentury, regular epidemics swept the colony. In 1872, it was reported that diphtheria killed six hundred people annually (the epidemic also hit Britain, Europe, the Americas, and China). Most victims were children.

Medicine in the colony was plural and idiosyncratic: indigenous Aboriginal healers (who largely treated their own communities), allopaths, homeopaths, pharmacists, dentists, herbalists, naturopaths, and traditional Chinese medical practitioners (referred to as "Chinese herbalists"). As diphtheria swept the colony, some of these herbalists entered the limelight following the success of treatments using their diphtheria powder. The news spread like wildfire. In response, on August 13, 1874, the Victoria Parliament debated and later accepted a proposal to run a trial testing the powder's efficacy. It was proposed, too, that Chinese herbalist Ah Sue conduct the trial and administer the remedy. However, the actual responsibility of "ascertaining the value" of the powder fell to Dr. John Blair, a surgeon from Melbourne's Alfred Hospital.

Blair secured four packets of the powder. Using laboratory facilities at the Technology Museum, he had the contents "qualitatively examined" and reported that the "Chinaman powder contains nothing new." It is "composed of alum, carbonate of lime, nitrate of potash, sulphate of sodium, sulfate of copper, nitrate, and chlorate of potash with camphor and mush added to give them odor" (Blair 1874, 294–295). Speaking before the Medical Society of Victoria, he boasted, "We know the nature of their composition, and can easily comprehend the mode of their action. . . . That when the powder is blown into the fauces [throat] the preparation can act as astringents, caustics, or escharotics." In the hands of an ignorant man, he added, these local preparations would cause grievous harm (Blair 1874, 294–295).

Blair followed his "expert technical interpretation" of the "facts" with ad hominem racist attacks against the Chinese herbalists. He called Ah Sue an "ignorant pretender" who had "received no medical Chinese education whatsoever," and claimed that the powder consisted only of substances used on an everyday basis for throat disease and picked up from local pharmacies. Following the "trial," Ah Sue reportedly returned to China. Other Chinese herbalists faced legal action for calling themselves "doctor," a title biomedical physicians reserved for themselves.

Biomedicine dominated until 2000, when the Victoria Parliament passed the Chinese Medicine Registration Bill, legitimizing the practice of Chinese medicine and establishing the Chinese Medicine Registration Board for practitioners. To date, in Victoria, only practitioners registered by the board can use

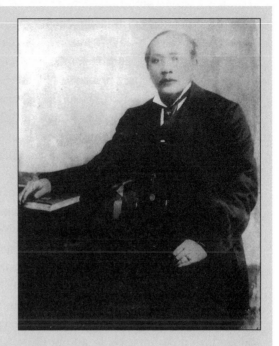

Figure 10.3. Dr. Luo Kwoi Sang, one of the Chinese herbalists who treated diphtheria sufferers during the 1870s in Victoria, Australia. He was eventually made to stand trial for using the title "doctor of medicine." Courtesy of Joseph P. L. Sang.

the titles "traditional Chinese medicine (TCM) practitioner," "Chinese medicine practitioner," "acupuncturist," or "Chinese herbalist."

Blair and his supporters doubtless saw themselves as promoting necessary standards for medical practice in the developing colony (although many also admitted those same standards to be self-interested and biased). It was not that Chinese practice did not have standards or was indifferent to them. Rather, there was no official openness to incorporating Chinese standards into those regulating medicine of the day. To incorporate standards from another tradition in ways that would have satisfied all parties would have required cross-translation. The testimonies of satisfied patients effectively promoted the herbalists' work, eliciting a parliamentary response. However, a different kind of response undermined that popular experience of Chinese standards. That was the pernicious effect of Blair's "trial."

In contrast, C. K. Ah Fong settled in Boise, Idaho, in 1889 and by 1893 had set up an herb store. Although he was initially refused a medical license, a local judge reversed the decision. Eventually Ah Fong became one of the only Chinese herbal doctors in the country to secure an American medical license based on his practice of Chinese medicine. He passed his practice on to his son Herbert, who transmitted it to his own son Gerald. Each received his training in China, the son and grandson going back for that purpose and then returning to work in the family herb practice in Idaho (Buell and Muench 1984; see also Ford and Jacox 1996). By 1964, the former Chinese community had disappeared except for C. K. Ah Fong's great-grandson Billy Fong, who departed unwillingly, and only when a wrecking ball was about to demolish his building as part of a redevelopment initiative. One factor that affected the Ah Fong business—as it had other Chinese American herbalists—involved the impact on the herb trade of the founding of the People's Republic of China. Trade restrictions made it increasingly difficult to import herbs that had previously been available.

In the United States, it also became complicated to assert one's Chinese identity too openly in a Cold War environment in which McCarthyism ran rampant. Families that had been in practice for generations found themselves unable to keep their businesses afloat, and felt more vulnerable if they promoted themselves outside of their own communities. Some opted not to work out of storefronts but rather to set up their practices in apartments on the second or third floor, invisible to all but those who knew the location through word of mouth. Such arrangements provided a variation (often a more economical one) on older versions in which an herbalist's family would live above or in the back of their herb store. These developments contributed to the wider perception that Chinese herbalists and acupuncturists served primarily their own communities.

Still, some family businesses survived. For example, Hen Sen Chin immigrated to Seattle, Washington, in 1923, opened an herb store, and passed on his learning to his daughter Juliana. She went from tasting and smelling herbs at the age of five to eventually carrying on her father's practice, Hen Sen Herbs. Or there is Dr. Carl Shan Leung, who founded Kamwo Herbal Pharmacy in New York in 1973. His son Thomas grew up helping out in the store, went on to study and practice biomedical pharmacology, and then gradually returned to the family business, at which point he got a degree in acupuncture and herbal medicine. He has integrated business practices used in American pharmacies and designed a Web-based program that enables practitioners to submit prescriptions for their patients, and to order herbs. These most recent iterations of multigenerational practices parallel ones found in Chinese immigrant communities around the world.

TCM and Chinese Immigrants with Tuberculosis in New York City's Chinatown: A Case Study

Ming Ho

Many studies of the integration of biomedicine and Chinese medicine focus on mainstream populations. But what occurs among Chinese immigrants? The following case study involves sixty Chinese immigrant patients recruited from New York City Department of Health chest clinics and directly observed therapy programs in order to gather information about their tuberculosis management (Ho 2003, 2004a, 2004b). Twelve of the sixty said they not only were on antituberculosis (TB) medication but also took Chinese medicine, generally using formulas with three types of function.

The first function involved symptom relief. For instance, one patient saw a traditional Chinese doctor, who prescribed herbal medicine for coughing and excessive phlegm. Another patient's husband worked in a grocery shop, where he got herbs to relieve her cough. Patients generally said they did not use Chinese medicine to *cure* tuberculosis, but only to alleviate its symptoms. (Only one claimed to have been cured with Chinese medicine alone, in China some twenty years earlier.)

The second frequently reported function addressed the side effects of biomedicine (Ho 2006). Many patients perceived biomedicine to be more potent than Chinese medicine and more effective in treating acute diseases or eliminating bacterial infection. However, they also felt it was not as good for chronic conditions because it was too strong for prolonged use. Many expressed the concern that taking antituberculosis medicine for as long as six months would harm their bodies and general health, some even indicating that they could not have adhered to biomedicine regimens had they not also been using Chinese medicine to ease the side effects.

The third function included supplementing their diet, nurturing their lungs, boosting their general resistance, and restoring their health. The meaning of the term "lungs" sometimes derived from Chinese medicine and sometimes corresponded more closely to the biomedical sense. One way in which kin might contribute to the patient's adherence to the therapeutic regimen was by providing the patient with recipes or actual food items that would help to restore general health. Many patients reported that their families or they themselves cooked *baotang* (nutritious, medicinal soup) to nurture their lungs.

Public health officials and biomedical doctors often consider Chinese traditional medicine a barrier to antituberculosis treatment. In addition to fearing the possibility of adverse drug interactions, they are likely to assume that patients believe either in biomedicine or in Chinese medicine, leading to the exclusive use of one system. That is, they anticipate that patients who choose Chinese medicine will not use biomedicine.

In reality, however, Chinese immigrant patients themselves generally used the two concurrently. They expressed the view that Chinese medicine does not replace but rather complements biomedicine. Some even stressed that it works in tandem with biomedicine and is therefore not simply complementary but also a necessary factor in returning to good health. Others explained that they could not use biomedicine if they did not relieve its side effects with Chinese medicine. On the whole, these patients experienced the positive effects of traditional Chinese medicine in alleviating unpleasant symptoms, reducing adverse reactions to biomedicine, and restoring their general health. The somewhat surprising finding, therefore, was that some patients utilize traditional Chinese medicine as a way of supporting their use of and adherence to the biomedical interventions offered through the Department of Health's directly observed therapy programs.

Generally, however, herbalists—both Chinese and non-Chinese—write prescriptions, and when herb stores are available, patients go there to have them filled. Some practitioners dispense herbs from their clinics. But practitioners in general also regularly cite patients' reluctance to cook up the herbs at home—a process that requires two rounds of simmering them in water until they reach a concentrated state, then blending the batches. Not only does this take time, but the cooking herbs also have a pronounced smell and, until one gets used to the taste, are often quite bitter.

A regular alternative involves formulas distilled into pill form, often referred to as "patent remedies." Sometimes a concentrated tincture of the herbs is sold mixed with alcohol (used as a preservative) and dispensed into hot water with an eyedropper. In the United States, herbs in a variety of forms are also available through herb stores, health food stores, groceries and supermarkets serving Asian customers and, increasingly, in mainstream pharmacies, supermarkets, discount department stores, and large wholesale clubs.

Although practitioners regularly agree that decocted herbs are best, they also agree that a decoction does little good if the patient never takes it—in which case pills or tinctures are the better course. An intermediate option involves reducing the distillation to a powder, a measure of which can be stirred into hot water, reconstituted, and drunk. Therefore, schools that teach herbal medicine must familiarize their students with the principles and composition of herbal formulas, the related uses of granular herbs, and appropriate substitutions with patent remedies.

Herbs have been exported from Taiwan, Hong Kong, mainland China, and other countries, often shipped in large drums and then repackaged by the stores that sell them. Differing international approaches to regulation and quality control have resulted in questions regarding possible contaminants from such sources as polluted waterways or water passing through aging lead pipes. Moreover, some overseas manufacturers can and do add pharmaceuticals. Such practices have caused concerns over the safety of some—though clearly far from all—herbal imports. In response, manufacturers have emerged in some countries in the West, with some supporting growers in their own country. To do so affords greater knowledge of and control over the sources, manufacturing procedures, and adherence to regulatory measures.

Demand for certain ingredients deriving from animals have led to poaching and smuggling. The illegal hunting and trapping of tigers for their bones, rhinoceroses for their horns, black bears for their paws and gallbladders, musk deer for their glands, and seahorses, for example, have reduced these and other species populations to the point of endangerment. Although many governments have passed laws to reserve land as protected habitats, such laws are not always enforced. Indeed, government officials themselves are sometimes complicit in turning a blind eye to, and even profiting from, the smuggling (Baum and Vincent 2005; St. Clair 2007; Bell 2009).

In the United States, problems such as these have led federal regulators to raid herb stores (sometimes claiming to look for illegal drugs), sending the store owner, workers, and customers onto the street during a search of the premises. Some herbalists report that investigators break open drums of herbs and, although they don't recognize most of the contents, pour shampoo over them to saturate and destroy them. In addition to the financial loss, there is an accompanying loss of face, particularly because the raiders rarely apologize. Similar raids have occurred in Chinese medicine stores in Canadian cities including Toronto and Vancouver.

Some practitioners who purchase herbs from mainland China have undertaken their own reforms. Dr. P. Q. Kang of San Francisco presents an uncommon example. Having inherited a *tuina* and herbal lineage from his family, he went to Shanghai Medical University, graduating in 1970 and eventually becoming the chief medical officer of the Department of Traditional Chinese Medicine at Shanghai Hospital. He came to the United States in 1985, to teach at the American College of Traditional Chinese Medicine (ACTCM). During his time in San Francisco, he and his wife have cultivated a network of farmers in China whom they have trained in organic herbiculture. They therefore import their own herbs, incorporating them into the formulas dispensed by Dr. Kang.

Another small circle of practitioners and botanists have initiated a network to engage in the experimental growing of organic Chinese herbs. In the United States, such a project began in 1987 with a collaborative exchange between the ACTCM in San Francisco and the University of California Botanical Garden. Professor Xu Hong-hua came from the Guangzhou College of Traditional Chinese Medicine, bringing plants and seeds and spending six months designing and planting a medicinal herb garden with eighteen sections that corresponded to treatment approaches. Following Xu's return to China, an ACTCM student, Robert Newman, worked for five years to expand the collection, collaborating with conservators from around the world. He also spent a year and a half as a curator at the Chinese herb garden at Nanjing Institute of Botany in China. When he finally left ACTCM in 1997, he distributed species to eight conservators in different regions of the United States and left behind a fully developed garden for student learning (Giblette 2009b).

Gardens such as the one at High Falls, New York, under the direction of Jean Giblette, now constitute part of a national network. Each garden is in a different region of the United States, making it possible to test how well different plants grow in each region. In addition, following the example of ACTCM, at least fifteen acupuncture and Oriental medicine colleges in the United States have herb gardens. High Falls Gardens has also identified farmers in New York and Pennsylvania who grow ginseng under conditions that mimic growth in the wild (Giblette 2009a).

Is Vietnamese Medicine Chinese Medicine?

Laurence Monnais

When one asks Vietnamese Canadians about their use of traditional medicine, they are often slow to respond. Not because they have nothing to say on the subject, but rather because they wonder *which* traditional medicine we are asking about: *thuốc bắc* or *thuốc nam*. Although the word *thuốc* can mean "tobacco," "folk remedy," or "medicine," Vietnamese in the diaspora differentiate between Chinese drugs (from the north, or *bắc*) and Vietnamese drugs (from the south, or *nam*).

The vocabulary for discussing Vietnamese medicine has changed over time, especially during the twentieth century. During French colonization (1858–1954), colonial administrators and health authorities, along with some Vietnamese doctors trained in Western medicine, disparaged what they called "Sino-Vietnamese medicine." They saw it as without scientific basis, and hence inefficient and dangerous. Such criticism combined with colonial attempts to control and even dismantle this other field of expertise by outlawing, for example, all therapeutic substances the French administration saw as toxic.

Several associations of traditional medical practitioners reacted in the 1920s and 1930s. They not only emphasized the indispensable nature of a medicine close to the people, able to fill daily gaps in an underfinanced and essentially urban colonial health care system, but also sought to promote the scientific and professional character of their practice, paving the way for a future independent and modern health care system for the country.

In this period of heightened nationalism, these practitioners found it equally important to remove Chinese influences from their practice and utilize an extraordinary local biodiversity to create a therapeutic system completely adapted to "Vietnamese constitutions." The idea of differentiating Vietnamese from Chinese medicines was hardly new—the distinction between *thuốc bắc* and *thuốc nam* dates to as early as the fourteenth century—but traditional practitioners saw the 1920s and the 1930s as an ideal occasion to complete the separation. Hence was born the concept of *thuốc ta,* or "our medicine" (Marr 1987, 179–180).

As a highly politicized, reinvented tradition, Vietnamese medicine took its place first in the Democratic Republic (1954–1975) and then in the Socialist Republic of Vietnam (1975–) (Huong et al. 1965), as part of a health care system dubbed "integrative" by the World Health Organization. The system is based on a combination of biomedicine and traditional medicine, or *y học cổ truyền.* Taken literally, the phrase means "the study of medicine passed down from antiquity"; however, it is usually translated into English as "Vietnamese traditional medicine" (VTM), the analogue of traditional Chinese medicine in China.

The identity of Vietnamese medicine as well as the field of intervention reserved for it remain ambiguous in practice. The expression *đông y,* distinguishing an "Eastern medicine" from "Western medicine" (Hoang et al. 1993), is still frequently used. But for many, Vietnamese medicine is defined

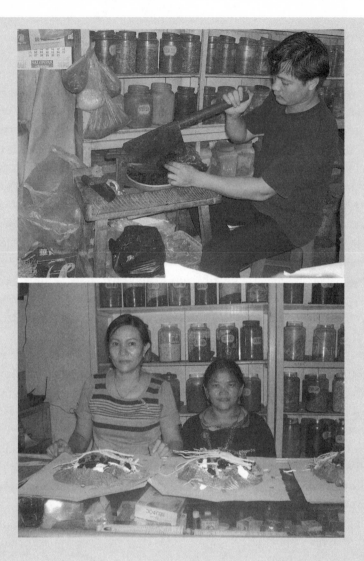

Figure 10.4. Herbal pharmacy in Hoi An, Vietnam. *Top:* Chopping herbs. *Bottom:* Contents for making medicinal rice wine. Courtesy of Martin Kolner.

almost exclusively by its pharmacopoeia, which has been updated (Wahlberg 2006). Yet this *material medica* cannot in and of itself provide an autonomous identity to Vietnamese medicine. Consequently, VTM is often relegated to the secondary status of "complementary" and "syncretic" medicine (Banh 1952).

In an era of globalization, Vietnamese immigrants in Canada are aware of these limits. Their use of Vietnamese medicine is generally limited to a number of minor, chronic health problems. It is often consumed in combination with Chinese medicine and, above all, biomedicine (Blanc and Monnais 2007). At the same time, its use by immigrant Vietnamese practitioners and pharmacists, alongside drugs produced by the Vietnamese pharmaceutical industry, illustrates that this national medicine is alive and ever changing. As in Vietnam (Craig 2002), it is constantly renegotiating its uses and its identity.

In Germany, Chinese herbs are generally imported from different Asian countries by specialized retailers and then resold to qualified practitioners. The challenge, however, is that Germany regulates the sale of herbs, requiring documentation of the plants' origin and production process—information often missing with imported herbs. In response, a collaborative field cultivation experiment has undertaken to grow sixteen herbs under controlled and documented conditions in order to improve their safety and quality. Unlike earlier generations, however, who were primarily interested in plants that were already a part of their pharmacopoeia, this group has expanded their list to include herbs commonly used in Chinese medicine (Bomme et al. 2007).

In contrast, in Cairo, Egypt, the marketplace carries ginseng tablets from the United States and other capsules and tablets from mainland China. Vendors must register—a process that can take from months to two or three years—and must agree to sell fewer than four kinds of medicines (WFCMS 2009). In Tanzania, patients may use local herbs, talismans from the Qu'ran, holy water, biomedical pharmaceuticals, and the intervention of elders, ancestors, and spirits. They turn to Chinese doctors for "formula drugs," which include powdered *materia medica* that sometimes may also incorporate vitamins or steroids, and which may call for simmering the substances, dissolving them in water, or directly swallowing them as pills (Hsu 2007, 22). As Michael Jennings puts it, "Healing in Tanzania—within Africa—consists of these multiple agents: coexisting and competing systems all granted legitimacy through use" (2005, 459).

South Africa legalized traditional Chinese medicine in April 2001 in response to practitioner petitions. At the same time, the legislation recognized traditional African and Ayurvedic medicines (Editorial Staff 2001). Practitioners themselves come from different ethnic backgrounds, including not only those of Chinese descent but also Indian- and European-descended South

Africans. Online companies have sprung up to provide Chinese herbal medicine and acupuncture supplies, along with texts and reference books, with sections dedicated to practitioners and others to patients. In 2003, registered practitioners established the National Acupuncture and Chinese Medicine Association of South Africa.

Further Worlds of *Qi*

Early Jesuit missionaries in China recognized that their effort to convert Chinese literati would fail if it included pressing for the rejection of ancestor traditions in particular. The Jesuits therefore adopted the strategy of representing the Confucian tradition to Rome as a philosophy and not a religion—a representation that has continued in the West over the centuries. Another legacy of this strategy has been the assumption that the terms "religion" and "religious" refer to Christianity. Not to be religious, therefore, can be a way of saying that one is not Christian—not that there are no religious dimensions to one's life.

The People's Republic of China (PRC) condemnation of religions in general and the Confucian tradition in particular, accompanied by the closing or destruction of thousands of temples, further buttressed the reluctance to identify openly with any of the traditions. At the same time, Confucian, Buddhist, Daoist, and gods- or ancestor-based religious influences have so permeated Chinese culture that they have persisted despite years of government opposition. During the 1980s and 1990s, temples and ancestor halls were rebuilt, spirit mediums and exorcists resurfaced, and various divination practices awakened new interest (Smith 2006). Some cab drivers in Beijing routinely wear Buddhist meditation beads around their wrists. Daoist temples have been renovated, such as the Baiyun Guan (White Cloud Temple) in Beijing (where offerings of red tassels are piled high before the diorama representing the Hell that awaits corrupt officials). In other countries with large Chinese populations or communities, the full range of such practices have long-standing roots, with new adaptations and expressions.

Anthropologist Thomas Csordas asks which aspects of religious practices and worldviews are most likely to travel. In part, he suggests, it depends on how "portable" they are—how easy it is to learn the rites, how much esoteric knowledge or paraphernalia one has to have, and the extent to which one can engage in the practice without having to buy into specific ideologies or institutions. Csordas cites *fengshui* as an example of a practice with characteristics that enable it to travel well. He goes on to propose that *how* practices travel also matters, whether it is through missionization (which utilizes various means to deliberately spread a tradition) or through migration (which includes both involuntary and voluntary movements of people around the globe). (See Csordas 2007a.) One could add as well the emergence of technologies that have expedited communication, encouraged the spread of information, and facilitated travel. Csordas suggests, too, that as religious tenets move across different cultural and linguistic settings, they are like a piece of music transposed into a different key: one continues to recognize the music but also hears the differences.

Many of these tenets are enacted through day-to-day activities—ones widely assumed to be secular, an assumption contributing to the illusion that secularization has increased. But it may be a case of what Andrew Kim calls "nonofficial religion" or Meredith McGuire characterizes as "religious and quasi-religious beliefs and practices that are neither accepted nor controlled by official religious groups" (Kim 2005; McGuire 2002, 113). In popular frames of reference, it often includes practices described as "spiritual" rather than "religious."

During the past sixty years, the migration of Chinese traditions met with seekers looking into worldviews that had grown up in China and spread out into the world. Insofar as these were the same traditions in which many of the movement-based practices were grounded, the distinction is often artificial. Other seekers studied with Chinese Buddhist or Daoist teachers, the latter including such key figures in the United States as Share K. Lew, Moy Lin-shin, Eva Wong, Hua-ching Ni, Mantak Chia, and Hsien Yuen. Some taught *taiji* or *gongfu (kungfu)*; some were ordained priests or monks, or students authorized to transmit the traditions.

In other instances, non-Chinese individuals went abroad, as happened for Charles Belyea, who—following years of training and practice—was first ordained as a Buddhist monk in Taiwan and then, after apprenticing with a number of Daoist masters, was given ordination and succession in the Liu Daoist family lineage, through which he took the name Liu Ming (for a detailed discussion of Daoism in North America, see Komjathy 2004). Sometimes the master-student relationship remained active throughout the teacher's lifetime; in other cases, after a period of apprenticeship students struck out on their own, with or without the teacher's full endorsement. Thus we are talking about a complex mixing of Chinese and non-Chinese; migration, conscious dissemination, and active pursuit; acculturation and adoption; and the influences of different markets, all in shifting configurations.

Visualizing Qi

Nancy N. Chen

> "Watch as I move my brush how it follows my body and breath." Master
> Wang, a wushu instructor, demonstrated by writing the character for *qi*
> using an ink brush on rice paper. With deft, fluid brush strokes he traced
> the character on paper that mirrored his martial art movements. *(Beijing,*
> *July 1991)*

Qi is described as a universal form of energy, life force, breath, or flow that can
be cultivated in human bodies through specific forms. Practitioners of Asian
calligraphy, medicine, martial arts, and even cooking now learn about it as a
central element of their training. As part of an embodied experience of healing, however, *qi* is also both represented visually and visualized. Indeed, the
healing traditions in particular offer insight into different ways in which visualization of *qi* is central to embodiment and transformation.

A common starting point is through written language and how the concept
of *qi* is visually represented in characters. The older ideogram for *qi* included
"rice" *(mi),* under the larger cognate form that connoted "vapor" or "breath."
In the simplified version of the character, the ideogram retains the upper component, which is also used in other compound terms, such as those for "breath,"
"atmosphere," "mood," "complexion," "car," or even "soda pop." Some of the
earliest visual portrayals of body cultivation are linked to drawings on silk of
figures engaged in a range of different poses that were found in the Mawangdui
excavation (no. 3 tomb) at Changsha (Harper 1998). Contemporary martial art
and *qigong* manuals that circulated in China during the 1990s claimed these
images to be the earliest recordings of *qi* exercise. We see how these images
suggest that *qi* is linked to bodies in motion rather than to static postures.

Chinese medical texts also provide visual representations of *qi*. Acupuncture
points superimposed on charts or three-dimensional anatomical body models
literally map the channels where *qi* moves or gathers in the body. The ancient
text *Huangdi neijing suwen* suggests more nuanced notions of *qi* visualization.
Paul Unschuld's analysis, for example, frames how ancient naturalists considered the role of *qi* as nearly inseparable from that of blood (2003). Their explorations extended beyond notions of *qi* as vapor. Elaborate descriptions of *qi*
movement from atmosphere to organs, or from food to the body, suggest that

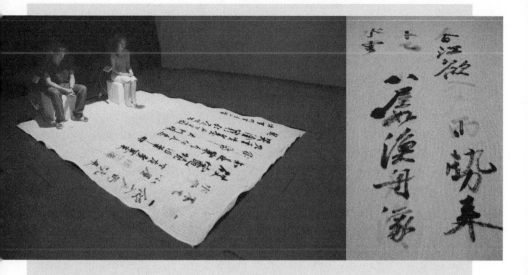

Figure 10.5. The "Flow of Qi" exhibit, staged by the Industrial Technology Research Institute (ITRI) Creativity Lab in the National Palace Museum, Taiwan, in 2007. The exhibit utilized ultra-wide-band technology to let participating observers orient their breathing in relation to the spirit of famous works of calligraphy from the National Palace Museum in Taiwan, and thereby establish personal contact with these cultural treasures. *Left:* Participants in the exhibit. *Right:* The rate and pulse of viewers' breathing interacted with the sound of digital music for their *qi* to influence the calligraphy. Photographs by Cheng-Ya Liu. Courtesy of the ITRI Creativity Lab, Taiwan.

qi permeates a body and gets distributed. Emotional states become possible endpoints for its flow. Rather than relying on more static visual representations that specify locations of *qi,* this text envisions an ongoing, interactive flow between organs and external elements such as atmosphere and internalized forms such as food.

Indeed, flow might be characterized as the main aspect of *qi* that practitioners of various forms of self-cultivation have come to recognize. The "Flow of Qi" exhibit staged by the ITRI Creativity Lab in the National Palace Museum in 2007 tried to capture this aspect. Participants sat side by side, two at a time. Sensors attuned to the patterns and movement of their breath fed related measures into a machine, which then generated calligraphic images. This technological feat replicated what Master Wang had demonstrated in his martial-art-influenced calligraphy, cited above. These examples illustrate how the visualization of *qi,* as it moves within or outside a body, manifests as a central component of cultivation and healing practices.

Harmonizing Practices

As earlier chapters have shown, movement-based practices that combine meditative and kinetic dimensions date back to early Chinese history, while their use in varied forms and ways has continued through to the present. As early morning visitors to parks not only in China but also in Chinese communities around the world know, people gather each day, year round, to practice *taijiquan* and other related movement forms. In Manhattan's Columbus Park, for example, people identify an individual whose *taiji* they like, and begin to follow what that person is doing. To walk the perimeter of the park is to observe different styles and approaches—some with music, some with fans, swords, or long red streamers. Gradually a group forms with that person as its teacher, and participants may congregate daily for years. A number of these teachers move on to find a more formal location, and in some cases they establish actual *taiji* schools.

Others arrive in the receiving country already having taught elsewhere, with the intention of seeking students. Although Chinese practitioners of movement-based practices have been migrating around the world for centuries, these more recent developments were further inspired by the popularity of martial arts films (and particularly those from Hong Kong). Although these action movies were first produced beginning in the 1930s and went through a series of genre conventions, the movies produced in the 1970s were disseminated worldwide, developing a passionate fan base. As a result, new generations of students of all different nationalities studied the different schools of practice, seeking anything from physical discipline to a technique for self-defense to spiritual growth.

At the same time, growing numbers of spiritual seekers around the world questioned the religious traditions with which they had been raised, and looked to new sources. As they became aware of the meditative dimensions of practices such as *taijiquan,* they looked for teachers in Taiwan, in Hong Kong, and among exiles from the PRC. Masters like Bow Sim Mark came to the United States, where she founded the Chinese Wushu Research Institute in Boston to teach *taijiquan* and *wushu.* She trained her son, Donnie Yen, who then went to Hong Kong, where he became an internationally known actor in martial arts films. But her other students come from many cultural backgrounds.

Taiji in America

Elijah Siegler

Although there is no record of the first *taiji* class taught in America, it is doubtful that Chinese immigrants arriving in the mid-nineteenth century practiced what we know today as *taiji*. They were mostly from south China, while *taiji* was centered in the north. Moreover, this first generation arrived between the 1850s and the 1880s, yet *taiji* gained public popularity in China only in the late nineteenth and early twentieth centuries, thanks to Yang Chengfu (1886–1935), to whom most of the original Yang-style *taiji* instructors in the United States trace their lineage. (Indeed, Yang remains the most popular style of *taiji* in the United States.) The first visual representation of *taiji* in America may be a 1930s newsreel depicting Chinese immigrants in California practicing it en masse.

European American authors Sophia Delza (1903–1996) and Edward Maisel (1937–2008) published the first American *taiji* books in English. A modern dancer from New York City, Delza wrote *Body and Mind in Harmony* (1961) as a straightforward guide to the practice. Maisel published *Tai Chi for Health* the following year. Maisel, who founded the Tai Chi Institute of America in New York City in 1961, attempts to excise anything overtly Chinese from *taiji*. While Delza uses simple line drawings to illustrate positions, Maisel's photographs show white men in loafers, slacks, shirt, and tie—everything but a sport jacket. His language recalls cheerful 1950s physical fitness boosterism, with chapter subheadings such as "A Way to Remain Youthful," "Never a Feeling of Strain," and "Tai Chi Prevents Freak Injuries."

Indeed, Maisel's conception of spiritual achievement owes more to Norman Vincent Peale's "power of positive thinking" than to Chinese thought. Maisel writes that *taiji* can give you "greater mental powers," acts as a "safe tranquilizer," and "furnishes strong motivation." Expert testimony comes not from Chinese sources but from physicians working in New York City hospitals. For Maisel, *taiji* is compatible with the American values of optimism and activism.

One of the first Chinese to teach *taiji* to non-Chinese in North America was Cheng Man-ch'ing (Zheng Manqing, 1901–1975). Born in eastern China and a former bodyguard for the Nationalists, he taught *taiji* at the Military Academy in Shanghai. He was also a painter, a doctor of Chinese medicine and, according to those who knew him, a legendary colorful character. Although he wrote his first *taiji* book in Chinese in 1950, his first successful book in English was

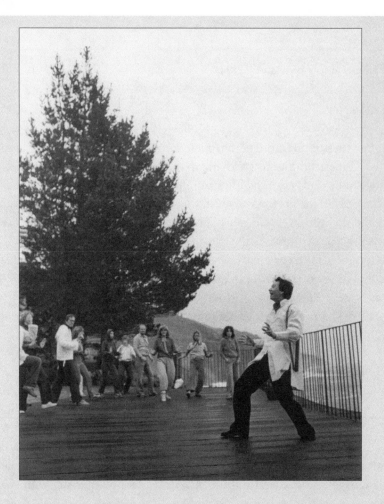

Figure 10.6. Taiji master Al Chungliang Huang performs at Esalen in the late 1970s. Courtesy of Kathleen T. Carr.

T'ai Chi: The Supreme Ultimate Exercise (1967), a collaboration with his American student Robert K. Smith.

Two important popularizers of *taiji* in America were both connected with Esalen, the retreat center in central California best known for giving birth to the human potential movement. *Taiji* "was the movement therapy that became most popular . . . chiefly through Gia-Fu Feng" (Taylor 1999, 245). Feng (1919–1985), a friend of Esalen founder Richard Price, was the only Chinese American on the full-time staff. The second figure, Al Chungliang Huang (b. 1937), has been a regular visitor, who often conducted seminars with his friend Alan Watts (1915–1973). Like Cheng and Feng, Huang was born into a privileged family in China.

Taiji spread quickly during the late 1960s; within just a year, Huang could write, "Recently a t'ai chi fad seems to be mushrooming in all the big cities" (Huang 1973, 58). Instructors came to include non-Chinese teachers as well as new generations of post-1965 immigrants from China and Taiwan, many of whom came to North America to attend graduate school and taught *taiji* at their universities. Today, *taiji* is part of American popular culture, depicted in television commercials and even featured in the For Dummies series of paperbacks.

Sometimes students find a teacher after seeing him or her practice or perform; others locate a teacher by word of mouth, by looking in telephone directories, or by searching the Internet. A number of these teachers have restricted the transmission of knowledge to their own family members, people known to them, or members of their own community, while others have opted to accept non-Chinese students—a move that sometimes is controversial and, for some, might require the permission of one's own teacher.

Temple Practices

Chinese immigrants built temples around the world. Some—like the temples in Oroville (built in 1863, for a local population of ten thousand Chinese residents) and Marysville in northern California—have remained active since the nineteenth century, providing spiritual homes to successive generations of Chinese immigrants. Whether Daoist or Buddhist, many of these temples also housed a shrine for the Medicine Buddha, or Medicine Master Buddha. This aspect recognizes the role of the Buddha and his teachings as the ultimate remedy for the sickness of suffering and ignorance. Petitioners ask for their own healing or that of others in their lives.

Temples dedicated to a particular deity often, in actuality, house multiple figures. For example, the Thien Hau Temple (Tianhou Gong) in Los Angeles, California, is dedicated to Mazu, goddess of the sea, patron of those whose livelihoods or ways of life are connected with the ocean, and source of help to those who hope to bear children. But other figures also have shrines in her temple: the earth god Tu Di (there called Fu De) and the bodhisattvas Guanyin (of compassion and mercy) and Dizang (Dayuan Dizang Pusa, or Dizang of the Great Vow). Some Buddhists view Mazu herself as one of Guanyin's reincarnations, and women turn to both when hoping to become pregnant. Each figure in the temple may be approached for matters related to illness, as well as to oversee the well-being of the larger community. Although built by a Vietnamese immigrant association—which included ethnic Chinese members—other Asian groups share the temple.

Newer temples have sprung up in more recent decades, some of them major complexes, as with the Hsi Lai Si (literally, "Coming to the West") temple of the Fo Guang Shan Buddhist order, which sits on fifteen acres of land in Hacienda Heights, California. The order, founded by the Venerable Master Hsing Yun (b. 1927), has been internationally recognized for introducing Humanistic Buddhism, a reformation movement that accepts all traditions and schools and works to promote unity between the different branches of Buddhism, as part of a larger aim to create a Pure Land here on earth. The order's temples are now an international presence. In 1992, Hsing also established the Guochü Foguang Hui (Buddha's Light International Association, or BLIA), a Buddhist monastic and lay organization headquartered at the Hacienda Heights temple. The group sponsors charitable efforts, taking as their example efforts by the founder, who has organized health initiatives in Taiwan, Thailand, the United States, and Japan.

Home and Business Practices

As in many traditions, the core acts of religious life may take place in homes, businesses, and other places not seen as overtly "religious." Historically, for example, home altars to the Stove Master (also known as the Kitchen God, Zao Shen) secured a moral and protective presence in the Chinese household. Such altars and cabinets, along with incense and figurines of Buddhas, bodhisattvas, Daoist immortals, Confucian venerables, gods and goddesses, continue to be sold in the housewares section of Chinese food markets (including the largest supermarkets), as well as in some herb stores.

Businesses like Lung An and Doc Hay's general store in John Day, Oregon, had a small altar where local people could make offerings. That practice has continued into the present, with many business and restaurant owners still putting up an altar to one of the deities—frequently Guan Gong—with daily gifts of incense and fruit, to oversee the health and good fortune of the business. Food markets and specialty stores also sell the goods needed for funerals, such as spirit money, incense, and the comforts of daily life fashioned from paper—houses, cars, appliances, clothes, jewelry—to burn, so that the smoke will transport them to the deceased. The point is to care for one's dead, maintain harmonious relations with them, and avoid their becoming disgruntled ghosts.

Clan Halls and Associations, and Civic Practices

Early Chinese immigrants—often merchants—organized clan-based benevolent societies *(gongsi)* in different parts of the world to help newcomers of the same family name, dialect, or place of origin. These societies provided social, legal, and job assistance. They loaned money and, when a member died, the association sent the deceased's bones back to China for burial. The associations also oversaw the local clan hall *(tanghao)*, which housed ancestral tablets for the dead. There could be thousands of such tablets, as in Singapore's Lin clan ancestral hall, and each could hold up to four names. Or families might choose instead to place such tablets in a Buddhist temple, to ensure perpetual chanting and care from the monks (Tong 2004).

The family associations also played a part in organizing annual New Year's festivals, a part of which involved firecrackers and the Lion Dance to drive out the *nianshou*, a mythical animal that lives in the jungle, the mountains, or under the ocean but emerges annually, posing a particular danger to children. Loud noises and the color red scare it off. The custom, which originated in Guangdong, attracted good luck and ensured community health. People with martial arts skills danced the lion—a tradition perpetuated by local martial arts schools.

New Organizations for Self-Cultivation and Service

During the second half of the twentieth century new groups focused on self-cultivation and service emerged—some in the PRC, some in Taiwan. They may have centers, but they are not temple-based. The members of these groups are primarily ethnic Chinese, many of them well-educated professionals with an interest in the cultivation of well-being. Participants are generally volunteers; they may exercise the option to donate but are not required to do so. Most activities are conducted in Chinese, sometimes with simultaneous translation. However, the role of non-Chinese members has grown insofar as groups have expanded in countries where ethnic Chinese are a minority, and to the extent that Chinese members have reached outside of their immediate circles.

The groups integrate Buddhist teachings and practices, charity, paradigms of the self rooted in Chinese and Buddhist thought (e.g., *qi*, karma, chakras), concepts drawn from the biomedical sciences, and a global orientation. These variables weave together in different ways to assist participants to find inner purification, harmonization with a larger cosmos, and the ability to heal themselves and their world.

The Tzu Chi Foundation grew out of the work of Dharma Master Cheng Yen (b. 1937) in Taiwan. When she was fifteen her mother faced surgery, and so the young woman turned to chanting "Compassion, Buddha," taking a vow to become vegetarian and sacrifice twelve years of her own life if the Buddha helped her mother—who recovered without need for surgery. In 1962, she took refuge in a small temple, shaved her hair, and began to live as a nun. A year later, she took refuge under the Venerable Master Yinshun (1906–2005), a reformer who advocated a this-worldly Buddhism (Huang 2008). He gave her the Buddhist name "Cheng Yen." Shortly thereafter she was ordained.

In 1966, she met nuns from a local Catholic high school, who talked with her about the Catholic Church's charitable activities around the world and asked what similar things Buddhism had done. The discussion led her to create such a charity, the Buddhist Tzu Chi Merit Association. She taught her followers to put aside fifty cents a day as a way to save, and to cultivate love—both as means of giving to others. The initiative inspired growing numbers of people, many of whom wanted to take refuge vows with her. Before allowing them to do so, she required that they first join the foundation and do charity work to help the poor and the sick.

Since its inception, the foundation has gone on to become the largest nongovernmental organization in Taiwan, with international chapters around the world and some ten million supporters. Its disaster relief work got under way in 1991 following flooding of the Yangzi River in the PRC. Volunteers pay their own way to reach disaster areas and are required to thank in person whomever they help, to ensure that aid does not get diverted by corrupt officials ("Help with a Bow" 2008).

Master Cheng Yen has characterized Buddhism as "principle," revealed through the implementation of the eight categories of charity, medicine, education, culture, international disaster relief, bone marrow donation, community volunteerism and environmental protection, or what she has referred to as "one step, eight footprints," echoing the Eightfold Path of Buddhism. Volunteers consciously view their work as bodhisattva practice.

FALUN GONG

One of the groups that has received the greatest public attention, because of a controversy in the PRC involving it, Falun Gong grew out of the country's large *qigong* movement during the 1990s. Founded in 1992 by Li Hongzhi (b. 1951), the approach became well known and widespread, attracting millions of followers. This led government authorities to become uneasy and Li to relocate to the United States in 1995. The government eventually cracked down on the group and has continued to classify it as a harmful cult, condemning it in the media and arresting followers.

Li Hongzhi has instructed Falun Gong participants to eschew leaders, bank accounts, property, or membership lists (Ackerman 2005). Group activities generally consist of practice sessions in public parks using a series of meditative exercises. People may also gather for study sessions of the founder's writings, spending the day reading and reciting together his major work, *Zhuan Falun,* or other pieces on *fa,* which emphasize a strict morality. They may also come together at periodic "experience-sharing" conferences (Ownby 2008a, 2008b, 2008c). Such gatherings have been held in countries as far-flung as Australia, India, Ethiopia, Pakistan, Iran, Guatemala, Canada, and the United States, along with countries with significant Chinese-descended populations. At such conferences, discussions focus on practitioners' personal experience of self-cultivation. The experiences shared are frequently health-related. Practitioners describe relief from suffering, further convincing them of the practice's power and efficacy.

In addition to individual predilections, the reasons for involvement may vary from country to country. In Malaysia, for example, middle-class seekers become aware of a group like Falun Gong in the context of a plethora of alternative possibilities. As Susan Ackerman notes, the group attracts "avid consumers of innovative, imported lifestyle products that promise enhanced mental and physical well-being" (Ackerman 2005, 496). In contrast, adherents in a country like Russia may be drawn to Falun Gong as an alternative to the dominance of atheism and to the rising cost of medical care (Kravchuk 2008).

CHANGSHENG XUE: LONGEVITOLOGY

Some other new groups, when defining their work, take pains to explain that they are "not Falun Gong." Such is the case with another development from Taiwan, reminiscent of older practices related to extending one's life *(changsheng).* Indeed, in Chinese it is called *changsheng xue,* or "the study of long life." Dr. Tom Lin, who had emigrated to California, practiced a form of healing that drew on what he conceptualized as a kind of universal energy. He taught the technique to his sister, Tzu-Chen Lin, back in Taiwan. She simplified the practice and began using it with friends and family members. They found it so beneficial that word spread, eventually leading Lin and her husband, Yu-Feng Wei, to found in 1993 what they call "Longevitology." They taught the system to growing numbers of people at no charge—a practice they have continued, now reaching an international audience. Although most participants and volunteers have been ethnic Chinese, the group has begun to attract students from other backgrounds.

Longevitology draws on the Buddhist concept of chakras (seven wheel-like energy or force centers in a person's subtle body). The first step in one's training involves the Master teacher first opening each student's chakras, and then teaching the process of returning to that state of openness on one's own. Adherents explain that the daily practice involves a deep meditative relaxation, enabling the universal energy channeled through the body to bring about the self-repair of cells and tissues, as well as the correction of wrongly arranged genetic codes. Practiced in a healthy state, it is understood to promote overall wellness.

Participants organize groups that come together on a regular but informal basis to practice and to provide "adjustments" to others in the group. Instruction focuses on how to address specific health issues, each defined in terms of biomedical categories. The organization makes no claims to cure any disease; rather, members suggest that by restoring an individual's energy balance, the body's ability to heal itself may be enhanced ("FREE Longevitology Class" 2009).

Preventive Spiritual Practices

The perception of spirits as posing a risk to health and life persists, both in the PRC and in the Diaspora. For example, in a study of one hundred ethnic Chinese patients in Singapore who sought psychiatric help, more of the women than the men attributed their problem to spirit possession. Half of the group or their relatives had first turned to a traditional healer for help. Nor was this explanation linked to their educational status (Kua, Chew, and Ko 1993). Longevitology treatments sometimes address the issue of such possession, with the adjustment intended to help clear the person of the presence of one or more spirits. Spirit possession also represents a diagnostic category in some schools of acupuncture (see Barnes 1998). For that matter, the phenomena of spirits and ghosts, along with their possession of the living, have filtered into the imagination of Chinese filmmakers, who create horror movies involving the possessed. Anecdotal evidence suggests that in countries like the United States, exorcisms may be performed by some immigrant practitioners (a number of them Daoist priests), although they do not publicize their services.

Protective amulets and talismans are still used. For example, the coin sword—a phenomenon dating back centuries—is made from brass coins (ideally with the same inscription) tied together with a lucky red string. It is used to challenge demons, cure illness, and extend the life of those who carried it or placed it in their home. Such talismans have different meanings for different audiences. For people seeking actual protection, they can—like any other amulet— assume a lived significance and power. If bestowed by a teacher within a larger framework, the talisman may carry the authority of both the teacher and the particular lineage or tradition. For some, it may represent an aspect of cultural nostalgia, in which case it may be viewed as a decorative element with a residue of authority that is not completely dismissed. For non-Chinese, it may constitute an aspect of cultural adoption, whether of a martial art, a form of divination, or an affinity for Chinese signs and symbols.

In addition to being gifted or sold by individual practitioners, coin swords and other talismans are also sold internationally in some Chinese supermarkets and souvenir shops. The swords have appeared in martial arts movies, sometimes hung over the bed of someone afflicted by a demon (Eagleton et al. 2007). More recently, they have made their way onto the Internet. Websites such as Fengshui Bestbuy sell them, for example, advertised as a "metal remedy" that deflects disasters and other evils and counteracts certain life-threatening illness. They are also described as warding off harmful spirits. Another item called a "martial arts exorcist Chinese sword" is identified with Daoism, related exorcistic practices, and *fengshui*.

There is no absolute divide between practitioners who identify themselves explicitly with "Chinese medicine" and those who focus on spiritual practices. For a practitioner of Chinese medicine who incorporates forms of divination into his or her work (e.g., *fengshui* or the *Classic of Changes*), amulet use may be recognized as one aspect of a more complex intervention. Some martial arts teachers may take such practices quite seriously as well, particularly if the practitioner trained outside of the PRC or with a teacher who comes from a family lineage in which such practices were accepted and transmitted.

Divination

The broad category of divination, in connection with Chinese healing arts, encompasses a range of practices intended to discern deeper patterns and processes related to *qi,* solicit the perspective of divine beings, and gain insight into the most timely and fitting human responses to specific situations. Historically, the full spectrum of Chinese social groups, from peasants to high-ranking officials, have engaged in such practices for personal, familial, and official purposes. More important, Chinese medicine physicians and other kinds of practitioners have incorporated all of them into their own practices in varying ways and degrees.

These practices include temple divination using numbered sticks *(shizhan),* dream interpretation, *fengshui,* face reading *(mianxiang),* the *Classic of Changes,* and the Three Cosmographies *(sanshi):* Six Water Cycles *(daliu ren),* Hidden

Period Irregular Opening *(qimen dunjia),* and Divine Emblem of the Great Unity *(taiyi shenshu).* Each of them is used directly in connection with preserving or restoring health.

Stalks and Sticks

The use of bamboo sticks or stalks *(lingqian)* is a long-standing practice in temples, whether Daoist, Buddhist, or dedicated to various gods. Divination by stalks *(shizhan)* involves formulating a question, the answer to which the petitioner views as requiring wisdom greater than his or her own or that of other individuals. In some temples, one writes out the question on red paper, along with one's "birth address" or "eight characters" *(bazi),* based on the time, day, month, and year of one's birth. These four factors converge to shape a person's destiny. One can also add any other information germane to the question.

To give the god time to consider the best answer to one's question, one places the paper on the god's altar (having first determined which deity is the likeliest to address the question effectively). One returns several days later, burns incense *(shaoxiang)* as an offering, and then takes a bamboo tube in which the divination sticks are stood upright, in order to seek the stick that holds an answer *(qiuqian).* One method of selecting a stick involves shaking the tube until a single bamboo stick falls out. Each stick has a number that corresponds to an answer, provided by the god through a medium.

One must then check to ensure that the answer is indeed the right one. This step involves throwing (*zhi,* or *bwa*) a pair of half-moon-shaped wooden or bamboo blocks (*jiao,* or *bwei*). After identifying oneself to the god, one lifts and then drops the blocks. If they fall with both rounded sides up or both rounded sides down, the answer associated with the divination stick is not correct and another must be chosen. Not only must one get a throw in which one rounded side is up and the other is down, but one must repeat that result three times to be sure of having secured the god's confirmation of the answer (Jordan 1982). Finally, one takes the stick to the temple attendant or selects the corresponding slip from a drawer. The answer may seem either straightforward or oblique; in the latter case one can solicit the advice of the attendant or one of the temple monks or priests. Insofar as temples are now present in sites around the world, pilgrims, petitioners, and tourists likewise may come from all backgrounds (see Matheson 2007).

The temple's reputation can depend in part on the degree to which visitors experience the god's answers as effective. Their testimony then attracts others, who may go on to help support the temple. New temples, therefore, try to secure an effective set of divination slips, sometimes turning to a parent temple.

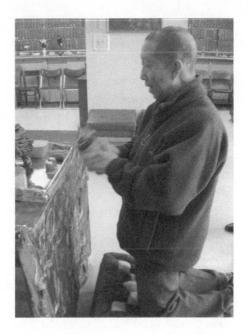

Figure 10.7. Demonstration of divination using bamboo sticks or stalks *(lingqian)* at Norras Temple, San Francisco. Courtesy of Linda L. Barnes.

This is the case with the temple to Huang Daxian (or Wong Tai Sin), a god popular not only in sections of the PRC but also in Hong Kong. Huang Daxian has immigrated to New York as well, with a temple now on the Bowery. A Daoist god, he is particularly associated with curing disease. His Hong Kong temple has historically had an herbal clinic, and the temple itself provides a special type of oracle sticks—medical prescription slips *(yaoqian),* which, although not as common as the regular divination sticks, hold a particular appeal for some visitors to the temple.

DREAM INTERPRETATION

The significance of dreams and their connection with insights into health and illness go back to early Chinese history, appearing in early texts such as the *Rites of Zhou (Zhouli),* the *Classic of Songs* [or *Poetry*] *(Shijing),* the *Inner Canon of the Yellow Emperor, Basic Questions* (see Unschuld 2003), and manuals like Chen Shiyuan's *Lofty Principles of Dream Interpretation* (*Mengzhan yizhi,* ca. 1562). The *Lofty Principles of Dream Interpretation* explained that each person has an ethereal soul *(hun)* and an earthly soul *(po),* joined during waking hours and freed from each other during sleep. Chen drew on a complex mix of sources with dream-related content, encompassing descriptions of practices, discussions from Daoist, Confucian, and Buddhist sources, biographies, literary sources, and dream manuals of the day (Chen 2008). Such manuals continue to be used at the grassroots level, as well as by specialists, even as different schools of practice developed different systems with which to classify dreams and determine whether they were lucky or unlucky (see Thompson 1988).

Chen's book posited nine categories of dreams, related to recommended methods of interpretation (Chen 2008). Other lists have included such features as heavenly bodies, parts of the body, different kinds of clothing, types of buildings (palaces, houses, warehouses), precious substances (gold, silver, jade, silk), food and drink, things related to death (cemeteries, graves, greeting or escorting coffins), religious figures (monks, nuns, spirits), animals (dragons, snakes, birds, beasts), and so on (Thompson 1988).

Dream classifications continue to appear on the Internet (although many sites appear to reproduce the same content). Popular audiences who conduct Internet searches on Chinese dream interpretation may accept this content uncritically. For example, one website says that the Chinese Almanac *(Tongshu)* contains a section on dream interpretation, "Grandmaster Zhou's Book of Dreams" *(Zhou Gong jiemeng).* The author of this Web page goes on to explain that the Duke of Zhou is also known as the "God of Dreams," and that "dreaming" or "seeing the Duke of Zhou" is an expression that refers to sleeping. The author traces the connection to Confucius's referring to a point at which he no longer dreamed of the Duke of Zhou, who in folk tradition alerts people of important events through their dreams (Fong 2009a, 2009b, 2009c).

It is indeed the case that the *Rites of Zhou* lays out six categories of bureaucratic functions. Officials in the Offices of Spring were responsible for state ritual affairs, which included divination. A grand diviner, who oversaw all divination, was in charge of four divining masters, as well as eight midlevel diviners *(Zhouli* 17.5). Another official, the examiner of dreams *(Zhouli* 17.6), was assigned the task of divining whether the six types of dreams—regular or restful, startling or disturbing, reflective, daydream, happy, and frightening—in their specific expressions, portended good or bad fortune (Brennan 1993). It is possible that the link between dream divination and the Duke of Zhou (to whom aspects of the *Classic of Changes* are also attributed) is a product of this section. To observe current efforts to introduce the Duke into the wider circle of popular culture, one has only to look on the social networking website Facebook to find that he now has his own page.

FENGSHUI

Divisions between *fengshui* practitioners date back to the Tang and Song periods, the most notable being the Form School *(xingshi pai)* and the Compass School *(fangzhi pai).* A more recent school, the Black Hat Sect, has gained adherents as well, although those of other schools repeatedly characterize it as

"Western." Differences entail uses of astrology, the trigrams of the *Classic of Changes,* the *luopan* compass, the topographical features of the landscape, and other variables. Even now, practitioners of each approach tend to place the others lower in the hierarchy of legitimacy (a recurring strategy across the different branches of Chinese medicine). One Canadian *fengshui* master, who estimated that there are some sixty thousand practitioners in North America, suggested that "what some of them are doing is to feng shui . . . as chop suey is to fine Chinese cuisine" (Walker 1999).

In official publications, some PRC authors still characterize *fengshui* as an obstacle to scientific development. On the other hand, it has continued to function as a popular health care modality not only in China but also in other countries. One school of practice, for example, refers to its interventions as "cures." A study of open-heart surgery patients in Hong Kong explored patients' perceptions of the placement of their beds, the management of their diets, and the movement therapies that had been recommended. It found that many of the patients would have preferred the implementation of *fengshui* in the intensive care unit but, given that this option was unavailable in the hospital setting, had to settle for practicing it at home (Murray 2002).

The issues for which people turn to consultants are, generally, eminently practical, as vernacular accounts attest. One individual noted, for example, that there were many car accidents in the street, until he (or she) positioned a mirror in the house "to reflect the 'killing atmosphere.'" After that, the people in the household felt better and the accidents stopped. A guard at a dockyard reported that the Westerners there subscribed to *fengshui.* "They changed the entrance to the place, because the old one was unlucky," he said. "They also put out a wok to deflect the bad luck, and a *fok dzi* [character for good fortune] upside down to bring luck in rather than out. All the workers feel a lot better now and in better health." Individuals attribute everything from depression to pain to factors such as poor furniture arrangement, their homes having the wrong directional exposure, or having a hill blocking favorable *fengshui* (Emmons 1992).

In southern California, in Hacienda Heights, a local McDonald's has redecorated, using *fengshui,* to appeal to Chinese and other Asian customers. The color red remains, but it now complements bamboo plants, a wall fountain, and curved lines rather than angled ones. All of the new features reinforce the good luck of being near the Hsi Lai temple. Decorations include examples of the five elements—earth, water, fire, metal and wood—to improve the flow of *qi.* The designer, Brenda Clifford, admitted to a near mistake when she initially planned for forty-four chairs, not realizing that the word for "four" in Chinese *(si)* sounds like the word for "death." (Associated Press 2008; Balla 2008). Ironically, McDonald's has also set up shop in the PRC, changing the menu to add

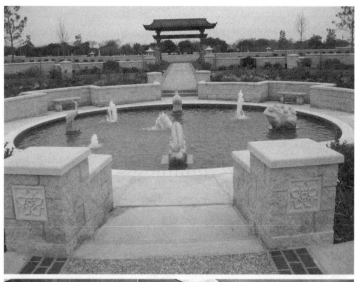

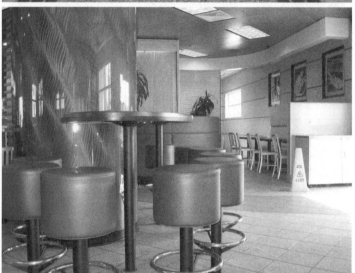

Figure 10.8. *Top:* Garden of Eternal Peace in the Forest Park Westheimer cemetery in Houston, Texas. *Bottom:* McDonald's designed using *fengshui,* Hacienda Heights, California. Courtesy of Linda L. Barnes.

chili garlic sauce, a New Year menu, pineapple and taro pies, and a walk-up window in addition to a drive-through (Griffith 2008).

In countries around the world, both Chinese and non-Chinese *fengshui* practitioners and consultants offer their services, often through the Internet. They form associations to represent the work of their teacher and/or their school of practice, and to disseminate information about both. Because there are few primary source materials in translation, association members can find themselves relying on popular source materials (Paton 2007), resulting in a variety of idiosyncratic hybrids. The practice has been represented as intersecting with different versions of Chinese cosmology, multiple forms of divination such as the *Classic of Changes*, holistic healing, Chinese folklore, quasi-scientific applications of electricity and magnets, and different approaches to meditation. The rationale for these links has been a connection based on "energy."

The general public in these countries may know little about the full range of issues addressed by *fengshui*. If they have heard of it at all, it is often in connection with interior decorating or architecture. Consequently, practitioners from non-Chinese groups may view the application of *fengshui* to the selection and positioning of burial sites as not only irrelevant but also not even real *fengshui*. Little do they realize that the term *fengshui* was defined early on in the *Book of Burial (Zangshu)* by Guo Pu (276–324), a Jin period scholar. Guo observed, for example, the way that *qi* follows the trunk of a hill and branches along its ridges (Paton 2007). Despite differences between schools of practice—particularly in their respective approaches to determining the positioning of *qi* and its various potential effects—the underlying commonality lies in this interest in tracing *qi,* Yin and Yang, and eventually the Five Phases *(wuxing),* the three cycles of nine periods *(sanyuan jiuyun),* and other astrological dynamics in the relationships between natural phenomena, things, and human beings.

Burial-related applications of *fengshui* remain strong in places with large Chinese populations, whether native or immigrant. Cities like New York and San Francisco, for example, have specialty funeral supply stores near Chinese funeral homes. Mourners can purchase paper replicas of all the material items the deceased might need in the afterlife—as noted earlier, spirit money, houses, servants, cars, appliances, clothing, jewelry and, more recently, paper replicas of medications like Viagra ("Replica Viagra" 2007)—to be incinerated in brick or masonry burners (Abraham 2010a, 2010b). The burning conveys the paper gifts to the departed, even as their spirits enjoy the essence of actual foods left at the grave to address their perpetual hunger and to deter their impulses to visit their frustrations on the living through bad luck and sickness.

Such practices continue to be carried out in "substantial [Chinese] cemeteries that are well marked, small rural cemeteries with few or no markers, Chinese sections of community cemeteries, and areas where local tradition claims a Chinese cemetery" (Abraham 2010c). Chinese families may prefer certain cemeteries because of the layout of the land—the presence of hills, bodies of running water, or certain rock configurations, for example. They may hire a *fengshui* specialist to help them identify a particularly favorable site.

More recently, large U.S. funeral chains have entered the picture. Apart from marketing aspects motivating these initiatives, the chains seek ways to adapt to the worldviews and needs of different immigrant and ethnic groups, and view the adoption of *fengshui* as one way to do so. For example, the Sunset Cemetery in Minneapolis, Minnesota, has installed a Garden of Eternal Peace. Cemetery staff used the Internet to identify *fengshui* consultant Andrew Hong, originally from Singapore, who first learned his practice from his grandmother before coming to the United States, where he attended the University of Chicago and New York University, becoming a financial advisor by day. The Garden of Eternal Peace has river rocks around a large tree, and granite headstones shaped like pagodas. The land stands somewhat higher than the other parts of the cemetery—an advantageous positioning that enables one to see and ward off any harmful influences that might be approaching. The Oak Hill Cemetery in San Jose, California, has installed a special ventilation system in its Sunshine Chapel to allow for the burning of incense, and it provides a kitchen where visitors can prepare food to place at the graves (Tim 2009; Yuen 2009).

The Forest Park Westheimer cemetery in Houston, Texas, has perhaps one of the richest examples of cemetery-based *fengshui* in the United States to date. Also called the Garden of Eternal Peace, it occupies a large corner section of the greater cemetery. The architects who designed the Garden drew on the advice of a local *fengshui* master, artist, and architect, C. C. Lee. Looking at it from above, one sees an octagonal garden surrounding a circular pool with fountains. One enters through one of four pagoda gateways, each with its own guardian—a turtle, a phoenix, a tiger, and a dragon, carved using stone from China. The plots face the eight different compass points, to ensure that a family can choose the most auspicious site for its needs. Every feature is designed to ensure harmony and good luck. A short distance from the burial grounds is the Chapel of Eternal Peace, with its own crematorium, and both Buddhist and Christian chapels (Ustinova 2007).

FACE READING

If a person's *qi* can be read through his or her pulses, it follows that it can also be read through other aspects of the body. Chinese physiognomy or face reading *(mianxiang)* dates back at least to the Northern Song period, and manuals explain how a person's fate and nature may be read through his or her face. Analysis can include not only the facial features but also the alignment of the ears, hair, and other bodily features, as well as movements and dispositions. One of the better-known foundational texts remains the *Complete Guide to Spirit Physiognomy (Shenxiang quanbian)*, compiled in the Ming period by physiognomist Yuan Zhongche (see Kohn 1986). It remains the basis for a pocket edition still used in Taiwan.

In one sense, face reading is a part of the diagnostic repertoire of Chinese medicine, which includes looking *(wang)*, listening and smelling *(wen)*, asking *(wen)*, and touching *(qie)*. The practitioner examines the patient's facial structure; the color tones of the face in natural light, along with its texture and sheen; the condition of the eyes and hair, and the person's body shape and posture. In some systems, different parts of the face correspond to different Channels. The face may also be looked at in three sections—upper (heaven), middle (earth), and lower (human)—with each of these having its own subdivisions.

Practitioners may be members of family traditions, may have been trained by someone from a family lineage, may have gained knowledge of face reading in the course of studying acupuncture and related diagnostic skills, or may have taught themselves by reading books, attending workshops, and using online resources (including courses). Lillian Garnier Bridges is an example of the first type. She grew up in a family in which face reading was a shared art, along with discussions of dreams. As she tells it, to bring home a friend was to invite commentary on his or her features, character, and potential future. She suggests that face reading contributes to self-discovery, to be complemented by discerning one's life purpose through dedicated workshops, adjusting one's surroundings with *fengshui* to support these discoveries, and rejuvenating oneself and cultivating longevity using contemporary versions of alchemy (Bridges 2003).

Face and palm reader John Moy sits on a folding chair across the street from Columbus Park in Manhattan's Chinatown, with posterboard signs behind him enlivened with photographs showing him at work or playing with other traditional Chinese musicians in the park on weekends. He says that he learned his divination skills from his master in Hong Kong. He uses a combination of observation and an almanac to determine what is likely to face his client during the current and upcoming year. For imbalances and difficulties that need rectification, he writes up talismans and inserts them in red paper envelopes to be either placed under one's pillow or carried in one's wallet. A steady stream of clients visit him—some local people, others curiosity-seeking tourists. Across the street, a cluster of older women offer similar services.

In contrast, Dr. John Shen, who trained in the Menghe-Ding lineage tradition from Shanghai, is usually recognized for his skills in pulse diagnosis. However, his training also included a face reading system that enabled one to detect which chronological phase of an illness was currently manifesting. Those who studied with him remember him arriving at diagnoses through what sometimes seemed an uncanny intuitive process (Rubio 2007). Shen, in turn, taught the method to his longtime student and eventual collaborator, Dr. Leon Hammer, who eventually decided not to include it in his own teaching after observing some students reduce it to an overly simplistic approach. Nonetheless, the plethora of self-help face-reading websites suggests a robust self-taught public, who may incorporate these strategies into everything from their daily lives to their practice of some other modality.

THE THREE STYLES OF DIVINATION

A core commonality underlying the different divinatory strategies involves the conviction that there are styles of discernment—technologies of timing, if you will—that enable the user to determine the best time, place, and way to act (or not act) in relation to particular categories of circumstance. For example, each of the Three Styles of divination was applied to a different order of events. Each involved the use of different boards, diagrams, and exploration of relationships between Yin and Yang, the Five Phases, and factors related to the Heavenly Stems and Earthly Branches.

Teachers in the PRC now offer to teach these systems to English-speaking students, advertising through the Internet. A site called DaMo Qigong and Taoist Internal Alchemy, with teachers based in northwest Hubei Province, says its objective is to promulgate "the study of ancient Chinese Taoism, Buddhism, Taoist Yoga, Taoist Kungfu, Taoist medicine and other subjects in relation to Taoism and Buddhism culture . . . to people who aspire for the spiritual development along a practical and correct path" ("HIV/AIDS Acupuncture" 2010). This phenomenon overlaps with the growing global practice of health tourism, nuanced by the pursuit of the exotic. Students can choose to attend workshops with master teachers in China, study with teaching assistants from England and Italy, or take the DaMo Qigong Home Study Course.

CLASSIC OF CHANGES

The underlying project of the *Classic of Changes* entails using divination techniques to detect the nature of the particular change in process. The purpose is to harmonize oneself with that change as effectively as possible, as a part of one's self-cultivation. The practice—like other Chinese forms of divination—assumes that discernible patterns of change characterize everything and connect everything. François Jullien refers to this dynamic as *shi*—a "configuration or disposition of things operating through opposition and correlation, and which constitutes a working system" (Jullien 1995, 17). That is, all phenomena involve a dynamic process, articulated through terms such as Yin and Yang (opposites, yet inextricably interrelated) or the Five Phases. Although no change is identical to any other, certain kinds of change tend to follow a certain course.

In the *Classic of Changes,* these different configurations of change-in-process are represented by diagrams called hexagrams—sixty-four combinations of broken and unbroken lines. (See "The Hexagram *Gu*" in Chapter 1.)

Outside of Chinese communities, the *Classic of Changes* had served primarily as a subject for scholars and historians (some of whom may also have used it privately). However, following the translation by Richard Wilhelm—first published in German in 1924 and then re-translated into English and published with a foreword by psychiatrist Carl G. Jung in 1950—the book seized the imaginations of seekers turning to the East for new cosmologies and practices (Wilhelm and Baynes 1950).

These readers experienced the *Classic of Changes* as a pivotal tool in their personal quest for deeper, mystical truths. For some of that generation, it was the possibility of harmonizing with other humans, the earth, and Heaven itself that attracted them to Chinese spiritual worldviews. These traditions seemed to promise the healing of rifts on every level.

Recent years have seen an explosion of translations. Some still emphasize the scholarly dimensions of the work, aiming for ever more definitive translations. Some present themselves as updates—"A Modern Interpretation of the Ancient Oracle" or "A New Interpretation for Modern Times"—emphasizing a popular theme of "timeless" wisdom. Some—in the vein of self-help books written in easy-to-access language—focus on the book's usefulness in everyday life, its role as a "guide to life's turning points," or its value as a tool in shaping one's personal and spiritual life or becoming one's authentic self. Some emphasize that their contribution lies in making the *Classic of Changes* accessible—a street-corner version in plain English, for example. In contrast, other translations position themselves in relation to the spiritual authority of the translator, as does the translation by Master Hua-Ching Ni, who transmitted his own lineage to his two sons, Daoshing and Mao Shing Ni, founders of Yo San University in Marina del Rey, California.

Translations have crossed other boundaries by coupling the *Classic of Changes* with Buddhism in general and Tibetan forms in particular, with Toltecan shamanism, or with Wiccan magic. It has even been interpreted in light of the genetic code. Moreover, translations are available not only in English but also in German, French, and Spanish. These translations are available on Amazon.com, making them as easy to acquire as *Classic of Changes* coins, workbooks, kits, beginner's versions, or gift sets. At the bottom of each related page on the Amazon website are links for online *Classic of Changes* readings. For that matter, YouTube has *Classic of Changes*-related videos in Portuguese, the *Changes* being popular in countries like Brazil.

Finally, explicit links to Chinese medicine per se have also been drawn (see Li Y. 1998). Then there is "the Yijing medical *qigong* system," which links Chinese medicine, the *Classic of Changes,* and *fengshui.*

Conclusion

The examples in these last two chapters point to ways in which migrations of practices have proved to be multidirectional, drawing on far more complex collections of influences than may at first meet the eye. They can no longer be neatly summarized within the boundaries of any of the nations—least of all mainland China itself. Likewise, the interface between these many branches and the surrounding culture of biomedicine has inflected the Chinese healing art in various ways. Some practitioners exhibit a felt need to construct an explicit link with biomedicine, as though doing so will confer greater legitimacy on the practice. One sees such changes in phrases such as "medical *qigong,*" "Chinese medical palmistry," "medical *I Ching* (medical *yijing*)," and "medical *fengshui.*"

As the preceding chapters have shown, the rich array of traditions related to healing arising from China provides the possibility for endless possible combinations and customized adaptations. We see continuities that trace down through the centuries; we also see how the very meanings of these continuities change in light of historical particulars and surrounding influences. It is not sufficient to draw a hard line between the practices of specialists and everyday folk, because the two so regularly cross-fertilize each other.

Religion scholar Joyce Flueckiger has used the concept of "vernacular Islam" to characterize the lived practice of everyday individuals, much as Vasudha Narayanan has employed the notion of customized practice. Yet even when common threads work their way through the many customized versions, resulting in grander weavings, Flueckiger reminds us also to focus on real people, in actual time, who work out their own ways to express and experience their engagement in particular branches of a larger, constantly changing world of traditions (Lee 2009).

Bibliography

Abraham, Terry. 2007. Other Burners, Other Fires. http://www.uiweb.uidaho.edu/special
-collections/papers/burners2.htm (accessed 2/12/10).

———. 2010a. Chinese Funerary Burners: A Bibliography. http://www.uiweb.uidaho.edu
/special-collections/papers/burners_bibliography.htm (accessed 2/12/10).

———. 2010b. Chinese Funerary Burners: A Census. http://www.uiweb.uidaho.edu/special
-collections/papers/burners.htm (accessed 2/12/10).

———. 2010c. Overseas Chinese Cemeteries. http://www.uiweb.uidaho.edu/special
-collections/papers/ch_cem.htm (accessed 2/12/10).

About the National Acupuncture Detoxification Association. 2010. http://acudetox.com
/about (accessed 2/14/10).

Academy of Traditional Chinese Medicine. 1975. *An Outline of Chinese Medicine.* Beijing:
Foreign Languages Press.

Accreditation Commission for Acupuncture and Oriental Medicine. 2012. Accredited
and Candidate Programs. http://www.acaom.org/find-a-school (accessed 8/9/12).

Ackerman, Susan. 2005. Falun Dafa and the New Age Movement in Malaysia: Signs of
Health, Symbols of Salvation. *Social Compass* 52(4):495–511.

Acupuncture.com.au. 2008. Acupuncture and TCM Events Calendar. http://www.acupunc
ture.com.au/events/eventdetails.html?id=171 (accessed 3/19/08).

Acupuncturists without Borders. 2009. AWB Floods Iowa with Support. *Acupuncture Today* 10(1). http://www.acupuncturetoday.com/mpacms/at/article.php?id=31870&no
_paginate=true&no_b=true (accessed 8/4/09).

———. 2010. Field Update: Haiti Disaster Recovery Project. Personal correspondence
(February 16).

Adachihara Akiko 安達原曄子. 1983. *Man'anpō no shōnimon ni tsuite* 万安方の小児門について.
Nihon ishigaku zasshi 日本医史学雑誌 29(4):353–367.

Adair, Alex, et al. n.d. Ghost Money: The Anthropology of Money in Southern California.
http://www.anthro.uci.edu/html/Programs/Anthro_Money/GhostMoney.htm
(accessed 2/8/10).

Ahmad, Lazgeen M. 2009. Acupuncture and Cesarean Section: Case Study from Iraq.
American Acupuncturist 47(March 31):19.

Allan, Sarah. 1981. *The Heir and the Sage: Dynastic Legend in Early China*. San Francisco: Chinese Materials Center.

——. 1991. *The Shape of the Turtle: Myth, Art, and Cosmos in Early China*. Albany: SUNY Press.

——. 1997. *The Way of Water and Sprouts of Virtue*. Albany: SUNY Press.

——, ed. 2005. *The Formation of Chinese Civilization: An Archaeological Perspective*. New Haven: Yale University and New World Press.

——. 2007. On the Identity of Shang Di 上帝 and the Origin of the Concept of a Celestial Mandate (*Tian Ming* 天命). *Early China* 31:1–46.

Allsen, Thomas T. 2001. *Culture and Conquest in Mongol Eurasia*. Cambridge: Cambridge University Press

American Association of Oriental Medicine. 2006. The Nomenclature Debates. http://www .aaom.info/2006_conf_nomenclature_binder.pdf (accessed 5/2/10).

American Presbyterian Mission. 1896. *The China Mission Hand-Book*. Shanghai: American Presbyterian Mission.

Amiot, Joseph-Marie. 1779. Notice du cong-fou des bonzes Tao-sée. In *Mémoires concernant l'histoire, les sciences, les arts, les moeurs, les usages, &c. des chinois*. Paris: Nyon l'aîné.

An Guanying 安冠英 et al., eds. 1993. *Zhonghua bainian laoyaopu* 中華百年老藥鋪. Beijing: Zhongguo wenshi chubanshe.

Anastasi, Joyce K., and Donald J. McMahon. 2003. Testing Strategies to Reduce Diarrhea in Persons with HIV Using Traditional Chinese Medicine: Acupuncture and Moxibustion. *Journal of the Association of Nurses in AIDS Care* 14(3):28–40.

Anderson, Eugene N. 1988. *The Food of China*. New Haven: Yale University Press.

——. 1996. *Ecologies of the Heart*. New York: Oxford University Press.

Andrews, Bridie J. 1996. The Making of Modern Chinese Medicine, 1895–1937. Ph.D. dissertation, Cambridge University.

——. 1997. Tuberculosis and the Assimilation of Germ-Theory in China, 1895–1937. *Journal of the History of Medicine and Allied Sciences* 52(1):114–157.

Announcer. 1992. On the History of the Use of Acupuncture by Revolutionary Health Workers to Treat Drug Addiction, and US Government Attacks under the Cover of the Counterintelligence Program (COINTELPRO): Interview with Dr. Mutulu Shakur. http://www.mutulushakur.com/interview-lompoc.html (accessed 1/2/10).

Arnold, Hans-Juergen. 1976. *Die Geschichte der Akupunktur in Deutschland*. Heidelberg: Haug.

Asakawa, Gil. n.d. Boulder's Chinese Kung Fu Connection. http://nikkeiview.com/nv/clips /shaolin.htm (accessed 4/2/10).

Asen, Daniel. 2009. "Manchu Anatomy": Anatomical Knowledge and the Jesuits in Seventeenth- and Eighteenth-Century China. *Social History of Medicine* 22(1):23–44.

Associated Press. 2008. McDonald's Aims to Boost Sales with Feng Shui. MSNBC.com.

Austin, Mary. 1975. *Textbook of Acupuncture Therapy*. Englewood, CO: ASI.

Baecker, Marcus, Iven Tao, and Gustav J. Dobos. 2007. *Acupuncture Quo Vadis?—On the Current Discussion around Its Effectiveness and "Point Specificity."* Stuttgart: Thieme.

Baker, Donald. 2003. Oriental Medicine in Korea. *Medicine Across Cultures: History and Practice of Medicine in Non-Western Cultures.* Helaine Sellin, ed. Dordrecht: Kluwer Academic Publishers.

Baker, Patricia A., and Gillian Carr. 2002. *Practitioners, Practices and Patients: New Approaches to Medical Archaeology and Anthropology.* Oxford: Oxford University Press.

Balla, Lesley. 2008. Only in SoCal: The Country's First Feng Shui McDonald's. Eater LA, February 13. http://la.eater.com/archives/2008/02/13/only_in_socal_the_countrys_first_feng_shui_mcdonalds.php (accessed 2/12/10).

Balme, Harold. 1921. *China and Modern Medicine: A Study in Medical Missionary Development.* London: United Council for Missionary Education.

Banh, Duong Ba. 1952. The Influence of Western Medicine on the Traditional Medicine of Vietnam. *Journal of the History of Medicine* 7:79–84.

Baptandier, Brigitte. 2006. Le rhizome et la perle. In *Penser/rêver: Revue de psychanalyse* 9:179–188.

Barbanel, Josh. 1981a. 3 Killed in Armored Car Holdup: 2 Officers and Guard Slain after Rockland Holdup. *New York Times* (October 21).

———. 1981b. 3 More Suspects Identified in Holdup of Brink's Truck. *New York Times* (October 26).

Barnes, Linda L. 1998. The Psychologizing of Chinese Healing Practices in the United States. *Culture, Medicine and Psychiatry* 22:413–443.

———. 2003a. Healing. In *Encyclopedia of Religion and Culture in the United States.* G. Laderman and L. León, eds. Pp. 627–630. Santa Barbara, CA: ABC-CLIO.

———. 2003b. The Acupuncture Wars: The Professionalizing of Acupuncture in the United States—A View from Massachusetts. *Medical Anthropology* 22:261–301.

———. 2005a. American Acupuncture and Efficacy: Meanings and Their Points of Insertion. *Medical Anthropology Quarterly* 19(3):239–266.

———. 2005b. *Needles, Herbs, Gods, and Ghosts: China, Healing, and the West to 1848.* Cambridge, MA: Harvard University Press.

———. 2007a. Religion and Spirituality in the Lives of Immigrants in the United States. In *Immigrant Medicine.* E. Barnett and P. Walker, eds. Pp. 681–692. Santa Barbara, CA: ABC-CLIO.

———. 2007b. Plural Health Systems: Meanings and Analytical Issues. In *A.R.H.A.P. International Colloquium.* J. Cochrane, ed. Pp. 46–54. Cape Town: African Religious Health Assets Programme.

———. 2007c. Five Ways of Rethinking the Normal: Reflections on the Preceding Comments. *Religion and Theology* 14:68–83.

———. 2009. Cultural Messages under the Skin: Practitioner Decisions to Engage in Chinese Medicine. *Medical Anthropology* 28(2):141–165.

Baum, Julia K., and Amanda C. J. Vincent. 2005. Magnitude and Inferred Impacts of the Seahorse Trade in Latin America. *Environmental Conservation* 32(4):305–319.

Baum, Richard. 1982. Science and Culture in Contemporary China: The Roots of Retarded Modernization. *Asian Survey* 22(12):1166–1186.

Be Well. n.d. Veteran Care/PTSD/Pain. http://bewell.omclinic.org/2009/01/19/veteran-care (accessed 9/20/09).

Beal, M. W., and L. Nield-Anderson. 2000. Acupuncture for Symptom Relief in HIV-Positive Adults: Lessons Learned from a Pilot Study. *Alternative Therapies in Health and Medicine* 6(5):33–42.

Beard, George M. 1869. Neurasthenia, or Nervous Exhaustion. *Boston Medical and Surgical Journal* 3:217–221.

———. 1881. *American Nervousness: Its Causes and Consequences.* New York: G. P. Putnam's Sons.

Beinfield, Harriet. 2001. Dreaming with Two Feet on the Ground: Acupuncture in Cuba. *Clinical Acupuncture and Oriental Medicine* 2. http://www.chinese-medicine-works.com/pdfs/dreaming_with_two_feet.pdf (accessed 2/22/09).

Beinfield, Harriet, and Efrem Komgold. 1991. *Between Heaven and Earth: A Guide to Chinese Medicine.* New York: Ballantine Books.

Bell, Alex. 2009. Zimbabwe: Another Government Official Implicated in Rising Poaching Crisis. http://allafrica.com/stories/printable/200907230919.html (accessed 7/28/09).

Bell, Mark R., and Taylor C. Boas. 2003. Falun Gong and the Internet: Evangelism, Community, and Struggle for Survival. *Nova Religio* 6(2):277–293.

Bemis, Ryan. 2010. Light and Dark in the Deep South, Part 1. http://acudetox.com/news/?p=34#more-34 (accessed 2/14/10).

Benedict, Carol. 1996. *Bubonic Plague in Nineteenth-Century China.* Stanford, CA: Stanford University Press.

Bennett, Adrian Arthur. 1967. *John Fryer: The Introduction of Western Science and Technology into Nineteenth-Century China.* Cambridge, MA: Harvard University Press.

Berger, Peter L. 2002. The Cultural Dynamics of Globalisation. In *Many Globalisations: Cultural Diversity in the Contemporary World.* Peter L. Berger and Samuel P. Huntington, eds. Pp. 1–16. Oxford: Oxford University.

Bi Yuan 畢沅 et al., eds. 1887. Jingxun tang congshu 經訓堂叢書. Shanghai: Datong shuju.

Bibeau, G. 1985. From China to Africa: The Same Impossible Synthesis between Traditional and Western Medicines. *Social Science and Medicine* 21(8):937–943.

Bisio, Tom. 2004. *A Tooth from the Tiger's Mouth: How to Treat Your Injuries with Powerful Healing Secrets of the Great Chinese Warriors.* New York: Fireside.

Bisio, Tom, and Frank Butler. 2007. *Zheng Gu Tui Na: A Chinese Medical Massage Textbook.* New York: Zheng Gu Tui Na.

Bivins, Roberta. 2000. *Acupuncture, Expertise, and Cross-Cultural Medicine.* London: Palgrave.

Blair, John. 1874. The Chinese Specifics for Diphtheria. *Australian Medical Journal* (October 7):288–296.

Blanc, Marie-Eve and Laurence Monnais. 2007. Culture, immigration et santé. La consommation de médicaments chez les Vietnamiens de Montréal. *Revue européenne des migrations internationales* 23(3):151–176.

Bloomberg, Brett. 2005. Acupuncture in India. *Acupuncture Today* 6(7). http://www.acupunc turetoday.com/mpacms/at/article.php?id=30154 (accessed 7/28/09).

Blow, David. 1994. The Acupuncture Treatment of Alcohol and Chemical Dependency. *Journal of Chinese Medicine* 45(May). http://www.whitelotusacupuncture.com/Articles /Alcohol%20and%20Chemical.pdf (accessed 7/29/09).

Blue, Gregory. 2000. Opium for China: The British Connection. In *Opium Regimes: China, Britain, and Japan, 1839-1952.* T. Brook and B. T. Wakabayashi, eds. Pp. 31–54. Berkeley: University of California Press.

Bogado Bordazar, L. L. 2003. *Influencia de la migración china en Argentina y Uruguay.* La Plata: University of La Plata.

Boileau, Gilles. 1998–1999. Some Ritual Elaborations on Cooking and Sacrifice in Late Zhou and Western Han Texts. *Early China* 23–24:89–123.

———. 2002. Wu and Shaman. *Bulletin of the School of Oriental and African Studies* 65(2):350–378.

Bokenkamp, Steven. 2002. Record of the Feng and Shan. In *Religions of Asia in Practice: An Anthology.* D. S. Lopez, ed. Pp. 386–395. Princeton, NJ: Princeton University Press.

Bokenkamp, Steven, and Peter Nickerson. 1997. *Early Daoist Scriptures.* Berkeley: University of California Press.

Boltz, Judith M. 1993. Not by the Seal of Office Alone: New Weapons in Battles with the Supernatural. In *Religion and Society in T'ang and Sung China.* P. B. Ebery and P. N. Gregory, eds. Pp. 241–305. Honolulu: University of Hawaii Press.

Bomme, Ulrich, Rudolf Bauer, Fritz Friedl, Heidi Heuberger, Günther Heubl, Paula Torres-Londoño, and Josef Hummelsberger. 2007. Cultivating Chinese Medicinal Plants in Germany: A Pilot Project. *Journal of Alternative and Complementary Medicine* 13(6):597–601.

Borsarello, Jean-François. 2005. *Traité d'acupuncture.* Paris: Masson.

Boym, Michael. 1682. *Specimen medicinae sinicae sive. Opuscula medica ad mentem sinensium.* Frankfurt am Main: Zubrodt.

Boym, Michael, and Andreas Cleyer. 1686. *Clavis medica ad Chinarum doctrinam de pulsibus.* Norimbergae.

Brandstätter, Christine. 2000. Elias in China: "Civilising Process," Kinship, and Customary Law in the Chinese Countryside. In *Max Planck Institute for Social Anthropology: Working Paper No. 6.* Halle/Saale.

Brashier, Kenneth E. 1996. Han Thanatology and the Division of "Souls." *Early China* 21:125–158.

Braun, Kelly. 2004. The Tzu Chi Foundation and the Buddha's Light International Association: The Impact of Ethnicity in the Transmission of Chinese Buddhism to Canada. Master's thesis, University of Alberta.

Bray, Francesca. 1997. *Technology and Gender: Fabrics of Power in Late Imperial China.* Berkeley: University of California Press.

———. 2008. Tales of Fertility: Reproductive Narratives in Late Imperial Medical Cases. In *Variantology 3: On Deep Time Relations of Arts, Sciences and Technologies.* S. Zielinski and E. Fürlus, eds. Pp. 93–114. Cologne: Walther König.

———, Vera Dorofeeva-Lictmann, and Georges Métailié, eds. 2007. *Graphics and Text in the Production of Technical Knowledge in China: The Warp and the Weft.* Leiden: Brill.

Brennan, John. 1993. Dreams, Divination, and Statecraft: The Politics of Dreams in Early Chinese History and Literature. In *In the Dream and the Text: Essays on Literature and Language.* C. S. Rupprecht, ed. Pp. 73–102. Albany: SUNY Press.

Breuer, Gabriel S., Hedi Orbach, Ori Elkayam, Yaakov Berkun, Dafna Paran, Michal Mates, and Gideon Nesher. 2006. Use of Complementary and Alternative Medicine among Patients Attending Rheumatology Clinics in Israel. *Israeli Medical Association Journal* 8(March):184–187.

Bridges, Lillian. 2003. *Face Reading in Chinese Medicine.* Oxford: Churchill Livingstone.

Bridgman, R. F. 1955. *La médecine dans la Chine antique.* Brussels: n.p.

Brody, Jane E. 1971. Acupuncture Demonstrated at Medical Parley Here. *New York Times* (December 15).

Brokaw, Cynthia J. 1991. *The Ledgers of Merit and Demerit: Social Change and Moral Order in Late Imperial China.* Princeton, NJ: Princeton University Press.

———. 2007. *Commerce in Culture: The Sibao Book Trade in the Qing and Republican Periods.* Cambridge, MA: Harvard University Press.

Brook, Timothy, and Bob Tadashi Wakabayashi. 2000. Opium's History in China. In *Opium Regimes: China, Britain, and Japan, 1839–1952.* T. Brook and B. T. Wakabayashi, eds. Pp. 1–27. Berkeley: University of California Press.

Buell, Paul D. 2011. Tibetans, Mongols and the Fusion of Eurasian Cultures. In *Islam and Tibet, Interactions along the Musk Route.* A. Akasoy, C. Burnett, and R. Yoeli-Tlalim, eds. Pp. 189–208. Burlington, VT: Ashgate.

Buell, Paul D., Eugene N. Anderson, and Charles Perry. 2000. *A Soup for the Qan: Chinese Dietary Medicine of the Mongol Era as Seen in Hu Szu-hui's Yin-shan Cheng-yao.* London: Kegan Paul International.

Buell, Paul D., and Christopher Meunch. 1984. Chinese Medical Recipes from Frontier Seattle. In *The Annals of the Chinese Historical Society of the Pacific Northwest.* P. D. Buell, D. W. Lee, and E. Kaplan, eds. Pp. 103–143. Bellingham, WA: Chinese Historical Society of the Pacific.

Bullock, Mary B. 1980. *An American Transplant: The Rockefeller Foundation and Peking Union Medical College.* Berkeley: University of California Press.

Bullock, Milton L., Patricia D. Culliton, and Robert T. Olander. 1989. Controlled Trial of Acupuncture for Severe Recidivist Alcoholism. *Lancet* June 24:1435–1439.

Burack, Jeffrey H., Misha R. Cohen, Judith A. Hahn, and Donald I. Abrams. 1996. Pilot Randomized Controlled Trial of Chinese Herbal Treatment for HIV-Associated Symptoms. *Journal of Acquired Immune Deficiency Syndromes and Human Retrovirology* 12(4):386–393.

Burton-Rose, Daniel. 1997. Interview with Dr. Mutulu Shakur. http://www.mutulushakur.com/interview-daniel.html (accessed 1/19/10).

Buyi leigong paozhi bianlan 補遺雷公炮製便覽. 2005. Shanghai: Cishu chubanshe.

Cai Jingfeng 蔡景峰, Li Qinghua 李慶華, and Zhang Binghuan 張冰浣, eds. 2000. *Zhongguo yixue tongshi: xiandai juan* 中國醫學通史: 現代卷. Beijing: Renmin weisheng chubanshe.

Call, Elizabeth. 2006. *Mending the Web of Life: Chinese Medicine and Species Conservation.* Gaithersburg, MD: Signature.

Campany, Robert F., and Ge Hong. 2002. *To Live as Long as Heaven and Earth: A Translation and Study of Ge Hong's Traditions of Divine Transcendents.* Berkeley: University of California Press.

Campbell, Cameron D., Feng Wang, and James Z. Lee. 2002. Pretransitional Fertility in China. *Population and Development Review* 28(4):735–750.

Canaves, Sky. 2008. In South Africa, Chinese Is the New Black. *Wall Street Journal* (June 19). http://blogs.wsj.com/chinajournal/2008/06/19/in-south-africa-chinese-is-the-new -black/?mod=googlenews_wsj (accessed 5/8/09).

Candelise, Lucia. 2008. La médecine chinoise dans la pratique médicale en France et en Italie, de 1930 à nos jours. Ph.D. dissertation, Sciences Sociales, École des Hautes Études.

Capitanio, Joshua. 2008. Dragon Kings and Thunder Gods: Rainmaking, Magic, and Ritual in Medieval Chinese Religion. Ph.D. dissertation, University of Pennsylvania.

Carlson, Alvar W. 1986. Ginseng: America's Botanical Drug Connection to the Orient. *Economic Botany* 40(2):233–249.

Cass, Victoria B. 1986. Female Healers in the Ming and the Lodge of Ritual and Ceremony. *Journal of the American Oriental Society* 106(1):233–245.

Cassidy, Clare M. 1998. Chinese Medicine Users in the United States: Part I. Utilization, Satisfaction, Medical Plurality. *Journal of Alternative and Complementary Medicine* 4:17–27.

———. 1998. Chinese Medicine Users in the United States: Part II. Preferred Aspects of Care. *Journal of Alternative and Complementary Medicine* 4:189–202.

Cell, Charles P. 1977. *Revolution at Work—Mobilization Campaigns in China.* New York: Academic Press.

Chalmers, Jim. n.d. Auriculotherapy: Modern Ear Acupuncture. http://www.auriculotherapy .info (accessed 2/14/10).

Chamfrault, Albert. 1954. *Traité de médecine chinoise.* Angoulème, France: Éditions Coquemard.

Chan Man Sing. 2012. Sinicizing Western Science: The Case of *Quanti xinlun* 全體新論. *T'oung Pao* 98(4–5): In press.

Chang Bide 昌彼得 et al., eds. 1984. *Songren zhuanji ziliao suoyin* 宋人傳記資料索引. 6 vols. Taipei: Dingwen shuju.

Chang Che-chia. 1998. The Therapeutic Tug of War: The Imperial Physician-Patient Relationship in the Era of Empress Dowager Cixi (1874–1908). Ph.D. dissertation, University of Pennsylvania.

Chang Chia-Feng 張嘉鳳. 1996a. Aspects of Smallpox and Its Significance in Chinese History. Ph.D. dissertation, School of Oriental and African Studies, University of London.

———. 張嘉鳳. 1996b. *Qing Kangxi huangdi caiyong rendoufa de shijian yu yuanyin shitan* 清康熙皇帝採人痘法的時間與原因試探. *Zhonghua yishi zazhi* 中華醫史雜志 26(1):30–32.

———. 2000. Dispersing the Foetal Toxin of the Body: Conceptions of Smallpox Aetiology in Pre-Modern China. In *Contagion: Perspectives from Pre-modern Societies.* L. Conrad and D. Wujastyk, eds. Pp. 23–38. Burlington, VT: Ashgate.

———. 2002. Disease and Its Impact on Politics, Diplomacy, and the Military. *Journal of the History of Medicine and the Allied Sciences* 57(2):177–197.

Chang Kwang-chih. 1983. *Art, Myth, and Ritual: The Path to Political Authority in Ancient China*. Cambridge, MA: Harvard University Press.

Chang, Pamela O'Malley. 2007. Acupuncture for All. *Yes! Magazine* (November 7). http://www.yesmagazine.org/issues/liberate-your-space/acupuncture-for-all (accessed 8/7/09).

Chang, Tsung-tung. 1970. *Der Kult der Shang-dynastie im Spiegel der Orakelinschriften: Eine paläographische Studie zur Religion im archaischen China*. Wiesbaden: Otto Harrassowitz.

Chao Yüan-ling. 2000. The Ideal Physician in Late Imperial China: The Question of Sanshi. *East Asian Science, Technology, and Medicine* (17):66–93.

———. 2009. *Medicine and Society in Late Imperial China: A Study of Physicians in Suzhou, 1600–1850*. New York: Peter Lang.

———. n.d. Patronizing medicine: From the Sanhuang Miao to the Yaowang Miao. Unpublished ms.

Chard, Robert L. 1999. The Imperial Household Cults. In *State and Court Ritual in China*. Joseph McDermott, ed. Pp. 237–266. Cambridge: Cambridge University Press.

Chau, Adam Yuet. 2003. Popular Religion in Shaanbei, North-Central China. *Journal of Chinese Religions* 31:39–79.

Chaudhry, Khalid. 2003. Fighting the War on Drugs. *The Review* (October 30). http://www.dawn.com/weekly/review/archive/031030/review5.htm (accessed 7/8/08).

Chen Bangxian 陳邦賢. 1936. *Zhongguo yixue shi* 中國醫學史. Shanghai: Shangwu yinshuguan.

Chen, C. C. 1989. *Medicine in Rural China: A Personal Account*. Berkeley: University of California Press.

Chen Chiu Hsueh. 1981. *Acupuncture: A Comprehensive Text*. John O'Connor and Dan Bensky, transl. Seattle: Eastland Press.

Chen Daojin 陳道瑾 and Xue Weitao 薛渭濤. 1985. *Jiangsu lidai yiren zhi* 江蘇歷代人物志. Suzhou: Jiangsu kexue jishu chubanshe.

Chen, H., G. Deng, Z. Li, G. Tian, Y. Li, P. Jiao, L. Zhang, Z. Liu, R. G. Webster, and K. Yu. 2004. The Evolution of H5N1 Influenza Viruses in Ducks in Southern China. *Proceedings of the National Academy of Sciences* 101(28):10452–10457.

Chen Jianmin 陳健民. 1990. Lu Yuanlei xiansheng de xueshusixiang 陸淵雷先生的學術思想. Zhonghua yishi zazhi 中華醫史雜志 20 (2), 91–95.

Chen Keji 陳可冀. 1990. *Qinggong yi'an yanjiu* 清宮醫案研究. Beijing: Zhongyi guji chubanshe.

Chen, Nancy N. 2003. *Breathing Spaces: Qigong, Psychiatry, and Healing in China*. New York: Columbia University Press.

Chen Shiyuan. 2008. *Wandering Spirits: Chen Shiyuan's Encyclopedia of Dreams*. R. E. Strassberg, trans. Berkeley: University of Califonia Press.

Chen Xinqian 陳新謙. 1996. Qingdai si da yaodian 清代四大藥店. *Zhongguo zhongyao zazhi* 中國中藥雜誌 21(1):56–60.

Chen Xizhong 陳曦鐘, Hou Zhongyi 侯忠義, and Lu Yuchuan 魯玉川, eds. 1998. *Shuihuzhuan huipingben* 水滸傳會評本. Beijing: Beijing daxue chubanshe.

Chen Yinke 陳寅恪. 1934. Tianshidao yu binhai diyu zhi guanxi 天師道與濱海地域之關係. *Zhongyang yanjiuyuan lishi yuyan yanjiusuo jikan* 中央研究院歷史語言研究所集刊 3:43–466.

Chen Yuanpeng 陳元朋. 1997. *Liang Song de "Shangyi shiren" yu "ruyi"—jianlun qi zai Jin-Yuan de liubian* 兩宋的「尚醫士人」與「儒醫」—兼論其在金元的流變. Taipei: Taiwan National University.

Cheng Dan'an 承澹盦. 1932. *Xiuding Zhongguo zhenjiu zhiliaoxue* 修訂中國針灸治療學. Shanghai: Qianqingtang shuju.

Cheng Man-ching, and Robert K. Smith. 1967. *T'ai Chi: The Supreme Ultimate Exercise for Health, Sport, and Self-Defense.* Rutland, Vermont: Tuttle Publishing.

Cheng Wen-chien. 2003. Images of Happy Farmers in Song China (960–1279): Drunks, Politics, and Social Identity. Ph.D. dissertation, University of Michigan.

———. 2011. Antiquity and Rusticity: Images of the Ordinary in the *Farmers' Wedding* Painting. *Journal of Song-Yuan Studies* 41:67–106.

Cheng Yingqi. 2012. First TCM medicine OK'd for EU market. China Daily.com.cn 中國日報網. April 19. http://www.chinadaily.com.cn/china/2012-04/19/content_15085051.htm (accessed 4/6/12).

Cherniack, Susan. 1994. Book Culture and Textual Transmission in Sung China. *Harvard Journal of Asiatic Studies* 54(1):5–125.

Choo, Jessey J.C. 2012. That "Fatty Lump": Discourses on the Fetus, Fetal Development, and Filial Piety in Early Imperial China. *Nan Nü: Men, Women and Gender in Early and Imperial China* 14(2).

Chia, Lucille. 2002. *Printing for Profit: The Commercial Publishers of Jianyang, Fujian (11th–17th centuries).* Cambridge, MA: Harvard University Asia Center for Harvard-Yenching Institute.

Childs-Johnson, Elizabeth. 1983. Excavation of Tomb No. 5 at Yinxu, Anyang. *Chinese Sociology and Anthropology* 15(3).

———. 1987. The Jue and Its Ceremonial Use in the Ancestor Cult of China. *Artibus Asiae* 48(3/4):171–196.

———. 1995. The Ghost Head Mask and Metamorphic Shang Imagery. *Early China* 20:79–92.

———. 1998. The Metamorphic Image: A Predominant Theme in the Ritual Art of Shang China. *Bulletin of the Museum of Far Eastern Antiquities* 70:5–171.

———. 2002. *Enduring Art of Jade Age China: Chinese Jades of Late Neolithic through Han Periods,* Vol. 2. New York: Throckmorton Fine Art.

Chinese Medicine Database. 2006–. *The Chinese Medicine Database.* http://www.cm-db .com (accessed August 3 2011).

Chu Ping-yi 祝平一. 1996. Linghun, shenti, yu tianzhu: Mingmo Qingchu xixue zhong de renti shengli zhishi 靈魂、身體與天主: 明末清初西學中的人體生理知識. *Xinshixue* 新史學 7(2):47–98.

City Is Trying to Destroy Lincoln Detox: Defend the Program! 1975. Mimeographed flyer.

Clark, Hugh R. 1991. *Community, Trade, and Networks: Southern Fujian Province from the Third to the Thirteenth Century.* Cambridge: Cambridge University Press.

Clunas, Craig. 1991. *Superfluous Things: Material Culture and Social Status in Early Modern China*. Urbana: University of Illinois Press.

Cohen, Misha R., Thomas F. Mitchell, Peter Bacchetti, Carroll Child, Sherrill Crawford, Andrew Gaeddert, and Donald I. Abrams. 1999. Use of a Chinese Herbal Medicine for Treatment of HIV-Associated Pathogen-Negative Diarrhea. *Integrative Medicine* 2(2/3):79–84.

Cohen, Misha R., and Robert G. Gish, with Kalia Doner. 2007. *The Hepatitis C Help Book: A Groundbreaking Treatment Program Combining Western and Eastern Medicine for Maximum Wellness and Healing*. New York: St. Martin's Griffin.

Cohen, Paul A. 1997. *History in Three Keys: The Boxers as Event, Experience, and Myth*. New York: Columbia University Press.

Cohn, Sherman L. 2008. Acupuncture and OM in the US: History as a Passport to Now. American Association of Acupuncture and Oriental Medicine, Chicago.

Cook, Constance A. 1990. *Auspicious Metals and Southern Spirits: An Analysis of the Chu Bronze Inscriptions*. Department of Oriental Languages, University of California, Berkeley.

———. 1995–1996. Scribes, Cooks, and Artisans: Breaking Zhou Tradition. *Early China* 20:241–269.

———. 1997. Wealth and the Western Zhou. *Bulletin of the School of Oriental and African Studies* 60(2):253–294.

———. 2003. Bin Gong Xu and Sage King Yu: Translation and Commentary. In *The X Gong Xu (燹公盨): A Report and Papers from the Dartmouth Workshop*. Xing Wen, ed. Special Issue of *International Research on Bamboo and Silk Documents: Newsletter*, 3:23–28. Hanover, NH: Dartmouth College.

———. 2005. Moonshine and Millet: Feasting and Purification Rituals in Ancient China. In *Of Tripod and Palate: Food, Politics, and Religion in Traditional China*. R. Sterckx, ed. Pp. 9–23. New York: Palgrave Macmillan.

———. 2006a. From Bone to Bamboo: Number Sets and Mortuary Ritual. *Journal of Oriental Studies* 1:1–40.

———. 2006b. *Death in Ancient China: The Tale of One Man's Journey*. Leiden: Brill.

———. 2007. Ritual, Politics, and the Issue of *Feng* (封). In *Shi Quan Xiansheng Jiushi Danchen Jinian Wenji* 石泉先生九十誕辰紀念文集. Wuhan Daxue Lishi Dili Yanjiu Suo, ed. Pp. 215–267. Wuhan: Hubei renmin chubanshe.

———. 2009. Ancestor Worship During the Eastern Zhou. In *Early Chinese Religion, Part One: Shang through Han (1250 B.C.–220 A.D.)*. J. Lagerwey and M. Kalinowski, eds. Pp. 237–279. Leiden: Brill.

Cook, Constance A., and John S. Major, eds. 1999. *Defining Chu: Image and Reality in Ancient China*. Honolulu: University of Hawaii Press.

Craig, David. 2002. *Familiar Medicine: Everyday Health Knowledge and Practice in Today's Vietnam*. Honolulu: University of Hawaii Press.

Crain, Liz. 2007. Sharp Thinking Applied to Health Care. *Portland Tribune* (January 16). http://www.portlandtribune.com/sustainable/print_story.php?story_id=116890618799445600 (accessed 8/13/09).

Croizier, Ralph C. 1968. *Traditional Medicine in Modern China: Science, Nationalism and the Tensions of Cultural Change.* Cambridge, MA: Harvard University Press.

Csordas, Thomas J. 2007a. Global Religion and the Re-enchantment of the World: The Case of the Catholic Charismatic Renewal. *Anthropological Theory* 7:295–313.

———. 2007b. Introduction: Modalities of Transnational Transcendence. *Anthropological Theory* 7:259–272.

Cui Xiuhan 崔秀漢. 1996. *Chaoxian yiji tongkao* 朝鮮醫籍通考. Beijing: Zhongguo zhongyiyao chubanshe.

Cui Yueli 崔月梨, ed. 1997. *Zhongyi chensi lu* 中醫沉思錄. Beijing: Zhongyi guji chubanshe.

Culin, Stewart. 1887. Chinese Drug Stores in America. *American Journal of Pharmacy* 59(December):593–598.

Cunningham, Andrew. 1992. Transforming Plague: The Laboratory and the Identity of Infectious Disease. In *The Laboratory Revolution in Medicine.* Andrew Cunningham and Perry Williams, ed. Pp. 209–244. Cambridge: Cambridge University Press.

DaMo Qigong and Taoist Internal Alchemy. 2010. http://www.taoiststudy.com/about (accessed 2/12/10).

Daode zhenjing jizhu 道德真經集注. In *Zhengtong Daozang* 706–707.

Darby, Meriel. 2003. Professor J. R. Worsley—A Personal Tribute. *European Journal of Oriental Medicine* 4(3). http://www.ejom.co.uk/vol-4-no-3/featured-articles/professor-j-r-worsley-a-personal-tribute.html (accessed 2/12/10).

Davis, Edward L. 2001. *Society and the Supernatural in Song China.* Honolulu: University of Hawaii Press.

Delza, Sophia. 1961. *T'ai Chi Ch'uan: Body and Mind in Harmony.* North Canton, OH: Good News Publishing.

Deng Tietao 鄧鐵濤. 1999. *Zhongyi jindai shi* 中醫近代史. Guangzhou: Guangdong gaodeng jiaoyu chubanshe.

Deng Yunte 鄧雲特. 1937. *Zhongguo jiuhuangshi* 中國救荒史. Shanghai: Shangwu yinshuguan.

Deshpande, Vijaya. 2000. Ophthalmic Surgery: A Chapter in the History of Sino-Indian Medical Contacts. *Bulletin of the School of Oriental and African Studies* 63:370–388.

———. 2001. Ancient Indian Medicine and Its Spread to China. *Economic and Political Weekly* 36(13):1078–1081.

———. 2007. The Body Revealed: The Contribution of Forensic Medicine to Knowledge and Representations of the Skeleton in China. In *Graphics and Text in the Production of Technical Knowledge in China: The Warp and the Weft.* F. Bray, V. Dorofeeva-Lichtmann and G. Métailié, eds. Pp. 635–684. Leiden and Boston: Brill.

Despeux, Catherine. 1990. *Immortelles de la Chine ancienne. Taoïsme et alchimie feminine.* Puiseaux: Pardès.

———. 1994. *Taoïsme et corps humain: Le xiuzhen tu.* Paris: Guy Tredaniel.

———. 2001. The System of the Five Circulatory Phases and the Six Seasonal Influences (Wuyun Liuqi), a Source of Innovation in Medicine under the Song (960–1279). In *Innovation in Chinese Medicine.* E. Hsu, ed. Pp. 121–165. Needham Research Institute Studies, Vol. 3. Cambridge: Cambridge University Press.

Despeux, Catherine, and Livia Kohn. 2003. *Women in Taoism.* Cambridge: Three Pine Trees.

DeWoskin, Kenneth J. 1983. *Doctors, Diviners, and Magicians of Ancient China: Biographies of Fang-shih,* New York: Columbia University Press.

Dharmananda, Subhuti. n.d. Chinese Medicine in Italy: Integrated into the Modern Medical System. http://www.itmonline.org/arts/italy.htm (accessed 9/12/09).

Diaz, Maria Dolores. 2001. The Honduras Healing Recovery Project: Second Yearly Report. *Acupuncture Today* 2(5). http://www.acupuncturetoday.com/archives2001/may /05honduras.html?no_b=true (accessed 8/4/09).

———. 2003. Update on the Honduras Healing Recovery Project. *Acupuncture Today* 4(9). http://www.acupuncturetoday.com/mpacms/at/article.php?id=28281&no _paginate=true&no_b=true (accessed 8/4/09).

Dikötter, Frank. 1998. *Imperfect Conceptions: Medical Knowledge, Birth Defects, and Eugenics in China.* New York: Columbia University Press.

———, Lars Laaman, and Xun Zhou. 2004. *Narcotic Culture: A History of Drugs in China.* London: Hurst.

Ding Zhongying 丁仲英. 1936. Zhongyiyao zhi qianzhan 中醫藥之前瞻. *Guanghua yiyao zazhi* 光華醫藥雜誌 4(9):8.

Dong Jianhua 董建華, Hou Dianyuan 侯點元, and Zhang Xijun 張錫君, eds. 1990. *Dangdai zhongyi* 當代中醫. Chongqing: Chongqing chubanshe.

Dongzhen taishang qingya shisheng jing 洞真太上青牙始生經. *Zhengtong Daozang* 1349.

DuBois, Thomas David. 2005. *Sacred Village: Social Change and Religious Life in Rural North China.* Honolulu: University of Hawaii Press.

Dunstan, Helen. 1975. The Late Ming Epidemics: A Preliminary Survey. *Ch'ing-shih wen-t'i* 3(3):1–59.

Dương, Bá Bành. 1947–1950. *Historie de la medécine dù Việt-Nam.* Hanoi: Faculté de Médecine de Hanoi.

Eadie, Gail A., and Denise M. Grizzell. 1979. China's Foreign Aid, 1975–78. *China Quarterly* 77:217–234.

Eagleton, Catherine, Jonathan Williams, Joe Cribb, and Elizabeth Errington. 2007. *Money: A History.* Richmond Hill, Ontario: Firefly Books.

Ebrey, Patricia Buckley. 1986. The Early Stages in the Development of Descent Group Organization. In *Women and the Family in Chinese History.* P. B. Ebrey and R. Watson, eds. Berkeley: University of California Press.

———. 1988. The Dynamics of Elite Domination in Sung China. *Harvard Journal of Asiatic Studies* 48(2):493–520.

———. 1991. *Confucianism and Family Rituals in Imperial China: A Social History of Writing about Rites.* Princeton, NJ: Princeton University Press.

———. 1993. The Response of the Sung State to Popular Funeral Practices. In *Religion and Society in T'ang and Sung China.* P. B. Ebrey and P. N. Gregory, eds. Honolulu: University of Hawaii Press.

———. 2003. *Women and the Family in Chinese History.* London: Routledge.

Ebrey, Patricia Buckley, and Maggie Bickford, eds. 2006. *Emperor Huizong and Late Northern Song China: The Politics of Culture and the Culture of Politics*. Cambridge, MA: Harvard University Press.

Ebrey, Patricia Buckley, and James L. Watson. 1986. Introduction. In *Kinship Organization in Late Imperial China 1000–1940*. P. B. Ebrey and J. L. Watson, eds. Pp. 1–15. Berkeley: University of California Press.

Echenberg, Myron. 2007. *Plague Ports: The Global Urban Impact of Bubonic Plague, 1894–1901*. New York, N.Y.: New York University Press.

Editorial Staff. 2001. News in Brief: South Africa Legalizes TCM. *Acupuncture Today* 2(8). http://www.acupuncturetoday.com/mpacms/at/article.php?id=27721 (accessed 7/28/09).

———. 2005. Relief Effort Update. *Acupuncture Today* (September 1). http://www.acupuncturetoday.com/mpacms/at/article.php?id=31242&no_paginate=true&no_b=true (accessed 8/4/09).

Edwards, William M., Jr. 1974. Acupuncture in Nevada. *Western Journal of Medicine* 120(June):507–512.

Eisenberg, David, Roger Davis, Susan Ettner, Scott Appel, Sonja Wilkey, Maria Van Rompay, and Ronald Kessler. 1998. Trends in Alternative Medicine Use in the United States, 1990–1997. *Journal of the American Medical Association* 280(18): 1569–1575.

Elman, Benjamin A. 1984. *From Philology to Philosophy: Intellectual and Social Aspects of Change in Late Imperial China*. Cambridge, MA: Harvard University Press.

———. 2000. *A Cultural History of Civil Examinations in Late Imperial China*. Berkeley: University of California Press.

———. 2005. *On Their Own Terms: Science in China, 1550–1900*. Berkeley: University of California Press.

Emad, Mitra C. 2006. The Debate over Chinese-Language Knowledge among Culture Brokers of Acupuncture in America. *ETC* (October):408–421.

Emmons, Charles F. 1992. Hong Kong's Feng Shui: Popular Magic in a Modern Urban Setting. *Journal of Popular Culture* 26(1):39–49.

Engelhardt, Ute. 1989. Translating and Interpreting the Fu-Ch'i Ching-I Lun: Experience Gained from Editing a T'ang Dynasty Taoist Medical Treatise. In *Approaches to Traditional Chinese Medical Literature*. P. U. Unschuld, ed. Pp. 129–138. Dordrecht: Kluwer Academic.

Eno, Robert. 2008. Shang State Religion and the Pantheon in the Oracle Bone Texts. In *Early Chinese Religion: Part One: Shang through Han (1250 B.C.–220 A.D.)*. J. Lagerwey and M. Kalinowski, eds. Pp. 41–102. Leiden: Brill.

Epler, D. C., Jr. 1980. Bloodletting in Early Chinese Medicine and Its Relation to the Origin of Acupuncture. *Bulletin of the History of Medicine* 54(3):337–367.

Ergil, Marnae C. n.d. Considerations for the Translation of Traditional Chinese Medicine into English. http://www.paradigm-pubs.com/resources/Translation (accessed 5/2/10).

Falkenhausen, Lothar Von. 1995. Reflections on the Political Role of Spirit Mediums in Early China: The Wu Officials in the Zhou Li. *Early China* 20:279–300.

———. 2006. *Chinese Society in the Age of Confucius (1000–250 B.C.): The Archaeological Evidence.* Los Angeles: Cotsen Institute of Archaeology, University of California.

Family and Friends of Dr. Mutulu Shakur. N.d. Mutulu Shakur: Black Liberation Army and People's Warrior. Leaflet.

Fan Ka-wai 范家偉. 2004a. On Hua Tuo's Position in the History of Chinese Medicine. *American Journal of Chinese Medicine* 32:313–320.

———. 2004b. Jiao Qi Disease in Medieval China. *American Journal of Chinese Medicine* 32:999–1011.

———. 2004c. *Liuchao Sui Tang yixue zhi chuancheng yu zhenghe* 六朝隋唐醫學之傳承與整合. Hong Kong: Chinese University Press.

———. 2005. Couching for Cataract and Sino-Indian Medical Exchange from the Sixth to the Twelfth Century A.D. *Clinical and Experimental Ophthalmology* 33:188–190.

———. 2007a. Acupuncture or Trepanation? A Study of Qin Minghe, a Skilled Physician of Tang China. In *Thieme Almanac: Acupuncture and Chinese Medicine.* Pp. 4–9. Stuttgart: Thieme.

———. 2007b. *Dayi jingcheng: Tangdai guojia, xinyang yu yixue* 大醫精誠 : 唐代國家、信仰與醫學. Taipei: Dongda Publishing House.

Fan Shi 范適. 1942. *Mingji xiyang chuanru zhi yixue* 明季西洋傳入之醫學 [China]: Zhonghua yishi xuehui Junshi chuban jijin weiyuanhui.

Fan Xingzhun 范行準. 1953. *Zhongguo yufang yixue sixiang shi* 中國預防醫學思想史. Shanghai: Huadong yiwu shenghuo she.

———. 1986. *Zhongguo yixue shi lüe* 中國醫學史略. Beijing: Zhongyi guji chubanshe.

Farquhar, Judith. 1994a. Multiplicity, Point of View, and Responsibility in Traditional Chinese Healing. In Body, Subject and Power in China. A. Zito and T. E. Barlow, eds. Pp. 78–99. Chicago, IL: University of Chicago Press.

———. 1994b. Knowing Practice: The Clinical Encounter in Chinese Medicine. Boulder: Westview Press.

———. 1995. Re-writing Traditional Medicine in Post-Maoist China In Knowledge and the Scholarly Medical Traditions. D. G. Bates, ed. Pp. 251–76. Cambridge: Cambridge University Press.

———. 1996a. "Medicine and the Changes are One": An Essay in Divination Healing. Chinese Science 16:107–34.

———. 1996b. Market Magic: Getting Magic and Getting Personal in Medicine after Mao. *American Ethnologist* 23(2):239–257.

Felt, Bob. 2006a. A Guided Tour of the Term Debate. http://www.paradigm-pubs.com/references/TourBook (accessed 5/2/10).

———. 2006b. Professional Papers on Translation, Linguistics and Lexicography. http://www.paradigm-pubs.com/references/Proffesional (accessed 8/2/09).

———. 2006c. Publisher's Comment on Chinese Acupuncture by George Soulié de Morant. http://www.paradigm-pubs.com/catalog/detail/ChiAcuDeMor (accessed 8/2/09).

Felton, Ann. n.d. Ah Fong Office. Second Chinatown: Its Rise and Fall, 1901–1972. http://www
.boisestate.edu/history/cityhistorian/galleries_city/galleries_chinatown/chinatown7
_fongoffice.html (accessed 5/8/09).

Feng, H. Y., and J. Shryock. 1935. The Black Magic in China Known as Ku. *Journal of the American Oriental Society* 55:1–30.

Fidler, Simon. n.d. The Successful Use of Auricular Acupuncture in the Supported Withdrawal and Detoxification of Substance Abusers. http://www.acupuncture.com
/conditions/addictres.htm (accessed 2/10/10).

Field, Stephen L. 2004. Review: Fengshui in China: Geomantic Divination between State Orthodoxy and Popular Religion. *Journal of Chinese Religions* 32:187–189.

Fitch, K. 1998. *Speaking Relationally: Culture, Communication, and Interpersonal Communication.* New York: Guilford.

———. 1999. Pillow Talk? *Research on Language and Social Interaction* 32:41–50.

Fixler, Marian, and Oran Kivity. 2002. Japanese Acupuncture: A Review of Four Styles. *European Journal of Oriental Medicine* 3(3):4–16.

Flaws, Bob. 1995a. *The Book of Jook: Chinese Medicinal Porridges—A Healthy Alternative to the Typical Western Breakfast.* Boulder, CO: Blue Poppy Press.

———. 1995b. *The Tao of Healthy Eating: Dietary Wisdom According to Traditional Chinese Medicine.* Boulder, CO: Blue Poppy Press.

Fong, Henry. 2009a. Chinese Dreams Dictionary. http://www.absolutelyfengshui.com/others
/dreams-grandmaster-zhou.php (accessed 12/3/09).

———. 2009b. Dreams Interpretation Chinese Style. http://www.selfgrowth.com/articles
/Dreams_Intepretation_Chinese_Style.html (accessed 12/3/09).

———. 2009c. The Chinese Almanac (a.k.a. Tong Sing). http://www.absolutelyfengshui.com
/others/tong-sing-tung-shu.php (accessed 12/3/09).

Foo and Wing Herb Company. 1897. *The Science of Oriental Medicine: A Concise Discussion of Its Principles and Methods.* Los Angeles: G. Rice and Sons.

Ford, Guila, and Elizabeth Jacox. 1996. Ah Fong—1845–1927. Idaho State Historical Society Reference Series, 1130 (January). http://www.idahohistory.net/Reference%20Series
/1130.pdf (accessed 12/8/09).

Franzini, Serge. 1992. 1935: Un premier écho chinois d'une acupuncture française. *Revue française d'acupuncture* 70:20–24.

Frank, Byron L., and Nader Soliman. 1998/1999. Shen Men: A Critical Assessment through Advanced Auricular Therapy. *Medical Acupuncture* 10(2). http://www.medicalacu-
puncture.org/aama_marf/journal/vol10_2/shenmen.html (accessed 9/12/09).

Frank, Robert, and Gunnar Stollberg. 2004a. Medical Acupuncture in Germany—Patterns of Consumerism among Physicians and Patients. *Sociology of Health and Illness* 26:353–372.

———. 2004b. Conceptualizing Hybridization: On the Diffusion of Asian Medical Knowledge to Germany. *International Sociology* 19(1):71–88.

Franzini, Serge. 1992. 1935: Un premier écho chinois d'une acupuncture française. *Revue française d'acupuncture* 70:20–24.

Fratkin, Jake. 1999. The Emergence of Japanese Style Acupuncture. http://www.drjakefratkin .com/pdf/hja.pdf (accessed 5/2/10).

FREE Longevitology Class Is Coming to Boston in September! 2009. Advertising flyer.

Freedberg, David. 2002. *The Eye of the Lynx: Galileo, His Friends, and the Beginning of Modern Natural History*. Chicago: University of Chicago Press.

Freiden, Betina. 2008. Acupuncture Worlds in Argentina: Contested Knowledge, Legitimation Processes, and Everyday Practices. Ph.D. dissertation, Brandeis University.

Fried, Diana. 2009. Name Change for the Vets Project. April 15: e-newsletter.

Fruehauf, Heiner. 2010. Chinese Medicine in Crisis: Science, Politics, and the Making of "TCM." http://chineseclassics.org/j/images/tcmcrisis.pdf.

Fu Weikang 傅維康, ed. 1990. *Zhongguo yixue shi* 中國醫學史. *Zhongyi jichu lilun xilie congshu* 中醫基礎理論系列叢書. Shanghai: Shanghai zhongyi xueyuan chubanshe.

Fuma Susumu 夫馬進. 1997. *Chūgoku zenkai, zendō shi kenkyū* 中國善會善堂史研究. Kyoto: Dōhōsha shuppan.

Furth, Charlotte. 1994. Rethinking van Gulik: Sexuality and Reproduction in Traditional Chinese Medicine. In *Engendering China: Women, Culture, and the State*. C. K. Gilmartin, G. Hershatter, R. Rofel, and T. White, eds. Pp. 125–146. Cambridge, MA: Harvard University Press.

———. 1999. *A Flourishing Yin: Gender in China's Medical History, 960–1665*. Berkeley: University of California Press, Berkeley.

———. 2006. The Physician as Philosopher of the Way: Zhu Zhenheng (1282–1358). *Harvard Journal of Asiatic Studies* 66(2):423–459.

———. 2007. Producing Medical Knowledge through Cases: History, Evidence, and Action. In *Thinking with Cases: Specialist Knowledge in Chinese Cultural History*. C. Furth, J. T. Zeitlin, and P.-C. Hsiung, eds. Pp. 125–151. Honolulu: University of Hawaii Press.

———. 2011. Becoming Alternative? Modern Transformations of Chinese Medicine in China and in the United States. *Canadian Bulletin of Medical History* 28(1):5–41.

Furth, Charlotte, and Angela Ki Che Leung, eds. 2010. *Health and Hygiene in Chinese East Asia: Policies and Publics in the Long Twentieth Century*. Chapel Hill, NC: Duke University Press.

Gao Wei 高偉. 1994. *Jin-Yuan yixue renwu* 金元醫學人物. Lanzhou: Lanzhou daxue chubanshe

Gao Wenjin 高文晉. 1856. *Waike tushuo* 外科圖說. [China]: Punan shensi tang.

Gao Xi 高晞. 2009. *De Zhen zhuan: Yi ge Yingguo chuanjiaoshi yu wan Qing yixue jindaihua* 德貞傳:一個英國傳教士與晚清醫學近代化. Shanghai: Fudan daxue chubanshe.

Garrett, Frances. 2006. Buddhism and the Historicising of Medicine in Thirteenth-Century Tibet. *Asian Medicine: Tradition and Modernity* 2(2):204–224.

Gates, Hill. 1987. Money for the Gods. *Modern China* 13(3):259–277.

Giblette, Jean. 2009a. High Falls Gardens e-newsletter.

———. 2009b. High Falls Gardens: Programs Overview. http://www.highfallsgardens.net /botanicalstudies/program/index.html (accessed 2/26/09).

Glahn, Richard von. 1987. *The Country of Streams and Grottoes: Expansion, Settlement, and the Civilizing of the Sichuan Frontier in Song Times*. Cambridge: Council on East Asian Studies, Harvard University.

Glaser, Shirley. 1971. Let Me Tell You about My Acupuncture. *New York Magazine* (September 27):64–65.

Gleditsch, Jochen. 2001. 50 Jahre DÄGfA. Zur Geschichte der deutschen Ärztegesellschaft für Akupunktur. *Deutsche Zeitschrift für Akupunktur* 2a:176–191.

Goble, Andrew Edmund. 2009. The Medical Silk Road: Chinese and Arabic Influences on Medieval Japanese Medicine. In *Tools of Culture: Japan's Cultural, Intellectual, Medical and Technological Contacts in East Asia, 1000s–1500s.* A. E. Goble, K. R. Robinson, and H. Wakabayashi, eds. Pp. 231–257. Ann Arbor: Association for Asian Studies.

———. 2011. *Confluences of Medicine in Medieval Japan: Buddhist Healing, Chinese Knowledge, Islamic Formulas, and Wounds of War.* Honolulu: University of Hawaii Press.

Goldschmidt, Asaf Moshe. 2009. *The Evolution of Chinese Medicine: Song Dynasty, 960–1200.* London: Routledge.

Gori, Luigi, and Fabio Firenzuoli. 2007. Ear Acupuncture in European Traditional Medicine. *Evidence Based Complementary and Alternative Medicine* 4(Supplement 1):13–16.

Grant, Joanna. 2003. *A Chinese Physician: Wang Ji and the Stone Mountain Medical Case Histories.* London: RoutledgeCurzon.

Graziani, Romain. 2008. The Subject and the Sovereign: Exploring the Self in Early Chinese Self-Cultivation. In *Early Chinese Religion: Part One: Shang through Han (1250 B.C.–220 A.D.).* J. Lagerwey and M. Kalinowski, eds. Pp. 495–517. Leiden: Brill.

Griffith, Wally. 2008. McDonald's has a big appetite for China. CNBC August 15: http://www.msnbc.msn.com/id/26226387/ns/business-cnbc_tv//print/1/displaymode/1098/ (accessed 4/14/10).

Guimarães, Sergio Botelho. 2007. Acupuncture in an Outpatient Clinic in Fortaleza, Brazil: Patients' Characteristics and Prevailing Main Complaints. *Journal of Alternative and Complementary Medicine* 13(3):308–310.

Gumenick, Neil. 2003. Oriental Medical World Mourns Professor J. R. Worsley. *Acupuncture Today* 4(8). http://www.acupuncturetoday.com/mpacms/at/article.php?id=28270&no_paginate=true&no_b=true (accessed 8/14/09).

Guo Licheng 郭立誠. 1979. *Zhongguo shengyu lisu kao* 中國生育禮俗考. Taipei: Wenshizhe chubanshe.

Guoyu 國語. 1983. Wei Zhao 韋昭 (204–273), ann. Yingyin *Wenyuange Sikuquanshu* 影印文淵閣四庫全書, vol. 406. Taipei: Taiwan shangwu yinshuguan.

Guy, R. Kent. 1987. *The Emperor's Four Treasuries: Scholars and the State in the Late Ch'ienlung Era.* Cambridge, MA: Harvard University Press.

Hacker, Edward, Steve Moore, and Lorraine Patsco. 2002. *I Ching: An Annotated Bibliography.* New York: Routledge.

Hammer, Leon I. 2005. *Chinese Pulse Diagnosis: A Contemporary Approach.* Seattle: Eastland Press.

Hammers, Roslyn L. 2002. The Production of Good Government: Images of Agrarian Labor in Southern Song (1127–1279) and Yuan (1272/79–1368) China. Ph.D. dissertation, University of Michigan.

Han Fei 韓非 (d. 233 b.c.) Wang Xianshen 王先慎 (1859–1922). 1991. *Han Feizi jijie* 韓非子集解. In *Zhuzi jicheng* 諸子集成, vol. 5. Reprint. Shanghai: Shanghai guji.

Hansen, Valerie. 1990. *Changing Gods in Medieval China*. Princeton, NJ: Princeton University Press.

Hanshu 漢書. 1975. Ban Gu 班固 (32–92 c.e.), Yan Shigu 顏師古 (581–645), ed. Beijing: Zhonghua shuju.

Hanson, Marta. 2003. The Golden Mirror in the Imperial Court of the Qianlong Emperor. *Early Science and Medicine* 8(2):111–147.

———. 2006. The Significance of Manchu Medical Sources in the Qing. In *Proceedings of the First North American Conference on Manchu Studies* (Portland, or, May 9–10, 2003). S. Wadley, C. Naeher, and K. Dede, eds. Pp. 131–175. Weisbaden: Harrassowitz Verlag.

———. 2010. Conceptual Blind Spots, Media Blindfolds: The Case of SARS and Chinese Medicine. In *Health and Hygiene in Chinese East Asia: Policies and Publics in the Long Twentieth Century*. C. Furth and A. K. C. Leung, eds. Pp. 228–254. Chapel Hill, NC: Duke University Press.

———. 2011. *Speaking of Epidemics in Chinese Medicine: Disease and the Geographic Imagination in Late Imperial China*. New York: Routledge.

Hare, Martha L. 1993. The Emergence of an Urban U.S. Chinese Medicine. *Medical Anthropology Quarterly* 7:30–49.

Harper, Donald. 1985. A Chinese Demonography of the Third Century b.c. *Harvard Journal of Asian Studies* 45:459–498.

———. 1995. The Bellows Analogy in *Laozi* V and Warring States Macrobiotic Hygiene. *Early China* 20:381–391.

———. 1998. *Early Chinese Medical Literature: The Mawangdui Medical Manuscripts*. Sir Henry Wellcome Asian Series, Vol. 2. London: Kegan Paul.

———. 1999. Warring States Natural Philosophy and Occult Thought. In M. Loewe and E. Shaughnessy, ed. *The Cambridge History of Ancient China: From the Origins of Civilization to 221 b.c.* Pp. 813–884. Cambridge: Cambridge University Press.

———. 2001. Iatromancy, Diagnosis, and Prognosis in Early Chinese Medicine. In *Innovation in Chinese Medicine*. E. Hsu, ed. Pp. 99–120. Cambridge: Cambridge University Press.

———. 2002. Spellbinding. In *Religions of Asia in Practice: An Anthology*. D. S. Lopez, ed. Pp. 376–385. Princeton, NJ: Princeton University Press.

———. 2005a. Ancient Medieval Chinese Recipes for Aphrodisiacs and Philters. *Asian Medicine: Tradition and Modernity* 1(2):91–100.

———. 2005b. Dunhuang Iatromantic Manuscripts: P. 2856 R° and P. 2675 V°. In *Medieval Chinese Medicine: The Dunhuang Medical Manuscripts*. V. Lo and C. Cullen, eds. Pp. 134–164. London: Routledge Curzon.

———. 2010. The Textual Form of Knowledge: Occult Miscellanies in Ancient and Medieval Manuscripts, Fourth Century b.c. to Tenth Century a.d. In *Looking at It from Asia: The Processes That Shaped the Sources of History of Science*. F. Bretelle-Establet, ed. Pp. 37–80. New York: Springer.

Harrington, Anne. 1999. *The Placebo Effect: An Interdisciplinary Exploration.* Cambridge, MA: Harvard University Press.

Hartwell, Robert M. 1982. Demographic, Political, and Social Transformations of China, 750–1550. *Harvard Journal of Asiatic Studies* 42(2):365–442.

Hattori Toshirō 服部敏郎. 1964. *Kamakura jidai igakushi no kenkyû* 鎌倉時代医学史の研究. Tokyo: Yoshikawa Kōbunkan.

He Shixi 何時希. 1997. Jindai yilin yishi 近代醫林軼事. Shanghai: Shanghai zhongyiyao daxue chubanshe.

He Zhiguo 何志國. 1995. *Xi Han renti jingmo qidiao kao* 西漢人體經脈漆雕考. Daziran tansuo 大自然探索 3:116–120.

Heinrich, Larissa N. 2008. *The Afterlife of Images: Translating the Pathological Body between China and the West.* Durham: Duke University Press.

Helms, Joseph. 1995. *Acupuncture Energetics: A Clinical Approach for Physicians* Berkeley: Medical Acupuncture Publishers.

Help with a Bow. 2008. *Economist* 387(8582):46–47.

Henderson, Gail. 1989. Issues in the Modernization of Medicine in China. In *Science and Technology in Post-Mao China.* D. F. Simon and M. Goldman, eds. Pp. 199–221. Cambridge, MA: The Council of East Asian Studies/Harvard University.

Hessel, Erin. 2009. Broken Bones. ESEMA (East Side Eastern Medicine Associates) Healing Arts http://www.erinhessel.com/tag/zheng-gu-tui-na (accessed 1/5/10).

Highfield, Ellen S., Linda L. Barnes, Lisa Spellman, and Robert Saper. 2008. If You Build It, Will They Come? A Free-Care Acupuncture Clinic for Minority Adolescents in an Urban Hospital. *Journal of Complementary and Alternative Medicine* 14(6):629–636.

Hinrichs, TJ. 1998. New Geographies of Chinese Medicine. *Osiris,* 2nd Series 13:287–325.

———. 2003. The Medical Transforming of Governance and Southern Customs in Song China (960–1279 C.E.). Ph.D. dissertation, History and East Asian Languages, Harvard University.

———. 2009. Medical Learning, Literati Culture, and the Contested Role of the Physician in the Song (960–1279 C.E.). Paper presented at Reconsidering Chinese History: Ideas, Places, and Social Networks, June 7–8, at Harvard University, Cambridge, MA.

———. 2011. Governance through Medical Texts and the Role of Print. In *Transmission and Transformation of Knowledge in China, Tenth-Fourteenth Centuries.* Pp. 217–238. L. Chia and H. D. Weerdt, eds. Leiden: Brill.

———. Forthcoming. The Catchy Epidemic: Theorization and Its Limits in Han to Song Period Medicine. *East Asian Science, Technology, and Medicine.*

History of the Lincoln Hospital Acupuncture/Detox Clinic: A Lesson in Community Health Organizing. n.d. Mimeographed pamphlet.

HIV/AIDS Acupuncture Treatment for Massachusetts Residents. 2010. http://www.mass resources.org/pages.cfm?contentID=114&pageID=31&subpages=yes&dynamic ID=902 (accessed 1/26/10).

Ho, Evelyn Y. 2009. Behold the Power of Qi: The Importance of Qi in the Discourse of Acupuncture. *Research on Language and Social Interaction* 39(4):411–440.

Ho, Ming-Jung. 2003. Migratory Journey and Tuberculosis Risk. *Medical Anthropology Quarterly* 17:442–424.

———. 2004a. Health-Seeking Patterns among Chinese Immigrant Patients Enrolled in the Directly Observed Therapy Program in New York City. *International Journal of Tuberculosis and Lung Diseases* 8:1355–1359.

———. 2004b. Sociocultural Aspects of Tuberculosis: A Literature Review and a Case Study of Immigrant Tuberculosis. *Social Science and Medicine* 59:753–762.

———. 2006. Perspectives on Tuberculosis among Traditional Chinese Medical Practitioners in New York City's Chinatown. *Culture, Medicine and Psychiatry* 30:105–122.

Ho, Ping-ti. 1962. *The Ladder of Success in Imperial China: Aspects of Social Mobility, 1368–1911*. New York: Columbia University Press.

Hoang Bao Chau, Pho Duc Thao, and Huu Ngoc. 1993. Overview of Vietnamese Traditional Medicine. In *Vietnamese Traditional Medicine*. Pp. 3–28. Hanoi: Thế Giới.

Hoang, Bao Chau. 1993. Overview of Vietnamese Traditional Medicine. In *Vietnamese Traditional Medicine*. B. C. Hoang and H. Ngoc, eds. Hanoi: Thế Giới.

Hobsbawm, Eric, and Terence Ranger. 1983. *The Invention of Tradition*. Cambridge: Cambridge University Press.

Hobson, Benjamin. 1851a. *Quanti xinlun* 全體新論. Canton: Hui'ai yiguan.

Hobson, Benjamin. 1851b. *Quanti xinlun*. 全體新論. Third ed. Shanghai: Mohai shuguan.

Hoover, Craig. 2003. Response to "Sex, Drugs and Animal Parts: Will Viagra Save Threatened Species?" by von Hippel and von Hippel. *Environmental Conservation* 30:317–318.

Horn, Joshua S. 1969. *Away with All Pests—An English Surgeon in People's China 1954–1969*. New York: Monthly Review Press.

Hou Hanshu 後漢書. 1965. Fan Ye 范曄 et al., ed. Beijing: Zhonghua shuju.

Hou Naifeng 侯乃峰. 2005. *Qin Yin daobing yuban mingwen jijie* 秦駰禱病玉版銘文集解. *Wenbo* 文博 6:69–75.

Hsiung, Ping-chen. 2005. *A Tender Voyage: Children and Childhood in Late Imperial China*. Stanford, CA: Stanford University Press.

Hsu, Elisabeth. 1992. The History and Development of Auriculotherapy. *Acupuncture in Medicine* 10(Supplement): 109–118.

———. 1996. Innovations in Acumoxa: Acupuncture Analgesia, Scalp and Ear Acupuncture in the People's Republic of China. *Social Science and Medicine* 42(3):421–430.

———. 1999. *The Transmission of Chinese Medicine*. Cambridge: Cambridge University Press.

———, ed. 2001. *Innovation in Chinese Medicine*. Cambridge: Cambridge University Press.

———. 2002. "The Medicine from China Has Rapid Effects": Chinese Medicine Patients in Tanzania. *Anthropology and Medicine* 9(3):291–313.

———. 2006. Reflections on the "Discovery" of the Anti-malarial Qinghao. *British Journal of Clinical Pharmacology Special Issue: Future Developments in Clinical Pharmacology* 61(6):666–670.

———. 2007. Chinese Medicine in East Africa and Its Effectiveness. *IIAS Newsletter* 45(Autumn):22.

————. 2008. Medicine as Business: Chinese Medicine in Tanzania. In *China Returns to Africa: A Rising Power and a Continent Embrace*. C. Alden, D. Large, and R. Soares de Oliveira, eds. Pp. 221–235. http://afrikastudiecentrum.nl/Pdf/paper10mei.pdf. London: Hurst.

————. 2009. Chinese Propriety Medicines: An "Alternative Modernity"? The Case of the Anti-Malarial Substance Aretmisinin in East Africa. *Medical Anthropology Special Issue: Globalizing Chinese Medicine* 28(2):111–140.

Hsu, Elisabeth, and Erling Høg. 2002. Countervailing Creativity: Patient Agency in the Globalisation of Asian Medicines. *Anthropology and Medicine* 9(3):205–363.

Hu, Shiu-Ying. 2005. *Food Plants of China*. Hong Kong: Chinese University of Hong Kong Press.

Hu Houxuan 胡厚宣, ed. 1978–82. *Jiaguwen heji* 甲骨文合集. Beijing: Zhonghua Shuju.

Hu Shijie 胡世杰, ed. 1990. *Xin'an yiji congkan* 新安醫集叢刊. Anhui: Anhui kexue jishu chubanshe.

Huang, Al. 1973. *Embrace Tiger, Return to Mountain: The Essence of Tai Chi*. Moab Utah: Real People Press.

Huang, Bi Yun. 2009. Analyzing a Social Movement's Use of Internet: Resource Mobilization, New Social Movement Theories and the Case of Falun Gong. Ph.D. dissertation, Indiana University.

Huang, C. Julia. 2008. Gendered Charisma in the Buddhist Tzu Chi (Ciji) Movement. *Nova Religio* 12(2):29–47.

Huang, H. T. 2000. *Science and Civilization in China*, Vol. 6: *Biology and Biological Technology*, Part 6: *Medicine*. Cambridge: Cambridge University Press.

Huangdi neijing lingshu 黃帝內經靈樞. 1995. Wang Bing 王冰 (fl. 762), ed. Zhongyi yanjiuyuan Ming edition repr. Beijing: Zhongyi guji chubanshe.

Huangdi neijing suwen 黃帝內經素問. 1995. Wang Bing 王冰 (fl. 762), ed. Zhongyi yanjiuyuan Ming edition repr. Beijing: Zhongyi guji chubanshe.

Huard, Pierre, and Ming Wong. 1968. *Chinese Medicine*. B. Fielding, trans. New York: McGraw-Hill.

Hubei sheng bowuguan 湖北省博物館. 1989. *Zenghou yi mu* 曾侯乙墓. 2 vols. Beijing: Wenwu.

Hubei sheng Jingzhou shi Zhou Liang Yu Qiao yi zhi bowuguan, 湖北省荊州市周梁玉橋遺址博物館, ed. 2001. *Guanju Qin Hanmu jiandu* 關沮秦漢墓簡牘. Beijing: Zhonghua Shuju.

Hucker, Charles O. 1985. *A Dictionary of Official Titles in Imperial China*. Stanford, CA: Stanford University Press.

Hummel, Arthur W., ed. 1943. *Eminent Chinese of the Ch'ing Period*. Washington, DC: Government Printing Office.

Hunan Zhongyiyao yanjiusuo and John E. Fogarty International Center for Advanced Study in the Health Sciences. 1990. *A Barefoot Doctor's Manual: The American Translation of the Official Chinese Paramedical Manual*. Philadelphia: Running Press.

Hung Chang-tai. 1994. *War and Popular Culture—Resistance in Modern China, 1937–1945*. Berkeley: University of California Press.

Huong, Nguyen Van et al. 1965. *Health Organization in the Democratic Republic of Vietnam*. Hanoi: Xunhasaba.

Hutchison, Alan. 1975. *China's African Revolution*. London: Hutchinson.

Hymes, Robert P. 1986. *Statesmen and Gentlemen: The Élite of Fu-chou, Chiang-hsi, in Northern and Southern Sung*. Cambridge: Cambridge University Press.

——. 1987. Not Quite Gentlemen? Doctors in Sung and Yuan. *Chinese Science* 8(January):9–76.

——. 2002. *Way and Byway: Taoism, Local Religion, and Models of Divinity in Sung and Modern China*. Berkeley: University of California Press.

Hymes, Robert P., and Conrad Shirokauer, eds. 1993. *Ordering the World: Approaches to State and Society in Sung Dynasty China*. Berkeley: University of California Press.

Icon plc. 2012. Tasly Pharmaceuticals Selects ICON as it Seeks First FDA Approval of a Traditional Chinese Medicine. http://www.iconplc.com/news-events/news/tasly -pharmaceuticals-sel/index.xml (accessed May 31, 2012).

Idema, Wilt. 1977. Diseases and Doctors, Drugs and Cures: A Very Preliminary List of Passages of Medical Interest in a Number of Traditional Chinese Novels and Related Plays. *Chinese Science* 2:37–73.

In Memory of Richard Taft. 1974. Mimeographed flyer.

Is Feng Shui a Science or Superstition? 2005. *Beijing Review* 48(43):46–47.

Ishida Hidemi 石田秀実. 1992. *Chūgoku igaku shisōshi* 中国医学思想史: もう一つの医学. Tōkyō: Tōkyō Daigaku Shuppankai.

Ishihara Akira 石原明. 1986. Kajiwara Shōzen no shôgai to sono chosho 梶原性全の生涯とその 著書. In *Man'anpō* 萬安方. Pp. 1731–1752. Tokyo: Kagaku Shoin.

Ishizaki, Naoto, Tadashi Yano, and Kenji Kawakita. 2010. Public Status and Prevalence of Acupuncture in Japan. *eCAM* 7(4):493–500.

Itō Michiharu, Ken-ichi Takashima, and Gary F. Arbuckle. 1996. *Studies in Early Chinese Civilization: Religion, Society, Language, and Palaeography*. Osaka: Kansai Gaidai University Publication.

ITRI Creativity Laboratory. 2007a. ITRI Creativity Lab's Flow of Qi Exhibition September 5–11, 2007 at the National Palace Museum, Taipei, Taiwan. http://www.creativitylab. itri.org.tw/eng/press/Flow%20of%20Qi.asp (accessed 7/21/09).

——. 2007b. Flow of Qi offers a Unique Experience of Chinese Culture. *ITRI Today* 51(5). http://www.itri.org.tw/chi/lib/DownloadFile.aspx?AttNBR=844 (accessed 7/30/11).

Jack. n.d. The Duke of Zhou's Dream Dictionary. http://www.dreamdict.com (accessed 8/12/09).

Jennings, Michael. 2005. Chinese Medicine and Medical Pluralism in Dar es Salaam: Globalisation or Glocalisation? *International Relations* 19(4):457–473.

Jia Gongyan 賈公彥. 1980. *Zhouli zhushu* 周禮注疏. Beijing: Zhonghua Shuju.

Jia Hawk. 2006. New Strain of Bird Flu Found in China's Poultry Markets. *Proceedings of the National Academy of Sciences* http://www.scidev.net/en/agriculture-and-environment/livestock/news/new-strain-of-bird-flu-found-in-chinas-poultry-ma. html (accessed 1/3/10).

Jia Huanguang. 1997. Chinese Medicine in Post-Mao China: Standardization and the Context of Modern Science. Ph.D dissertation. University of North Carolina.

Jiangsu xinyi xueyuan 江蘇新醫學院. 1979. Zhongyao dacidian 中藥大辭典. Shanghai: Shanghai kexue jishu chubanshe.

Jiu Tangshu 舊唐書. 1975. Liu Xu 劉昫 et al., eds. Beijing: Zhonghua shuju.

Johnson, Susan. 2009. In Memoriam: Dr. Miriam Lee (1926–2009). *Acupuncture Today* 10(9). http://www.acupuncturetoday.com/mpacms/at/article.php?id=32021&no_paginate=true&no_b=true (accessed 12/7/10).

Jordan, David K. 1982. Taiwanese Poe Divination: Statistical Awareness and Religious Belief. *Journal for the Scientific Study of Religion* 21(2):114–118.

Josephs, Gordon. n.d. How I First Learned about Sri Lankan-Style Acupuncture. http://www.chelationcare.com/newpage1.htm (accessed 3/14/08).

Jullien, François. 1995. *The Propensity of Things: Toward a History of Efficacy in China.* J. Lloyd, trans. New York: Zone.

Jütte, Robert. 2005. *A History of the Senses: From Antiquity to Cyberspace.* T. Lynn, trans. Oxford: Polity Press.

Kaempfer, Engelbert. 1712. *Amoenitatum exoticarum politico-physico-medicarum fasciculi V.* Lemgoviæ: Meyer.

Kalinowski, Marc. 2005. Mantic Texts in Their Cultural Context. In *Medieval Chinese Medicine: The Dunhuang Medical Manuscripts.* V. Lo and C. Cullen, eds. Pp. 109–133. London: Routledge Curzon.

———. 2008. Diviners and Astrologers under the Eastern Zhou: Transmitted Texts and Recent Archaeological Discoveries. In *Early Chinese Religion: Part One: Shang through Han (1250 B.C.–220 A.D.).* J. Lagerwey and M. Kalinowski, eds. Pp. 341–396. Leiden: Brill.

Kane, Lou Ann. 2007. Acupuncture at Sea. http://www.cruisemates.com/articles/feature/acupuncture-at-sea.cfm (accessed 6/23/08).

Kapferer, Bruce. 1991. *A Celebration of Demons: Exorcism and the Aesthetics of Healing in Sri Lanka.* Oxford: Berg.

Kaptchuk, Ted J. 1983. *The Web That Has No Weaver: Understanding Chinese Medicine.* New York: Congdon and Weed.

———. 1998a. Intentional Ignorance: A History of Blind Assessment and Placebo Controls in Medicine. *Bulletin for the History of Medicine* 72:389–435.

———. 1998b. Powerful Placebo: The Dark Side of the Randomized Controlled Trial. *Lancet* 351:1722–1725.

———. 2002. Acupuncture: Theory, Efficacy and Practice. *Annals of Internal Medicine* 136:374–383.

Kaptchuk, Ted J., John M. Kelley, Lisa A. Conboy, R. B. Davis, Catherine E. Kerr, Eric E. Jacobson, I. Kirsch, Rosa N. Schyner, Bong-Hyun Nam, Long T. Nguyen, Andrea L. Rivers, Claire McManus, Efi Kokkotou, Douglas A. Drossman, Peter Goldman, and Anthony L. Lembo. 2008. Components of Placebo Effect: Randomized Controlled Trial of Patients with Irritable Bowel Syndrome. *British Medical Journal* 226(998–1003).

Kaptchuk, Ted J., William B. Stason, Roger B. Davis, Anna T. R. Legedza, Rosa N. Schyner, Catherine E. Kerr, David A. Stone, Bong-Hyun Nam, Irving Kirsch, and R. H. Goldman. 2006. Sham Device V Inert Pill: Randomized Controlled Trial of Two Placebo Treatments. *British Medical Journal* 332:391–397.

Karchmer, Eric I. 2004. Orientalizing the Body: Postcolonial Transformations in Chinese Medicine. Ph.D. dissertation, University of North Carolina.

———. 2010. Chinese Medicine in Action: On the Postcoloniality of Medical Practice in China. *Medical Acupuncture* 29(3):226–252.

Katz, Paul. 1995. *Demon Hordes and Burning Boats: The Cult of Marshal Wen in Late Imperial China.* New York: SUNY Press.

Keightley, David. 1978. *Sources of Shang History: The Oracle-Bone Inscriptions of Bronze Age China.* Berkeley: University of California, Berkeley.

———. 2000. *The Ancestral Landscape: Time, Space, and Community in Late Shang China (ca. 1200–1045 B.C.).* Berkeley: Institute of East Asian Studies, University of California, Berkeley.

Kendall, Laurel. 2007. Does the Marketplace Disenchant Sacred Goods? In *Society for the Anthropology of Religion Annual Meeting.* Phoenix, AZ.

Kerber, Theodorus. 1832. *Dissertatio inauguralis medico-chirurgica de acupunctura.* Halis Saxonum: Heinrich Ruffius.

Khánh, Vũ Ngọc. 2004. Tuệ Tĩnh (1330–?) In *Renowned Vietnamese Intellectuals prior to the 20th Century.* Hanoi: Thế Giới.

Kim, Andrew Eungi. 2005. Nonofficial Religion in South Korea: Prevalence of Fortunetelling and Other Forms of Divination. *Review of Religious Research* 46(3):284–302.

Kim Ho. 2000. *Hŏ Chun ŭi Tongŭi pogam yŏn'gu.* Seoul: Ilchisa.

Kim Nam-il. 1999. Yi Kyu-jun's Study on *Huangdi neijing* in the Late Choson Era. *Current Perspectives in the History of Science in East Asia.* Yung Sik Kim and Francesca Bray, eds. Seoul: Seoul National University Press.

Kim Sin-gŭn. 2001. *Han'guk ŭiyaksa* 韓國醫藥事. Seoul: Seoul National University Press.

Kimber, Stephanie. 2005. Acupuncture at Sea. Acupuncture.com 3(12). http://www.accupuncture.com/newsletters/m_dec05/main3.htm (accessed 6/23/08).

Kimura Akifumi 木村明史 2001. Sōdai no minkan iryō to fugeki kan: Chihookan ni yoru fugeki torishimari no ichisokumen 宋代の民間醫療と巫覡觀—地方官による巫覡取締の一側面. *Tôhôgaku* 101:89–104.

Kleinman, Arthur. 1986. *Social Origins of Distress and Disease: Depression, Neurasthenia, and Pain in Modern China.* New Haven: Yale University Press.

———. 1995. *Writing at the Margin: Discourse between Anthropology and Medicine.* Berkeley: University of Califonia Press.

Kleinman, Arthur, Yunxiang Yan, Jing Jun, Sing Lee, Everett Zhang, Pan Tianshu, Wu Fei, and Guo Jinhua. 2011. *Deep China: The Moral Life of the Person—What Anthropology and Psychiatry Tell Us about China Today.* Berkeley: University of California Press.

Knoblock, John. 1988. *Xunzi: A Translation and Study of the Complete Works*, Vol. 1. Stanford, CA: Stanford University Press.

Knoblock, John, and Jeffrey Riegel. 2000. *The Annals of Lü Buwei: A Complete Translation and Study.* Stanford, CA: Stanford University Press.

Kobayashi, Akiko, Miwa Uefuji, and Washiro Yasumo. 2007. History and Progress of Japanese Acupuncture. eCAM doi:10.1093/ecam/nem155.

Kohn, Livia. 1986. *A Textbook of Physiognomy: The Tradition of the Shenxiang quanbian.* Asian Folklore Studies 45:227–258.

———. 1995. Kōshin: A Taoist Cult in Japan; Part I: Contemporary Practices, Part II: Historical Development; Part III: The Scripture—A Translation of the Kōshinkyō. *Japanese Religions* 18(1–2):113–139; 20(1):34–55; 20(2):123–142.

———. 2001. *Daoism and Chinese Culture.* Cambridge: Three Pines Press.

Kohn, Livia, and Yoshinobu Sakade. 1989. *Taoist Meditation and Longevity Techniques.* Ann Arbor: Center for Chinese Studies, University of Michigan.

Kolenda, John. 2000. A Brief History of Acupuncture for Detoxification in the United States. *Acupuncture Today* 1(9). http://www.acupuncturetoday.com/mpacms/at/article .php?id=27686&no_paginate=true&no_b=true (accessed 9/20/09).

Kominami, Ichirō. 2008. Rituals for the Earth. In *Early Chinese Religion: Part One: Shang through Han* (1250 B.C.–220 A.D.). J. Lagerwey and M. Kalinowski, eds. Pp. 201–234. Leiden: Brill.

Komjathy, Louis. 2004. Tracing the Contours of Daoism in North America. *Nova Religio* 8(2):5–27.

Kong S. Y. 江潤祥 et al. 1996. *Huihui yaofang* 回回藥方. Hong Kong: Hong Kong Zhongguo bianyi yinwu youxian gongsi.

Kong Yingda 孔穎達, ed. 1965. *Chunqiu Zuozhuan zhengyi* 春秋左傳正義. In *Shisanjing zhushu* 十三經注疏, vol. 6. Ruan Yuan 阮元 (1764–1849), ed. Taipei: Yiwen.

Kovacs, Jürgen, and Paul U. Unschuld. 1998. *Essential Subtleties on the Silver Sea: The Yin-hai jing-wei: A Chinese Classic on Ophthalmology.* Berkeley: University of California Press.

Köster, Anne-Dorothee. 2009. Das Gesundheitssystem der VR China: Gesundheitspolitik zwischen fragmentiertem Auoritarismus, Kaderkapitalismus und Familiarismus. WIP-Diskussionspapier 1/09. Wissenschaftliches Institut der PKV. Köln.

Imura Kōzen 井村哮全. 1936. Chihōshi ni kisai seraretaru Chūgoku ekirei ryakkō 地方史に 記載せられたる中國疫癘略考. *Chūgai iji shimpō* 中外醫事新報 1232(June):263–325.

Kradin, Richard. 2008. *The Placebo Response and the Power of Unconscious Healing.* London: Routledge.

Kravchuk, A. 2008. Activity of the Chinese Religious Movement Falun Gong in Russia. *Anthropology and Archeology of Eurasia* 46(3):36–50.

Kua, E. H., P. H. Chew, and S. M. Ko. 1993. Spirit Possession and Healing among Chinese Psychiatric Patients. *Acta Psychiatrica Scandinavica* 88(6):447–450.

Kubo Noritada 窪徳忠. 1956. *Kōshin shinkō* 庚申信仰. Tokyo: Yamagawa.

———. 1961. *Kōshin shinkō no kenkyū* 庚申信仰の研究. Tokyo: Nihon gakujutsu shinkō kai.

Kuhn, Philip A. 1990. *Soulstealers: The Chinese Sorcery Scare of 1768.* Cambridge, MA: Harvard University Press.

Kuriyama, Shigehisa. 1999. *The Expressiveness of the Body and the Diverence of Greek and Chinese Medicine.* New York: Zone.

Lagerwey, John, and Marc Kalinowski, eds. 2008. *Early Chinese Religion: Part One: Shang through Han* (1250 B.C.–220 A.D.). Leiden: Brill.

Lai Guolong. 2005. Death and Otherworldly Journey in Early China as Seen through Tomb Texts, Travel Paraphernalia, and Road Rituals. *Asia Major* 144(1):1–44.

Lampton, David L. 1977. *The Politics of Medicine in China: The Policy Process 1949–1977.* Westview Special Studies on China and East Asia. Folkestone, UK: Dawson/Westview Press.

Lang, Graeme, Selina Ching Chan, and Lars Ragvald. 2005. Temples and the Religious Economy. *Interdisciplinary Journal of Research on Religion* 1(1):1–27.

Langevin, Helene M., Nicole A. Bouffard, David L. Churchill, and Gary J. Badger. 2007. Connective Tissue Fibroblast Response to Acupuncture: Dose-Dependent Effect of Bidirectional Needle Rotation. *Journal of Alternative and Complementary Medicine* 13(3):355–360.

Langwick, Stacey. 2011. *Bodies, Politics, and African Healing: The Matter of Maladies in Tanzania.* Bloomington: Indiana University Press.

———. Forthcoming. Making Tanzanian Traditional Medicine. In *The Matter of Maladies: The Ontological Politics of Postcolonial Healing in Tanzania.* Stacey. Langwick, ed. Bloomington: Indiana University Press.

Laozi zhongjing 老子中經. In Yunji qiqian 雲笈七籤. *Zhengtong Daozang* 1032.

Lavier, J. 1966. *Histoire, doctrine, et pratique de l'acupuncture chinoise.* Geneva: Tchou.

———. 1974. *Points of Chinese Acupuncture.* P. M. Chancellor, trans. Rustington, Sussex: Health Science Press.

———. 1977. *L'acupuncture chinois.* Taiwan: Laffont Medecines et Traitements Naturels Parution.

Le Blanc, Charles, and Susan Blader, eds. 1987. *Chinese Ideas about Nature and Society: Studies in Honour of Derk Bodde.* Hong Kong: University of Hong Kong Press.

Lee Jen-der 李貞德. 1996. Han-Tang zhijian yishu zhong de shengchan zhi dao 漢唐之間醫書中的生產之道. *Zhongyang yanjiuyuan lishi yuyan yanjiusuo jikan* 中央研究院歷史語言研究所集刊 67(3):533–654.

———. 1997. Han-Tang zhijian qiuzi yifang shitan 漢唐之間求子醫方試探. *Zhongyang yanjiuyuan lishi yuyan yanjiusuo jikan* 中央研究院歷史語言研究所集刊 68(2):283–367.

———. 2000. Wet Nurses in Early Imperial China. *Nan Nü: Men, Women and Gender in China* 2(1):1–39.

———. 2003. Gender and Medicine in Tang China. *Asia Major* (Third Series) 16(2):1–29.

———. 2005. Childbirth in Early Imperial China. *Nan Nü: Men, Women and Gender in China* 7(2):216–286.

———. 2008. *Nüren de zhongguo yiliao shi: Han-Tang zhijian de jiankang zhaogu yu xingbie* 女人的中國醫療史: 漢唐之間的健康照顧與性別. Taipei: Sanming shuju.

———. 2011. Ishinpo and Its Excerpts from Chanjing: A Japanese Medical Text as a Source for Chinese Women's History. In *Overt and Covert Treasures: Essays on the Sources for Chinese Women's History.* Clara Wing-ching Ho, ed. Hong Kong: Chinese University Press.

Lee, Jonathan H. X. 2009. Transnational Goddess on the Move: Meiguo Mazu's Celestial Inspection Tour and Pilgrimage as Chinese American Culture Work and Vernacular Chinese Religion. Ph.D. dissertation, University of California, Santa Barbara.

Lee, James Z., and Wang Feng. 1999. *One Quarter of Humanity: Malthusian Mythology and Chinese Realities, 1700–2000.* Cambridge, MA: Harvard University Press.

Lee, Miriam. 1992. *Insights of a Senior Acupuncturist*. Boulder, CO: Blue Poppy Press.

Lee, Sing. 1999. Diagnosis Postponed: Shenjing Shuairuo and the Transformation of Psychiatry in Post-Mao China. *Culture, Medicine and Psychiatry* 23(3):349–380.

———. 2011. Depression: Coming of Age in China. In *Deep China, The Moral Life of the Person, What Anthropology and Psychiatry Tell Us about China Today*. A. Kleinman, Y. Yan, J. Jun, and S. Lee, eds. Pp. 177–212. Berkeley: University of California Press.

Lee, Sing, and Arthur Kleinman. 2007. Are Somatoform Disorders Changing with Time? The Case of Neurasthenia in China. *Psychosomatic Medicine* 69(6):846–849.

Legge, James, and Ming Tso-ch'iu (Ming Zuoqiu). 1972. *The Ch'un ts'ew, with the Tso chuen*. *The Chinese Classics*, Vol. 5. Taipei: Wen shi zhe chubanshe.

Lei, Sean Hsiang-Lin. 1999. When Chinese Medicine Encountered the State: 1910–1949. Ph.D. dissertation, University of Chicago.

———. 2002. How Did Chinese Medicine Become Experiential? The Political Epistemology of Jingyan. *Positions: East Asia Cultures Critique* 10(2):333–364.

Lessa, William A. 1968. *Chinese Body Divination: Its Forms, Affinities, and Functions*. Los Angeles: United World.

Leung, Angela Ki Che (Liang Qizi 梁其姿). 1985. L'accueil des enfants abandonnés dans la Chine du Bas-Yangzi aux XVIIe et XVIIIe siècles. *Études Chinoises* 4(1):15–54.

———. 1987. Organized Medicine in Ming-Qing China: State and Private Medical Institutions in the Lower Yangzi Region. *Late Imperial China* 8(1):134–166.

———. 1995. Zhongguo jinshi yiliao yu shehui 中國近世醫療與社會. Research project report, Taipei, NSC 84-2411-H-001-009. Taipei: Academia Sinica.

———. 1996. Variolation and Vaccination in Late Imperial China. In *Vaccinia, Vaccination, Vaccinology – Jenner, Pasteur and their Successors*. S. A. Plotkin and B. Fantini, eds. Pp. 65–71. Paris: Elsevier.

———. 1997. *Shishan yu jiaohua: Ming-Qing de cishan zuzhi* 施善與教化: 明清的慈善組織. Taipei: Lianjing chuban shiye gongsi.

———. 1999. Women Practicing Medicine in Pre-modern China. In *Chinese Women in the Imperial Past: New Perspectives*. H. Zurndorfer, ed. Pp. 101–134. Leiden: Brill.

———. 2001. Song-Yuan-Ming de difang yiliao ziyuan chutan 宋元明的地方醫療資源初探. *Zhongguo shehui lishi pinglun* 中國社會歷史評論 3:219–237.

———. 2002. Fangtu yu jibing: Yuan zhi Qing yijia de kanfa 方土與疾病: 元至清醫家的看法. In *Xingbie yu yiliao* 性別與醫療. Huang Kewu 黃克武, ed. Taipei: Institute of Modern History, Academia Sinica.

———. 2003a. Mafeng geli yu jindai Zhongguo 麻風隔離與近代中國. *Lishi yanjiu* 歷史研究 5:3–14.

———. 2003b. Medical Instruction and Popularization in Ming-Qing China. *Late Imperial China* 24(1):130–152.

———. 2003c. Medical Learning from the Song to the Ming. In *The Song-Yuan-Ming Transition in Chinese History*. P. J. Smith and R. von Glahn, eds. Pp. 374–512. Harvard East Asian Monographs, Vol. 221. Cambridge, MA: Harvard University Asia Center.

———. 2005. Recent Trends in the Study of Medicine for Women in Imperial China. *Nan Nü: Men, Women and Gender in China* 7(2):110–126.

———. 2009. *Leprosy in China: A History*. New York: Columbia University Press.

———. Forthcoming. Ming-Qing shehui zhong de yixue fazhan 明清社會中的醫學發展. In *Zhongguo shixin lun* 中國史新論. Li Jianmin 李建民, ed. Taipei: Lianjing.

Lewis, I. M. 1971. *Ecstatic Religion: A Study of Shamanism and Spirit Possession*, 2nd edition. London: Routledge.

Lewis, Mark E. 1990. *Sanctioned Violence in Early China*. Albany: SUNY Press.

———. 1999. *Writing and Authority in Early China*. Albany: SUNY Press.

———. 2006a. *The Construction of Space in Early China*. Albany: SUNY Press.

———. 2006b. *The Flood Myths of Early China*. Albany: SUNY Press.

Li Bozhong 李伯重. 1994. Kongzhi zengzhang, yi bao fuyu—Qingdai qianzhongqi Jiangnan de renkou xingwei 控制增長, 以保富裕—清代前中期江南的人口行為. *Xin shixue* 新史學 5(3):25–70.

Li Feng. 2006. *Landscape and Power in Early China: The Crisis and Fall of the Western Zhou 1045-771 B.C.* Cambridge: University of Cambridge.

Li Fengmao 李豐楙. 1993. *Daozang* suoshou zaoqi daoshu de wenyiguan: yi *Nüqing guilü* and *Dongyuan shenzhou jing* weizhu 《道藏》所收早期道書的瘟疫觀—以《女青鬼律》及《洞淵神咒經》為主. *Zhongyang yanjiuyuan Zhongguo wenzhe yanjiu jikan* 中央研究院中國文哲研究集刊 3(March):417–454.

———. 1995. Xingwen yu songwen: daojiao yu minzhong wenyi guan de jiaoliu he fenqi 行瘟與送瘟—道教與民眾瘟疫觀的交流和分歧. *In* Minjian xinyang yu Zhongguo wenhua guoji yantaohui lunwenji 民間信仰與中國文化國際研討會論文集. Hanxue yanjiu zhongxin 漢學研究中心, ed. Pp. 373–422. Taipei: Hanxue yanjiu zhongxin.

Li Hongzhi. 2000. Zhuan Falun (English Version). Internet Version, Third Translation. http://www.falundafa.org/book/eng/zflus.html (accessed 4/12/10).

Li Hui-Lin. 1979. *Nan-fang ts'ao-mu chuang: A Fourth Century Flora of Southeast Asia, Introduction, Translation, Commentaries*. Hong Kong: Chinese University Press.

Li Haowen 李好文. 1970. *Chang'an zhitu* 長安志圖: Zhongguo fangzhi conshu.

Li Jianmin. 2008. *They Shall Expel Demons*: Etiology, the Medical Canon and the Transformation of Medical Techniques before the Tang. In *Early Chinese Religion: Part One: Shang through Han (1250 B.C.–220 A.D.)*. J. Lagerwey and M. Kalinowski, eds. Pp. 1103–1150. Leiden: Brill.

——— 李建民. 2011. *Hua Tuo yincang de shoushu: Waike de zhongguo yixue shi* 華佗隱藏的手術: 外科的中國醫學史. Taipei: Dongda tushu gongsi.

Li Jiren 李濟仁. 1990. *Xin'an mingyi kao* 新安名醫考. Hefei: Anhui kexue jishu chubanshe.

Li Jingwei 李經緯. 1988. *Zhongyi renwu cidian* 中醫人物詞典. Shanghai: Cishu chubanshe.

Li Jingwei 李經緯, and Lin Zhaogeng 林昭庚, eds. 2000. *Zhongguo yixue tong shi: gudai juan* 中國醫學通史 : 古代卷. Beijing: Renmin weisheng chubanshe.

Li Jun 力鈞. 1998. *Chongling bing'an* 崇陵病案. Beijing: Xueyuan chubanshe.

Li Junde 李俊德. 1996. *Ming laozhongyi tan yangsheng zhi dao* 名老中醫談養生之道. Huaxia chubanshe.

Li Li. 2003. Irresistable Scientization: Rhetoric of Science in Institutional Chinese Medicine. M.Phil. University of North Carolina.

Li Ling 李零. 1993. *Zhongguo fangshu kao* 中國方術考. Beijing: Renmin Zhongguo chubanshe.

———. 2001. *Zhongguo fangshu kao* 中國方術考. Beijing: Dongfang chubanshe.

———. 2006. *Zhongguo fangshu xu kao* 中國方術續考. Beijing: Zhonghua shuju.

Li Shizhen 李時珍. 1986. *Bencao gangmu* 本草綱目. Taipei: Taiwan shangwu yinshuguan.

Li Shunbao 李順保, ed. 2002. Wenbingxue quanshu 溫病學全書. Beijing: Xueyuan chubanshe.

Li Ting 李梴. 1999. *Yixue rumen* 醫學入門. Tianjin: Tianjin kexue chubanshe.

Li Xueqin 李學勤. 2001. *Jianbo yiji yu xueshu shi* 簡帛佚籍與學術史. Nanchang: Jiangxi jiaoyu chubanshe.

———, et al. 2003. The Earliest Writing? Sign Use in the Seventh Millennium B.C. in Jiahu, Henan, China (Research). *Antiquity* 77(295):31–41.

Li Yang. 1998. *Book of Changes and Traditional Chinese Medicine*. Beijing: Beijing Science and Technology Press.

Li Yang 李楊 and Liang Jing 梁晶. 2007. Zhongyi xianzhuang diaocha 中醫現狀調查. *Zhongguo xinwen zhoukan* 中國新聞周刊 No. 3. Re-posted at NetEase. http://news.163.com /07/0121/00/35AOPV7P00011SM9.html (accessed 6/6/2012).

Li Zhichong. 李致重 2004. *Zhongyi fuxing Lun* 中醫復興論. Beijing: Zhongguo yiyao keji chubanshe.

Liang Jun 梁峻. 1995. *Zhongguo gudai yizheng shilüe* 中國古代醫政史略. Hohhot: Nei Menggu renmin chubanshe.

Lienwand, Donna. 2007. States Seek to Get Grip on Wild Ginseng Market. *USA Today* (December 2). http://www.usatoday.com/news/nation/2007-12-02-Ginseng_N.htm (accessed 8/19/08).

Lin Fu-shih 林富士. 1987. Shilun Handai de wushu yiliao fa jiqi guannian jichu 試論漢代的巫術醫療法及其觀念基礎. *Shiyuan* 史原 16:29–53.

———. 1994. *Chinese Shamans and Shamanism in the Chiang-nan Area During the Six Dynasties Period (3rd–6th Century A.D.)*. Ph.D. dissertation, Princeton University.

———. 1999a. *Handai de wu zhe* 漢代的巫者. Taipei: Daoxiang, Qishiqi nian.

———. 1999b. Zhongguo Liuchao Shiqi De Wuxi Yu Yiliao 中國六朝時期的巫覡與醫療. *Zhongyang yanjiuyuan lishi yuyan yanjiusuo jikan* 中央研究院歷史語言研究所集刊 70(1):1–48.

———. 2002. Zhongguo zaoqi daoshi de yiliao huodong jiqi yishu kaoshi: yi Han Wei Jin Nan Bei Chao shiqi de zhuanji ziliao wei zhu de chubu tantao 中國早期道士的醫療活動及其醫術考釋：以漢魏晉南北朝時期的傳記資料為主的初步探討. *Zhongyang yanjiuyuan lishi yuyan yanjiusuo jikan* 中央研究院歷史語言研究所集刊 73:43–118.

———. 2008. The Image and Status of Shamans in Ancient China. In *Early Chinese Religion: Part One: Shang through Han (1250 B.C.–220 A.D.)*. J. Lagerwey and M. Kalinowski, eds. Pp. 397–458. Leiden: Brill.

Linde K., C. M. Witt, A. Streng, W. Weidenhammer, S. Wagenpfeil, B. Brinkhaus, S. N. Willich, D. Melchart. 2007. The Impact of Patient Expectations on Outcomes in Four Randomized Controlled Trials of Acupuncture in Patients with Chronic Pain. *Pain* 128:264–271.

Liu An 劉安 (d. 122 B.C.E.). 1936?. *Huainanzi* 淮南子. *Sibu beiyao* 四部備要, *(Zibu Zajia)*. Shanghai: Zhonghua shuju.

Liu Bingfan 劉炳凡 and Zhou Shaoming 周紹明, eds. 1999. *Huxiang mingyi dianji jinghua* 湖湘名醫典籍精華. Changsha: Hunan kexue jishu chubanshe.

Liu Boji 劉伯驥. 1974. *Zhongguo yixueshi* 中國醫學史. Taipei: Huagang chubanbu.

Liu Baonan 劉寶楠, ed. 1991. *Zhuzi jicheng* 諸子集成. Shanghai: Shanghai Shudian.

Liu Guohui. 2001. *Warm Diseases: A Clinical Guide.* Seattle: Eastland Press.

Liu Li. 2004. *The Chinese Neolithic: Trajectories to Early States.* Cambridge: Cambridge University Press.

Liu Lihong 劉力紅. 2006. *Sikao zhongyi* 思考中醫, 3rd ed. Guilin: Guanxi shifan daxue chubanshi.

Liu Zhenmin 劉振民 and Cui Wenzhi 崔文志 eds. 1998. *Shijian yu tansuo: Zhongguo gaodeng zhonyiyao jiaoyu sishi nian* 實踐與探索 ：中國高等中醫藥教育四十年. Beijing Zhongguo zhongyiyao chubanshe.

Liu Zhongyu 劉仲宇, Gao Yuqiu 高毓秋, and Shen Hong 沈紅, eds. 2000. *Zhongguo gudai yangsheng geyan* 中國古代養生格言. Shanghai: Shanghai renmin chubanshe.

Lloyd, Geoffrey, and Nathan Sivin. 2002. *The Way and the Word: Science and Medicine in Early China and Greece.* New Haven: Yale University Press.

Lo, Vivienne. 2000. Crossing the Neiguan "Inner Pass." *East Asian Science, Technology, and Medicine* 17:15–65.

——. 2001a. *Huangdi Hama Jing (Yellow Emperor's Toad Canon).* Asia Major 14(2):61–100.

——. 2001b. The Influence of Nurturing Life Culture on the Development of Western Han Acumoxa Therapy. In *Innovation in Chinese Medicine.* E. Hsu, ed. Pp. 19–50. Cambridge: Cambridge University Press.

——. 2002a. Lithic Therapy in Early Chinese Body Practices. In *Practitioners, Practices and Patients: New Approaches to Medical Archaeology and Anthropology.* P. A. Baker and G. Carr, eds. Pp. 195–220. Oxford: Oxbow Books.

——. 2002b. Spirit of Stone: Technical Considerations in the Treatment of the Jade Body. *Bulletin of the School of Oriental and African Studies* 65:99–128.

——. 2005. Pleasure, Prohibition and Pain: Food and Medicine in China. In *Of Tripod and Palate: Food, Politics, and Religion in Traditional China.* R. Sterckx, ed. Pp. 163–186. London: Palgrave MacMillan.

——. 2007. Imagining Practice: Sense and Sensuality in Early Chinese Medical Illustration. In *Graphics and Text in the Production of Technical Knowledge in China: The Warp and the Weft.* F. Bray, V. Dorofeeva-Lictmann, and G. Métailié, eds. Pp. 383–423. Leiden: Brill.

Lo, Vivienne, and Penelope Barrett. 2005. Cooking up Fine Remedies: On the Culinary Aesthetic in a Sixteenth-Century Chinese Material Medica. *Medical History* 49(4):395–422.

Lo, Vivienne, and Christopher Cullen, eds. 2005. *Medieval Chinese Medicine: The Dunhuang Medical Manuscripts.* London: RoutledgeCurzon.

Lo, Vivienne, and Zhiguo He 何志國. 1996. The Channels: A Preliminary Examination of a Lacquered Figurine from the Western Han Period. *Early China* 21:81–123.

Loewe, Michael. 2004. *The Men who Governed China in Han Times.* Leiden: Brill.

———. 1997. The Physician Chunyu Yi and His Historical Background. In *En suivant La voie royale: mélanges en hommage à Léon Vandermeersch*. Jacques Gernet, et al, eds. Pp. 297–313. Paris: École francaise d'Extrême-Orient.

Loewe, Michael, and Edward L. Shaughnessy, eds. 1999. *The Cambridge History of Ancient China: From the Origins of Civilization to 221 B.C.* Cambridge: Cambridge University.

Lohiya, P. B. 2009. Training Courses—Indian Academy of Acupuncture Science. http://www.acupunctureindia.org/train.html (accessed 7/28/09).

Lopez, Donald S., ed. 2002. *Religions of Asia in Practice: An Anthology.* Princeton, NJ: Princeton University Press.

Lora-Wainwright, Anna. 2006. Perceptions of Health, Illness and Healing in a Sichuan Village, China. Ph.D dissertation. Oxford University.

Lowe, Scott. 2003. Chinese and International Contexts for the Rise of Falun Gong. *Nova Religio* 6(2):263–376.

Lu Bosi 魯伯嗣. 1987. *Yingtong bai wen* 嬰童百問. Taipei: Xinwenfeng.

Lu Liancheng 盧連成, Hu Zhisheng 胡智生, and Baoji City Museum, eds. 1988. *Baoji Guo Mudi* 寶雞弓魚國墓地. Beijing: Wenwu.

Lu Shizhong 路時中 (*fl.* 1107–1158). 1926. *Wushang xuanyuan santian yutang dafa* 無上玄元三天玉堂大法 (1126). *Zhengtong Daozang*正統道藏 220, fasc. 100–104. Shanghai: Shangwu yinshuguan.

Lu Yanyao 陸炎垚 et al., eds. 1999. *Lu Shouyan xueshu jingyan ji* 陸瘦燕學術經驗集. Shanghai: Shanghai zhongyiyao daxue chubanshe.

Lu Yuanlei 陸淵雷. 1931. *Lu shi lun yi ji* 陸氏論醫集. Taipei: Ruisheng chubanshe.

———. 1934. *Shengli buzheng* 生理補証. Manuscript published by the author.

Lu Zonghan 盧崇漢. 2006. *Fuyang jiangji* 扶陽講記. Beijing. Zhongguo zhongyiyao chubanshe.

Luo Jing. 2006. Over Seventy Percent of City Dwellers Are in Subhealth (Qichengduo shimin yajiankang). http://ala.online.sh.cn.

Lupher, Mark. 1995. Revolutionary Little Red Devils: The Social Psychology of Rebel Youth, 1966–1967. In *Chinese Views of Childhood*. A. B. Kinney, ed. Pp. 321–344. Honolulu: University of Hawaii Press.

Lü Buwei 呂不韋. 1936?. *Lüshi chunqiu* 呂氏春秋. *Sibu beiyao* 四部備要, (*Zibu Zhou-Qin zhuzi*). Shanghai: Zhonghua shuju.

Ma Boying 馬伯英. 1993. *Zhongguo yixue wenhua shi* 中國醫學文化史. Shanghai: Shanghai People's Publishing House.

Ma Boying 馬伯英, Gao Xi 高晞, and Hong Zhongdi 洪中立. 1993. *Zhongwai yixue wenhua jiaoliu shi: Zhongwai yixue kua wenhua chuantong* 中外醫學文化交流史—中外醫學跨文化傳通. Shanghai: Wenhui chubanshe.

Ma Dazheng 馬大正. 1991. *Zhongguo fuchanke fazhan shi* 中國婦產科發展史. Xi'an: Shaanxi kexue jiaoyu chubanshe.

Ma Jixing 馬繼興. 1957. *Songdai de renti jiepou tu* 宋代的人體解剖圖. Yixueshi yu baojian zuzhi 醫學史與保健組織 1(2):125–128.

———. 1990. *Zhongyi wenxian xue* 中醫文獻學. Shanghai: Shanghai Kexue Jishu Chubanshe.

———. 1992. *Mawangdui guyishu kaoshi* 馬王堆古醫書考釋. Changsha: Hunan Kexue Jishu.

Ma, Laurence J. C. 1971. *Commercial Development and Urban Change in Sung China (960–1279)*. Ann Arbor: Department of Geography, University of Michigan.

MacFarquhar, Roderick. 1983. *The Origins of the Cultural Revolution, Vol. 2: The Great Leap Forward 1958–1960*. London: Royal Institute of International Affairs.

MacPherson, Kerrie L. 1998. Cholera in China, 1820–1930: An Aspect of the Internationalization of Infectious Disease. In *Sediments of Time: Environment and Society in Chinese History*. M. Elvin and T.U.-J. Liu, eds. Pp. 487–519. Cambridge: Cambridge University Press.

Main, Roderick. 1999. Magic and Science in the Modern Western Tradition of the I Ching. *Journal of Contemporary Religion* 14(2):263–275.

Mair, Victor. 1990. Old Sinitic *MyAG, Old Persion MAGUŜ, and English 'Magician.' *Early China* 15:27–47.

Maisel, Edward. 1963. *Tai Chi for Health*. New York: Holt Rinehart and Winston.

Major, John S. 1987. The Meaning of Hsing-te. In *Chinese Ideas about Nature and Society: Studies in Honour of Derk Bodde*. C. Le Blanc and S. Blader, eds. Pp. 281–291. Hong Kong: Hong Kong University Press.

———. Characteristics of Late Chu Religion. 1999. In *Defining Chu: Image and Reality in Ancient China*. Constance A. Cook and John S. Major, eds. Pp. 121–143. Honolulu: University of Hawaii Press.

Mak Hin Chung, Kwok Man Ho, and Angela Smith. 1986. *T'ung Shu, the Ancient Chinese Almanac*. M. Palmer, ed. Boston: Shambhala.

Manaka, Yoshio. 1980. *Layman's Guide to Acupuncture*. New York: n.p.

———. 1995. *Chasing the Dragon's Tail: The Theory and Practice of Acupuncture in the Work of Yoshio Manaka*. Cambridge, MA: Paradigm Publishers.

Mandell, Richard. 2002. The Pan African Acupuncture Project. *Acupuncture Today* 3(4). http://www.acupuncturetoday.com/mpacms/at/article.php?id=27955&no_paginate=true&no_b=true (accessed 8/4/09).

Manicom, Philippe. 2007. To Whom It May Concern. Undated personal correspondence.

Mann, Felix. 1962. *Meridians of Acupuncture*. London: William Heinemann Medical Books.

———. 1973a. *Acupuncture: The Ancient Chinese Art of Healing and How It Works Scientifically*. New York: Vintage Books.

———. 1973b. *Atlas of Acupuncture*. London: William Heinemann Medical Books.

———. 1985. *Acupuncture: Cure of Many Diseases*. London: Pan Books.

———. 1992. *Reinventing Acupuncture: A New Concept of Ancient Medicine*. London: Butterworth-Heinemann Medical.

Markson, Barry. 2006. Acupuncturists without Borders: Report from the Streets of New Orleans. *Acupuncture Today* 7(1). http://www.acupuncturetoday.com/mpacms/at/article.php?id=30294&no_paginate=true&no_b=true (accessed 8/4/09).

Marr, David. 1987. Vietnamese Attitudes Regarding Illness and Healing. In *Death and Disease in Southeast Asia: Explorations in Social, Medical and Demographic History*. N. G. Owen, ed. Pp. 162–186. Singapore: Oxford University Press.

Matheson, Richard. 2007. Bua Buei: Your Future in a Pair of Blocks. *Xpat Magazine* Fall:44–45, 47.

Mawangdui hanmu boshu 馬王堆漢墓帛書. 1984. Mawangdui Hanmu Boshu Zhengli Xiaozu 馬王堆漢墓帛書整理小組, ed. Beijing: Wenwu.

McCarthy, Patrician. 2008. *The Face Reader: Discover Anyone's Personality through the Chinese Art of Mien Shiang.* New York: Plume.

McCreery, John L. 1990. Why Don't We See Some Real Money Here? Offerings in Chinese Religion. *Journal of Chinese Religions* 18:1–24.

McCurley, Dallas. 2005. Performing Patterns: Numinous Relations in Shang and Zhou China. *The Drama Review* 49(3):135–156.

McDermott, Joseph P., ed. 1999. *State and Court Ritual in China.* Cambridge: Cambridge University Press.

McDonald, J. 1987. Chinese versus French Perspectives on the Channel System. *Australian Journal of Acupuncture* 3(2):22–38.

McFadden, Robert D. 1981a. Police Raid Apartments to Gather Evidence on Killings in Rockland. *New York Times* (October 23).

———. 1981b. Brink's Holdup Spurs U.S. Inquiry on Links among Terrorist Groups. *New York Times* (October 25).

McGovern, Patrick E., et al. 2004. Fermented Beverages of Pre- and Proto-Historic China. *Proceedings of the National Academy of Sciences of the United States of America* 101(51):17593–17598.

McGuire, Meredith B. 2002. *Religion: The Social Context.* Belmont, CA: Wadsworth.

Mendis, Githanjan. 2005. Prof. Anton Jayasuriya. http://www.openinternationaluniversity. org/more.jsp?massage=head (accessed 1/2/10).

Meng Qingyun 孟慶雲, ed. 1999. *Zhongguo zhongyiyao fazhan wushi nian* 中國中醫藥發展五十年. Zhengzhou: Henan yike daxue chubanshe.

Meng Shujiang 孟澍江, ed. 1989. *Wenbing xue* 溫病學. Beijing: Renmin weisheng chubanshe.

Mengzi (Mencius) and James Legge. 1972. *The Works of Mencius. The Chinese Classics,* Vol. 2. Taipei: Wen Shi Zhe.

Mianyang Shuangbao Shan hanmu 綿陽雙包山漢墓. 2006. Sichuan sheng wenwu kaogu yanjiusuo 四川省文物考古研究所, Mianyang bowuguan 綿陽博物館, eds. Beijing: Wenwu Chubanshe.

Miki Sakae 三木榮. 1962. *Chōsen igakushi oyobi shippeishi* 朝鮮醫學史及疾病史. Osaka: Shibun chuppansha.

Miyakawa Hisayuki 宮川尚志. 1955. An Outline of the Naito Hypothesis and Its Effects on Japanese Studies of China. *Far Eastern Quarterly* 14(4):533–553.

———. 1960. The Confucianization of South China. In *The Confucian Persuasion.* A. F. Wright, ed. Stanford, CA: Stanford University Press.

Miyashita Saburō 宮下三郎. 1967. Sō-Gen no iryō 宋元の医療. In *Sō-Gen jidai no kagaku gijutsu shi* 宋元時代の科学技術史. Yabuuchi Kiyoshi 薮内清, ed. Pp. 123–170. Kyoto: Kyoto daigaku kenkyujo.

———. 1979. Malaria (yao) in Chinese Medicine during the Chin and Yüan Periods. *Acta Asiatica* 36(September):90–112.

Moffett, Howard, Pat Sanders, Thomas Sinclair, and Kevin Ergil. 1994. Using Acupuncture and Herbs for the Treatment of HIV Infection. *Aids Patient Care* 8(4):194–199.

Moran, Elizabeth, and Master Joseph Yu. 2001. *The Complete Idiot's Guide to I Ching*. Exton, PA: Alpha.

Morgan, Carole. 1998. Old Wine in a New Bottle: A New Set of Oracle Slips from China. *Journal of Chinese Religions* 26(1–19).

Morris, Will, ed. 2009a. AAAOM Forums: CAN Community and FPD (January 11). http://forums.aaaomonline.org/viewtopic.php?f=25&t=130 (accessed 2/6/09).

———. 2009b. Integrative Medicine and Public Health. Acupuncture Today 10(6). http://www.acupuncturetoday.com/mpacms/at/article.php?id=31957&no_paginate=true&no_b=true (accessed 3/14/08).

Moskin, Julia. 2008. Let the Meals Begin: Finding Beijing in Flushing. *New York* (July 30). http://www.nytimes.com/2008/07/30/dining/30flushing.html?th=&emc=th&pagewanted=all (accessed 7/30/08).

Mote, Frederick W. 1977. Yuan and Ming. In *Food in Chinese Culture: Anthropological and Historical Perspectives*. K. C. Chang, ed. Pp. 193–258. New Haven: Yale University Press.

Murray, Barbara June. 2002. Feng Shui: Implications of Selected Principles for Holistic Nursing Care of the Open Heart Patient. Master's thesis, University of South Africa.

MutuluShakur.com. 2009. http://www.mutulushakur.com/about.html (accessed 9/12/09).

Nakagawa Tadateru 中川忠英. 1799. *Shinzoku kibun* 清俗紀聞. 13 vols. Tōto [Tokyo]: Nishinomiya Tasuke.

Nakamura Jihēi 中村治兵衛. 1992. *Chūgoku shamanismu no kenkyū* 中國シャーマニズムの研究. Tokyo: Tōsui shobō.

Nan Qishu 南齊書. Xiao Zixian 蕭子顯, ed. 1992. Beijing: Zhonghua shuju.

Nanjing Zhongyi xueyuan 南京中醫學院. 1958. *Zhongyixue ga lun* 中醫學概論. Beijing: Renmin weisheng chubanshe.

Napadow, Vitaly, Rupali P. Dhond, Jieun Kim, Lauren LaCount, Mark Vangel, Richard E Harris, Norman Kettner, and Kyungmo Park. 2009. Brain Encoding of Acupuncture Sensation—Coupling On-Line Rating with fMRI. *NeuroImage* 47:1055–1065.

Napolitano, Valentina, and Gerardo Mora Flores. 2003. Complementary Medicine: Cosmopolitan and Popular Knowledge, and Transcultural Translations—Cases from Urban Mexico. *Theory, Culture and Society* 20(4):79–95.

Nappi, Carla. 2009. *The Monkey and the Inkpot: Natural History and Its Transformations in Early Modern China*. Cambridge, MA: Harvard University Press.

Naquin, Susan. 1976. *Millenarian Rebellion in China: The Eight Trigrams Uprising of 1813*. New Haven: Yale University Press.

Narayanan, Vasudha. 2006. Shanti: Peace for the Mind, Body, and Soul. In *Teaching Religion and Healing*. Linda L. Barnes and Ines Talamantez, eds. Pp. 61–82. New York: Oxford University Press.

Nathan, Carl, F. 1967. *Plague Prevention and Politics in Manchuria, 1910–1931*. Cambridge, East Asian Research Center, Harvard University; distributed by Harvard University Press.

———. 1974. The Acceptance of Western Medicine in Early Twentieth-century China: The Story of the North Manchurian Plague Prevention Service. In *Medicine and Society in China.* John Z. Bowers and Elizabeth F. Purcell, eds. Pp. 55–81. New York: Josiah Macy, Jr. Foundation.

NADA (National Acupuncture Detoxification Association). 2008. *Acupuncture Detoxification Specialist Training Manual: A Handbook for Individuals Training in the National Acupuncture Detoxification Association's Five-Needle Acudetox Protocol.* Vancouver, WA: National Acupuncture Detoxification Association.

National Institutes of Health. 1997. Acupuncture. NIH Consensus Statement Online Nov. 3–5. 15(5):1–34. <http://consensus.nih.gov/1997/1997acupuncture107html.htm> (accessed June 7, 2012).

Needham, Joseph. 1956. *Science and Civilization in China,* Vol. 2, *History of Scientific Thought.* With the assistance of Wang Ling. Cambridge: Cambridge University Press.

———. 2000. *Science and Civilization in China.* Volume 6, *Biology and Biological Technology,* Part VI, *Medicine.* Cambridge: Cambridge University Press.

Newton, Douglas. 2009. Doctors under Fire: Practicing When Your Life Is at Risk (Interview with Dr. Lazgeen M. Ahmad). *American Acupuncturist* 47(March 31):21.

Nghi, Nguyên Van, with Emmanuel Picou. 1971. *Pathogénie et pathologie énergétiques en médecine chinoise: Traitement par acupuncture et massages.* Marseille: Impr. École technique Don Bosco.

Nghi, Nguyên Van, and Mark Seem. 1983. *Acupuncture Energetics: A Workbook for Diagnostics and Treatment.* Tamarac, FL: Raiko.

Ngo, Van Xuyet. 1976. *Divination, magie et politique dans la Chine ancienne.* Paris: Presses universitaires de France.

Nguyen, Johan. 2010. Nguyen Van Nghi (1909–1999): Retour sur l'acupuncture au XXe siècle. *Acupuncture and Moxibustion* 9(1):9–15.

Nguyen, Kiet Chi. 1986. Traditional Drugs of Vietnam in the Works of Tue Tinh. *Vietnamese Studies,* New Series 12:47–104.

Ni Hua-Ching. 1999. *I Ching: The Book of Changes and the Unchanging Truth.* Los Angeles: Sevenstar Communications.

Ni, Maoshing, and Cathy McNease. 2009. *The Tao of Nutrition.* Los Angeles: Sevenstar Communications.

Niemtzow, Richard C., Stephen M. Burns, Jared Cooper, Salvatore Libretto, Joan A. G. Walter, and John Baxter. Acupuncture Clinical Pain Trial in a Military Medical Center: Outcomes. *Medical Acupuncture* 20(4):255–261.

———. 2007. Battlefield Acupuncture. *Medical Acupuncture* 19(4):225–228.

Nogier, Paul F. M. 1956. Le pavillon de l'oreille. Zones et points réflexes. *Bulletin de la Société d'Acupuncture* (20/mai): n.p.

———. 1957. Über die Akupunktur der Ohrmuschel. *Deutsche Zeitschrift für Akupunktur* 6:25–35, 58–63 and 87–93

———. 1969. *Handbook to Auriculotherapy.* Sainte-Ruffine: Maisonneuve.

———. 1983. *From Auriculotherapy to Auricular Medicine.* Sainte-Ruffine: Maisonneuve.

Nogier, Paul F. M., and R. Nogier. 1985. *The Man in the Ear.* Sainte-Ruffine: Maisonneuve.

Nügong lianji huandan tushuo 女功煉己還丹圖說. 1906. In *Nüdan hebian* 女丹合編. He Longxiang 賀龍驤, ed. Chengdu: Erxianan.

Obituary: Benjamin Hobson. 1873. *British Medical Journal* 1:355–356.

Obituary: J. D. Van Buren. 2003. http://www.bestacupuncture.co.uk/van%20Buren%20 obituary.pdf (accessed 9/12/09).

Obringer, Frédéric. 1997. *L'aconit et l'orpiment: drogues et poisons en Chine ancienne et médiévale*. Paris: Fayard.

———. 2001. A Song Innovation in Pharmacology. In *Innovation in Chinese Medicine*. E. Hsu, ed. Pp. 192–213. Needham Research Institute Studies, Vol. 3. Cambridge: Cambridge University Press.

———. 2005. Fengshui, or the Search for a Very Human Dragon. *Diogenes* 207:55–63.

Okanishi Tameto 岡西為人. 1969. *Sō izen iki kō* 宋以前醫籍考. Taipei: Guting shuwu.

Ong, Aihwa. 1995. Anthropology, China and Modernities. In *The Future of Anthropological Knowledge*. H. L. Moore, ed. Pp. 60–92. London: Routledge.

———. 2006. *Neoliberalism as Exception: Mutations in Citizenship and Sovereignty*. Durham: Duke University Press.

Ong, C. K., et al., eds. 2005. *WHO Global Atlas of Traditional, Complementary and Alternative Medicine*. Geneva: WHO.

Organization Structure of the Program. 1975–1976. Mimeographed flyer.

Ordre des Acupuncteurs du Québec. 2009. L'acupuncture, des origines à la première decade de l'ordre des acupuncteurs du Québec: Les grandes lignes. http://www.ordre desacupuncteurs.qc.ca/public/main.php?s=1&l=fr (accessed 7/8/08).

Ōshima Ritsuko 大島立子. 1980. Gendai kokei to yōeki 元代戸計と徭役. *Rekishigaku kenkyū* 歴史学研究 484:23–32, 60.

Ots, Thomas. 1994. The Silenced Body: The Expressive *Leib*: On the Dialectic of Mind and Life in Chinese Cathartic Healing. In *Embodiment and Experience: The Existential Ground of Culture and Self*. T. J. Csordas, ed. Pp. 116–139. Cambridge: Cambridge University Press.

Oving, N. Herman. 2007. Terminology in Chinese Medicine: A Critique of the WHO Term List. http://www.paradigm-pubs.com/node/346 (accessed 4/19/10).

Ownby, David. 2008a. In Search of Charisma: The Falun Gong Diaspora. *Nova Religio* 12(2):106–120.

———. 2008b. *Falun Gong and the Future of China*. New York: Oxford University Press.

———. 2008c. In Search of Charisma: The Falun Gong Diaspora. *Nova Religio* 12(2):106–120.

Palmer, David A. 2007. *Qigong Fever: Body, Science, and Utopia in China*. New York: Columbia University Press.

Pankenier, David. 1999. Applied Field-Allocation Astrology in Zhou China: Duke Wen of Jin and the Battle of Chengpu (632 B.C.). *Journal of the American Oriental Society* 119(2):261–279.

———. 2004. A Brief History of Beiji 北極 (Northern Culmen), with an Excursus on the Origin of the Character di 帝. *Journal of the American Oriental Society* 124(2):211–236.

Parker, Laura. 1984. Chinese Herb Medicine Isn't History Yet. *Seattle Post-Intelligencer* (March 13).

Paton, Michael John. 2007. Fengshui: A Continuation of Art of Swindlers? *Journal of Chinese Philosophy* 427–445.

Pearson, Richard. 1981. Social Complexity in Chinese Coastal Neolithic Sites. *Science* 213(4512):1078–1086.

Peng Shengquan 彭勝權, ed. 2000. *Wenbing xue* 溫病學. Beijing: Renmin weisheng chubanshe.

Pershouse, Didi. 2000. An Acupuncturist's Visit to Cuba. *American Acupuncturist* 23(20):20–21.

Peterson, Willard J. 2002. Introduction: New Order for the Old Order. In *The Cambridge History of China*. W. J. Peterson, ed. Pp. 1–8, Vol. 9, *Part One: The Ch'ing Dynasty to 1800*. Cambridge: Cambridge University Press.

Phillips, Michael R., et al. 2009. Prevalence, Treatment, and Associated Disability of Mental Disorders in Four Provinces in China during 2001–05: An Epidemiological Survey. *Lancet* 373(9680):2041–2053.

Pi Guoli 皮國立. 2008. *Jindai zhongyi de shenti guan yu sixiang zhuan xing: Tang Zonghai yu zhong xi yi huitong shidai* 近代中醫的身體觀與思想轉型: 唐宗海與中西醫匯通時代. Beijing: Sanlian shudian.

Poo, Mu-chou. 2008. Ritual and Ritual Texts in Early China. In *Early Chinese Religion: Part One: Shang through Han (1250 B.C.–220 A.D.)*. J. Lagerwey and M. Kalinowski, eds. Pp. 281–313. Leiden: Brill.

Porter, Dorothy. 1994. *The History of Public Health and the Modern State*. Amsterdam: Rodopi.

Porter, Kristen, and Beth Sommers. 2004. Acupuncture: Part of the Public Health Equation. *Acupuncture Today* 5(3). http://www.acupuncturetoday.com/mpacms/at/article.php?id=28413 (accessed 8/4/09).

———. 2005. PanAfrican Acupuncture Project Continues to Train Ugandan Health Workers. *Acupuncture Today* 6(1). http://www.acupuncturetoday.com/mpacms/at/article.php?id=30011&no_paginate=true&no_b=true (accessed 8/4/09).

———. 2008. Refugees: Feeling at Home with Acupuncture. *Acupuncture Today* 9(5). http://www.acupuncturetoday.com/mpacms/at/article.php?id=31718&no_paginate=true&no_b=true (accessed 8/4/09).

Pregadio, Fabrizio. 2006. *Great Clarity: Daoism and Alchemy in Early Medieval China*. Stanford, CA: Stanford University Press.

Producing New Disciples Old-Fashioned Way. 2008. http://www.china.org.cn/health/2008-07/23/content_16053027_3.htm (accessed 2/12/10).

Puett, Michael J. 2002. *To Become a God: Cosmology, Sacrifice, and Self-Divinization in Early China*. Cambridge, MA: Harvard University Asia Center for the Harvard-Yenching Institute.

Qian Jinyang 錢今陽, ed. 1950. *Shanghai mingyi zhi* 上海名醫誌. Shanghai: Zhongguo yixue chubanshe.

Qian Xiuchang 錢秀昌. 1955. *Shangke buyao* 傷科補要. Shanghai: Qianqingtang shuju.

Qin Bowei 秦伯未. 1929. Jiaowu baogao 教務報告. *Zhongguo yixueyuan kan* 中國醫學院刊 1(1), Appendix 6–7.

Qing Xitai 卿希泰. 1994. *Zhongguo daojiao* 中國道教. Shanghai: Zhishi chubanshe.

Qiu Peiran 裘沛然 and Ding Guangdi 丁光迪, eds. 1992. *Zhongyi ge jia xueshuo* 中醫各家學說. Beijing: Beijing renmin weisheng chubanshe.

Qiu Zhonglin 邱仲麟. 2004. Mingdai shiyi yu Fuzhou xian yixue 明代世醫與府州縣醫學. *Hanxue yanjiu* 漢學研究 22(2):327–359.

Qu Limei 曲黎敏. 2008. *Huangdi neijing yangsheng zhihui* 黃帝內經·養生智慧. Xiamen: Lujiang chubanshe.

Raphals, Lisa. 1998a. *Sharing the Light: Representations of Women and Virtue in Early China.* Albany: SUNY Press.

———. 1998b. The Treatment of Women in a Second-century Medical Casebook. *Chinese Science:*7–28.

Rawson, Jessica, ed. 1996. *Mysteries of Ancient China: New Discoveries from the Early Dynasties.* London: British Museum.

———. 1999. Ancient Chinese Ritual as Seen in the Material Record. In *State and Court Ritual in China.* J. P. McDermott, ed. Pp. 20–49. Cambridge: Cambridge University Press.

Reid, Alexander. 1986. F.B.I. Captures a Key Fugitive in Brink's Case: Suspect in 1981 Holdup Is Held in Los Angeles. *New York Times* (February 13).

Reid, Erin M. 2008. Needling the Spirit: An Investigation of the Perceptions and Uses of the Term Qi by Acupuncturists in Quebec. Master's thesis, McGill University.

Remorini, P. G. 2005. Desarrollo de la Medicina Tradicional China en Argentina y sus perspectivas futuras. Paper presented at the First National Symposium of Traditional Chinese Medicine and the Third National Conference of Qi-Gong, Buenos Aires, Argentina, 2005.

Ren Yingqiu 任應秋. 1980. *Zhongyi ge jia xueshuo* 中醫各家學說, Revised ed. Shanghai: Shanghai kexue jishu chubanshe.

———. 1981. *Yixue liupai suhui lun* 醫學流派溯洄論. *Beijing zhongyi xueyuan xuebao* 北京中醫學院學報 (1):1–6.

———. 1984. *Ren Yingqiu lunyiji* 任應秋論醫集. Beijing: Renmin weisheng chubanshe.

Renshaw, Michelle. 2005. *Accommodating the Chinese: The American Hospital in China, 1880–1920.* New York: Routledge.

Replica Viagra Burnt for Afterlife Sex. 2007. *News Limited* (March 21).

Reston, James. 1971. Now, about My Operation in Peking. *New York Times* (July 26).

Rhijne, Willem. 1683. *Dissertatio de arthritide: mantissa schematica de acupunctura et orations.* London: Impensis R. Chiswell.

Rico Company. 2010. I Ching—The Magic Ancient Chinese Divination for iPhone, iPod touch, and iPad on the iTunes App Store. http://itunes.apple.com/us/app/i-ching -the-magic-ancient/id318774102?mt=8 (accessed 5/2/10).

Riegel, Jeffery. 1982. Early Chinese Target Magic. *Journal of Chinese Religions* 10:1–18.

Robinet, Isabelle. 1993. *Taoist Meditation: The Mao-Shan Tradition of Great Purity.* Albany: SUNY Press.

———. 1997. Taoism: Growth of a Religion. P. Brooks, trans. Stanford, CA: Stanford University Press.

Rogaski, Ruth. 1996. From Protecting Life to Defending the Nation: The Emergence of Public Health in Tianjin, 1858–1953 Ph.D. dissertation, Yale University.

———. 2002. Nature, Annihilation, and Modernity: China's Korean War Germ-Warfare Experience Reconsidered. *Journal of Asian Studies* 61(2):381–415.

———. 2004. *Hygienic Modernity: Meanings of Health and Disease in Treaty-Port China.* Berkeley: University of California Press.

Rohleder, Lisa. 2006. *The Remedy: Integrating Acupuncture into American Health Care.* Portland, OR: Working Class Acupuncture.

———. 2008. A Guide to Understanding CAN's Anger, for Any Member of the Acu-Establishment. Community Acupuncture Network. http://www.communityacupuncturenetwork.org/blog/guide-understanding-cans-anger-any-member-acu-establishment (accessed 3/18/09).

———. n.d. Love Your Micro Business: Marketing a Community-Based Acupuncture Practice. http://www.workingclassacupuncture.org/files/e-book.pdf (accessed 12/9/09).

———, et al. 2009. *Acupuncture Is Like Noodles: The Little Red (Cook) Book of Working Class Acupuncture.* Portland, OR: Working Class Acupuncture.

Rosen, George. 1958. *A History of Public Health,* rev. ed. Baltimore: Johns Hopkins University Press.

Rosen, Ross, and Brandt Stickley. 2007. An Introduction to Contemporary Chinese Pulse Diagnosis. *Chinese Medicine Times* 2(6):1–8.

Rossabi, Morris. 1983. *China among Equals: The Middle Kingdom and Its Neighbors, 10th–14th Centuries.* Berkeley: University of California Press.

Roth, Harold David. 1999. *Original Tao: Inward Training (nei-yeh) and the Foundations of Taoist Mysticism.* New York: Columbia University Press.

Rubio, Ray. 2007. Tribute: Dr. John H. F. Shen. In *AOM Pioneers and Leaders 1982–2007.* K. Reynolds, ed. Pp. 81–82. Sacramento: American Association of Acupuncture and Oriental Medicine, the National Certification Commission for Acupuncture and Oriental Medicine, the Council of Colleges for Acupuncture and Oriental Medicine, and the Accreditation Commission for Acupuncture and Oriental Medicine.

Sagli, Gry. 2001. Chinese Medical Concepts in Biomedical Culture: The Case of Acupuncture in Norway. In *Historical Aspects of Unconventional Medicine: Approaches, Concepts, Case Studies.* M. E. Robert Juette and Marie C. Nelson, eds. Pp. 211–226. Sheffield, UK: European Association for the History of Medicine and Health Publications.

Said, Edward. 1978. *Orientalism.* New York: Pantheon.

Sakade Yoshinobu. 2000. Divination as Daoist Practice. In *Daoism Handbook.* L. Kohn, ed. Pp. 541–566. Leiden: Koninklijke Brill.

Schafer, Edward. 1967. *The Vermilion Bird, T'ang Images of the South.* Berkeley: University of California Press.

———. 1985. *The Golden Peaches of Samarkand: A Study of T'ang Exotics.* Berkeley: University of California Press.

Scheid, Volker. 1993. Orientalism Revisited: Reflections on Scholarship, Research, and Professionalism. *European Journal of Oriental Medicine* 1(3):23–31.

———. 2000. *Chinese Medicine in Contemporary China: Plurality and Synthesis.* Chapel Hill, NC: Duke University Press.

———. 2001. Famous Contemporary Chinese Physicians: Professor Shen Zhong-Li. *Journal of Chinese Medicine* 65(February):33–39.

————. 2002a. Wujin Medicine Remembered. *Taiwanese Journal for Studies of Science, Technology, and Medicine* 2(March):122–184.

————. 2002b. Orientalism Revisited: Reflections on Scholarship, Research, and Professionalism. *Annals of the American Academy of Political and Social Sciences* 583(September):136–159.

————. 2004. Restructuring the Field of Chinese Medicine: A Study of the Menghe and Ding Scholarly Currents, 1600–2000 (Part 1). *East Asian Science, Technology, and Medicine* 22:10–68.

————. 2005. Restructuring the Field of Chinese Medicine: A Study of the Menghe and Ding Scholarly Currents, 1600–2000 (Part 2). *East Asian Science, Technology and Society: An International Journal* 23:79–130.

————. 2007. *Currents of Tradition in Chinese Medicine: 1626–2006.* Seattle: Eastland Press.

Schmidt-Herzog, Thomas. 2003. Fakt und Fiktion in chinesischer Kampfkunst: Untersuchung von Fakt und Fiktion in der Chinesischen Kampfkunst anhand eines Vergleichs von kontemporärer Kampfkunstpraxis in China mit ihrer Darstellung in den Romanen des Hongkong Autoren Jin Yong. Master's thesis, University of Heidelberg.

Schnyer, Rosa N., Lisa A. Conboy, Eric Jacobson, Patrick Mcknight, Thomas Goddard, Francesca Moscatelli, Anna T. R. Legedza, Catherine Kerr, Ted J. Kaptchuk, and Peter M. Wayne. 2005. Development of a Chinese Medicine Assessment Measure: An Interdisciplinary Approach Using the Delphi Method. *Journal of Alternative and Complementary Medicine* 11(6):1005–1013.

Schonebaum, Andrew. 2004. Fictional Medicine: Diseases, Doctors and the Curative Properties of Chinese Fiction. Ph.D. dissertation, Columbia University.

Schwartz, Robert. 1981. Acupuncture and Expertise: A Challenge to Physician Control. *The Hastings Center Report* 11(2):5–7.

Scogin, Hugh. 1978. Poor Relief in Northern Sung China. *Oriens Extremus* 25:30–46.

Seem, Mark. 1987. *Acupuncture Energetics: A Workbook for Diagnostics and Treatment.* Rochester, VT: Healing Arts Press.

————. 1993. *A New American Acupuncture: Acupuncture Osteopathy—The Myofascial Release of the Bodymind's Holding Patterns.* Boulder, CO: Blue Poppy Press.

————. 2002. *Acupuncture Physical Medicine.* Boulder, CO: Blue Poppy Press.

————. 2010. The Other Acupuncture: A Reflective Practicum with Dr. Mark Seem, Ph.D., L.Ac. Tri-State College of Acupuncture, New York City, Center for Acupuncture Educational Research. http://www.tsca.edu/site/other-acupuncture (accessed 08/19/ 11).

Seem, Mark, and Joan Kaplan. 1989. *Bodymind Energetics: Toward a Dynamic Model of Health.* Rochester, VT: Healing Arts Press.

Serrano, Ricardo B. n.d. Acupuncture Treatment for Chemical Dependency—An Overview. http://www.acutcmdetox.com/nada.htm (accessed 2/14/10).

Shachtman, Noah. 2008. Air Force to Use "Battlefield Acupuncture" for Pain Relief. Wired .com (December 11). http://blog.wired.com/defense/2008/12/air-force-turns.html (accessed 12/31/08).

Shakur, Matulu, and Michael Smith. 1977. The Use of Acupuncture to Treat Drug Addiction and the Development of an Acupuncture Training Program. In *National Drug Abuse Conference.*

Shanghai zhongyi xueyuan 上海中醫學院, ed. 1962. *Jindai zhongyi liupai jingyan xuanji* 近代中醫流派經驗選集. Shanghai: Shanghai kexue jishu chubanshe.

Shapiro, Hugh. 1998. The Puzzle of Spermatorrhea in Republican China. *Positions: East Asia Cultures Critique* 6(3):551–596.

———. 2003. How Different are Western and Chinese Medicine? The Case of Nerves. In *Medicine Across Cultures: History and Practice of Medicine in Non-Western Cultures.* H. Selin, ed. Pp. 351–372. Dordrecht: Kluwer Academic Publishers.

Shemo, Connie A. 2011. *The Chinese Medical Ministries of Kang Cheng and Shi Meiyu, 1872–1937: On a Cross-Cultural Frontier of Gender, Race, and Nation.* Bethlehem, PA: Lehigh University Press.

Shen, Gao-quan. 2003. Circular-Rubbing Manipulation. *Journal of Acupuncture and Tuina Science* 1(6):54–55.

Shen, John H. F. 1990. *Chinese Medicine.* New York: J.H.F. Shen.

Shenjing xitong 神經系統. 1933. Shanghai: Shanghai xueyou meishushe.

Shi Nai'an and Luo Guanzhong. 1993. *Outlaws of the Marsh.* 3 vols. Sidney Shapiro, trans. Beijing: Foreign Language Press.

Shiba Yoshinobu 斯波義信. 1970. *Commerce and Society in Sung China.* Mark Elvin, trans. Ann Arbor: University of Michigan.

———. 1988. *Sōdai Kōnan keizaishi no kenkyū* 宋代江南経済史の研究. Tokyo: Tōkyō Daigaku Tōyō Bunka Kenkyūjo.

Shin Dong-won. 2001. *Chosŏn saram Hŏ Chun.* Seoul: Hangyŏre sinmunsa.

———. 2010a. How Commoners Became Consumers of Naturalistic Medicine in Korea, 1600–1800. *East Asian Science, Technology and Society: An International Journal* 4(2):275–301.

———. 2010b. The Characteristics of Joseon Medicine: Discourses on the Body, Illustration and Dissection. *Review of Korean Studies* 13:7–240.

Shin Dong-won and Kim Yuseok. 2009. Korean Anatomical Charts in the Context of the East Asian Medical Tradition. *Asian Medicine: Tradition and Modernity* 5(1):186–207.

Shinno, Reiko. 2007. Medical Schools and the Temples for the Three Progenitors in Yuan China: A Case of Cross-Cultural Interactions. *Harvard Journal of Asiatic Studies* 67(1):67–89.

Shuihudi Qin mu zhujian 睡虎地秦墓竹简, 2nd ed. 2001. Shuihudi Qinmu zhujian zhengli xiaozu 睡虎地秦墓竹簡整理小组, ed. 7 vols. Beijing: Wenwu chubanshe.

Sima Qian 司馬遷. 1959. *Shiji* 史記. Beijing: Zhonghua shuju.

Simmons, Lee C., and Robert M. Schindler. 2003. Cultural Superstitions and the Price Endings Used in Chinese Advertising. *Journal of International Marketing* 11(2):101–111.

Simonds, Nina. 1999. *A Spoonful of Ginger: Irresistible Health-Giving Recipes from Asian Kitchens.* New York: Knopf.

Sivin, Nathan. 1968. *Chinese Alchemy: Preliminary Studies.* Cambridge, MA: Harvard University Press.

———. 1987. *Traditional Medicine in Contemporary China: A Partial Translation of Revised Outline of Chinese Medicine (1972) with an Introductory Study on Change in Present-Day and Early Medicine.* Ann Arbor: Center for Chinese Studies, University of Michigan.

———. 1993. Huang ti nei ching 黃帝內經. In *Early Chinese Texts: A Bibliographical Guide.* M. Loewe, ed. Pp. 196–215. Early China Special Monograph Series, Vol. 2. Berkeley: Society for the Study of Early China and the Institute of East Asian Studies, University of California.

———. 1995. Text and Experience in Classical Chinese Medicine. In *Knowledge and the Scholarly Medical Traditions.* D. G. Bates, ed. Pp. 177–204. Cambridge: Cambridge University Press.

Smith, G. J. D., X. H. Fan, J. Wang, K. S. Li, K. Qin, J. X. Zhang, D. Vijaykrishna, C. L. Cheung, K. Huang, J. M. Rayner, J. S. M. Peiris, H. Chen, R. G. Webster, and Y. Guan. 2006. Emergence and Predominance of an H5N1 Influenza Variant in China. *Proceedings of the National Academy of Sciences* 103(45):16936–16941.

Smith, Hilary. 2008. Foot Qi: History of a Chinese Medical Disorder. Ph.D. dissertation, History and Sociology of Science, University of Pennsylvania.

Smith, Joanna H. 1995. Opening and Closing a Dispensary in Shan-yin County: Some Thoughts about Charitable Associations, Organizations and Institutions in Late Ming China. *Journal of the Economic and Social History of the Orient* 38(3):371–392.

Smith, Michael O. 1979. Acupuncture and Natural Healing in Drug Detoxification. *American Journal of Acupuncture* 2(7):97–106.

———. 2009. Ear Acupuncture Protocol Meets Global Needs. *Medical Acupuncture* 21(2):75.

———, R. Squires, J. Aponte, Naomi Rabinowitz, and R. Bonilla-Rodriguez. 1982. Acupuncture Treatment of Drug Addiction and Alcohol Abuse. *American Journal of Acupuncture* 10:161–163.

Smith, S. A. 2006. Talking Toads and Chinless Ghosts: The Politics of "Superstitious" Rumors in the People's Republic of China, 1961–1965. *American Historical Review* April:405–427.

Snow, Philip. 1988. *The Star Raft: China's Encounter with Africa.* New York: Weidenfeld and Nicolson.

Sommers, Beth. 2010. The Role of Acupuncture as an Adjuvant Therapy in the Treatment of HIV/AIDS: Examining Disparities in Access, Cost-Effectiveness of Using Acupuncture as a Promoter of Adherence to Antiretroviral Treatment, and Public Health Considerations. Ph.D. dissertation, Boston University School of Public Health.

Sommers, Beth, and Kristen Porter. 2003. Acupuncture in the Global Village. *Acupuncture Today* 4(3). http://www.acupuncturetoday.com/mpacms/at/article.php?id=28169&no _paginate=true&no_b=true (accessed 7/28/09).

Sommers, Beth, Ahmad Al-Hadidi, and Kristen Porter. 2009. International Efforts toward Integrated Care: Acupuncture in Iraq. *American Acupuncturist* 48(Summer):36–37, 39.

Song Ci (Sung Tz'u, 1186–1249). 1981. *The Washing Away of Wrongs: Forensic Medicine in Thirteenth-Century China.* Brian E. McKnight, trans. Ann Arbor: Center for Chinese Studies, University of Michigan.

Song dazhaoling ji 宋大詔令集. 1962. Beijing: Zhonghua shuju.

Song Minqiu 宋敏求, Li Haowen 李好文. 1970. Chang'an zhitu 長安志圖. In *Zhongguo fang-zhi congshu* 中國方志叢書 290. Taipei: Chengwen chubanshe.

Song Xian 宋峴. 2001. *Gudai bosi yixue yu zhongguo* 古代波斯醫學與中國. Beijing: Jinggi ribao chubanshe.

Soulié de Morant, Georges. 1934. *Précis de la vraie acuponcture chinoise. Doctrine, diagnostic, thérapeutique.* Paris: Mercure de France.

———. 1994. *L'Acupuncture chinoise/Chinese Acupuncture.* Brookline, MA: Paradigm.

Southern Medicine for Southern People: Vietnamese Medicine in the Making. 2012. Monnais-Rousselot, Laurence, Claudia Michele Thompson, and Ayo Wahlberg, eds. Newcastle upon Tyne, UK: Cambridge Scholars Pub.

Spence, Jonathan. 1999. *The Search for Modern China.* 2nd ed. New York: W. W. Norton.

Spira, Alan. 2008. Acupuncture: A Useful Tool for Health Care in an Operational Medicine Environment. *Military Medicine* 173(7):629–634.

Spiro, Stanley R. 1973. This Is No Humbug.Gentlemen!! *Anesthesia Progress* January–February:23–26.

St. Clair, Gregg. 2007. Mending the Web of Life: Interview with Elizabeth Call. *Acupuncture Today* 8(11). http://www.acupuncturetoday.com/mpacms/at/article.php?id=31615&no_paginate=true&no_b=true (accessed 8/4/09).

Staden, Heinrich von. 1989. *Herophilus: The Art of Medicine in Early Alexandria: Edition, Translation, and Essays.* Cambridge: Cambridge University Press.

Stadlen, Pamela. n.d. Dr Johannes Diedericus van Buren (November 27, 1921–May 12, 2003). *European Journal of Oriental Medicine* 4(3). http://www.ejom.co.uk/vol-4-no-3/featured-articles/dr-johannes-diedericus-van-buren-november-27-1921-may-12-2003.html (accessed 1/3/10).

Standaert, Nicolas, ed. 2001. *Handbook of Christianity in China, Vol. 1: 635–1800.* Leiden: Brill.

Stange, Rainer, Robert Amhof, and Susanne Moebus. 2008. Attitudes and Patterns of Use by German Physicians in a National Survey. *Complementary and Alternative Medicine* 14(10):1255–1261.

Stollberg, Gunnar. 2006. Acupuncture in Western Europe. In *Hybridising East and West.* G. S. Dominique Schirmer and Christl Kessler, eds. Pp. 236–261. Muenster: Lit.

Strickmann, Michel. 2002. *Chinese Magical Medicine.* Stanford, CA: Stanford University Press.

Su Shi 蘇軾 (1036–1101). 1908–1909. *Dongpo ji* 東坡集. *Dongpo qiji* 東坡七集. China: Baohua an.

Su Shi 蘇軾 (1036–1101) and Shen Gua 沈括 (1031–1095). 1939. Su Shen liang fang 蘇沈良方. In *Congshu jicheng chubian* 叢書集成初編. Wang Yunwu 王雲五, ed. Shanghai: Shangwu yinshuguan.

Su Zhiliang 蘇智良. 1997. *Zhongguo dupin shi* 中國毒品史. Shanghai: Renmin chuban she.

Sui Lee, K. W. 1999. Los inmigrantes chinos en la Argentina M.A. thesis, Center of Advanced Studies, University of Buenos Aires.

Sui shu 隋書. 1973. Wei Zheng 魏徵 (580–643), et al., ed. Beijing: Zhonghua Shuju.

Summers, William C. 1995. Congruences in Chinese and Western Medicine from 1830–1911: Smallpox, Plague and Cholera. *Yale Journal of Biology and Medicine* 67:23–32.

Suh Soyoung. 2008. Herbs of Our Own Kingdom: Layers of the "Local" in the Materia Medica of Chosŏn Korea. *Asian Medicine: Tradition and Modernity* 4(2).

———. 2010. From Influence to Confluence: Positioning the History of Pre-Modern Korean Medicine in East Asia. *Korean Journal of Medical History* 19(2).

Sun Simiao 孫思邈. 1992. *Beiji qianjin yaofang* 備急千金要方. Collated and reprinted, based on an 1849 Japanese facsimile of a 1066 Bureau for Editing Medical Treatises edition. 30 *juan*. Beijing: Renming weisheng chubanshe.

———. 1995. *Yaowang quanshu* 藥王全書. Beijing: Huaxia chubanshe.

———. 1997. *Beiji qianjin yaofang jiaoshi* 備急千金要方校釋. Li Jingrong 李景榮 et al., eds. Beijing: Renmin Weisheng Chubanshe.

———. 2008. *Bei Ji Qian Jin Yao Fang: Essential Prescriptions worth a Thousand in Gold for Every Emergency.* S. Wilms, trans. The Chinese Medicine Database, Vols. 2–4. http://cm-db.com.

Sun Yikui 孫一奎. 1999. Sun shi yi'an 孫氏醫案. In *Sun Yikui yixue quanshu* 孫一奎醫學全書. Han Xuejie 韓學杰 and Zhang Yinsheng 張印生, eds. Beijing: Zhongguo Zhongyiyao chubanshe.

Suo Yanchang 索延昌, ed. 2000. *Jingcheng guoyi pu* 京城國醫譜. Beijing: Zhongguo zhongyiyao keji chubanshe.

Sutton, Donald S. 2000. From Credulity to Scorn: Confucians Confront the Spirit Mediums in Late Imperial China. *Late Imperial China* 21(2):1–39.

Sweeney, Jack. 1994. Qi Men Dun Jia Analysis of the Nicole Brown Simpson and Ronald Goldman Murders. http://philica.com/display_article.php?article_id=61 (accessed 4/12/09).

———. n.d. Traditional Chinese Medicine Divination. http://www.infoholix.net/category.php?mId=102 (accessed 9/8/09).

Tan, Tze-Ching. 2004. Father of Neurosurgery in Hong Kong. *Neurosurgery* 54:984–991.

Tan Xiaochun, and Koh Kok Kiang. 1993. *I Ching: An Illustrated Guide.* Singapore: Asiapac Books.

Tang Guangxiao 唐光孝. 1999. *Shixi mianyang yongxing shuangbao Shan xihan erhao mu muzhu shenfen* 試析綿陽永興雙包山西漢二號墓墓主身份. *Sichuan wenwu* 四川文物 2:6–18.

Tao Hongjing 陶弘景. 1994. *Ben cao jing ji zhu* 本草經集注. Beijing: Renmin Weisheng Chubanshe.

Tang huiyao 唐會要, 2 vols. 1991. Wang Pu 王溥, ed. Shanghai: Shanghai guji chubanshe.

Tao, Iven F. 2008. A Critical Evaluation of Acupuncture Research: Physiologization of Chinese Medicine in Germany. *East Asian Science, Technology and Society: An International Journal* 2(4):1875–2160.

Tao Yufeng 陶御風, Zhu Bangxian 朱邦賢, and Hong Pimo 洪丕謨. 1988. *Lidai biji yishi bielu* 歷代筆記醫事別錄. Tianjin: Tianjin kexue jishu chubanshe.

Taussig, Michael. 1986. *Shamanism, Colonialism, and the Wild Man: A Study in Terror and Healing.* Chicago: University of Chicago Press.

Taylor, Eugene. 1999. *Shadow Culture.* Washington, DC: Counterpoint.

Taylor, Kim. 1999. Paving the Way for TCM Textbooks: The Chinese Medical Improvement Schools. *The Ninth International Conference on the History of Science in East Asia.* Singapore: The East Asian Institute, National University of Singapore.

———. 2000. Medicine of Revolution: Chinese Medicine in Early Communist China 1945–1963. Ph.D dissertation. University of Cambridge.

———. 2005. *Chinese Medicine in Early Communist China, 1945–63: A Medicine of Revolution.* London: RoutledgeCurzon.

Teixeira, Marcus Zulian, Chin An Lin, and Milton de Arruda Martins. 2005. Homeopathy and Acupuncture Teaching at the University of São Paulo Medical School: The Undergraduates' Attitudes. *Journal of Alternative and Complementary Medicine* 11(5):787–788.

The Nation: Acupuncture in Nevada. 1973. http://www.time.com/time/magazine/article/0,9171,945215,00.html (accessed 9/8/09).

Theiss, Janet. 2004. *Disgraceful Matters: The Politics of Chastity in Eighteenth Century China.* Berkeley: California University Press.

Thompson, C. Michele. 2007. Tuệ Tĩnh. In *Dictionary of Medical Biography.* W. F. Bynum and H. Bynum, eds. Westport, CT: Greenwood.

———. 2010. Sinification as Limitation: Minh Mạng's Prohibition on Use of Nôm and the Resulting Marginalization of Nôm Medical Texts. In Looking at It from Asia: The Processes That Shaped the Sources of History of Science. Florence Bretelle-Establet, ed. Pp. 393–412. New York: Springer.

Thompson, Laurence G. 1988. Dream Divination and Chinese Popular Religion. *Journal of Chinese Religion* 16:73–82.

Thurston, Anne. 1987. *Enemies of the People.* New York: Knopf.

Tim. 2009. Finding A Final Resting Place. http://www.8asians.com/2009/07/06/finding-a-final-resting-place (accessed 2/12/10).

Tone, Andrea. 2001. *Devices and Desires: A History of Contraceptives in America.* New York: Hill and Wang.

Tonelli, M. R., and T. C. Callahan. 2001. Why Alternative Medicine Cannot Be Evidence Based. *Academic Medicine* 76:1213–1220.

Tong, Chee Kiong. 2004. *Chinese Death Rituals in Singapore.* New York: Routledge.

Tuệ Tĩnh 禅师. n.d. Hồng Nghĩa Giác Tư Y Thư 洪義覺斯醫書. N.p.

Twicken, David. 2003. I Ching Acupuncture. *Acupuncture Today* 4(10). http://www.acupuncturetoday.com/mpacms/at/article.php?id=28317&no_paginate=true&no_b=true (accessed 8/12/09).

———. 2005. Chinese Medicine and Feng Shui: I Ching and Nei Jing: The Roots of Feng Shui. *Acupuncture Today* 6(6). http://www.acupuncturetoday.com/mpacms/at/article.php?id=30149&no_paginate=true&no_b=true (accessed 8/12/09).

Twitchett, Denis. 1979. Population and Pestilence in T'ang China. In *Studia Sino-Mongolica: Festschrift fur Herbert Franke.* W. Bauer, ed. Pp. 35–68. Wiesbaden: Franz Steiner Verlag GmbH.

Twitchett, Denis, and Paul Jakov Smith. 2009. *The Sung Dynasty and Its Precursors, 907–1279.* New York: Cambridge University Press.

Umeh, B. 1988. Ear Acupuncture Using Semi-Permanent Needles: Acceptability, Prospects and Problems in Nigeria. *American Journal of Chinese Medicine* 16(1):67–70.

Unschuld, Paul U. 1979. *Medical Ethics in Imperial China: A Study in Historical Anthropology*. Berkeley: University of California Press.

———. 1985. *Medicine in China: A History of Ideas*. Berkeley: University of California Press.

———. 1986. *Medicine in China: A History of Pharmaceutics*. Berkeley: University of California Press.

———, ed. 1989. *Approaches to Traditional Chinese Medical Literature*. Dordrecht: Kluwer Academic Publishers.

———. 2000. *Medicine in China: Historical Artifacts and Images*. Munich: Prestel.

———, ed. 2003. *Huang Di Nei Jing Su Wen: Nature, Knowledge, Imagery in an Ancient Chinese Medical Text*. Berkeley: University of California Press.

———. 2008. China's Barefoot Doctor: Past, Present, and Future. *Lancet* 372 (November 29).

———. 2010. *Medicine in China: A History of Ideas*. Berkeley: University of California Press.

Two Anecdotes from Dr. John Shen. n.d. http://www.tcmaa.org/Resourses/anecdotes.html (accessed 1/14/10).

Ustinova, Anasastia. 2007. Houston Has Its First Feng Shui-Designed Cemetery. Houston Chronicle (April 18). http://www.chron.com/disp/story.mpl/business/4725090.html (accessed 2/12/10).

Valussi, Elena. 2008a. Blood, Tigers, Dragons: The Physiology of Transcendence for Women. Asian Medicine: *Tradition and Modernity* 4(1):46–85.

———. 2008b. Female Alchemy and Paratext: How to Read Nüdan in a Historical Context. *Asia Major* 21(2):153–193.

———. 2008c. Men and Women in He Longxiang's Nüdan hebian (Combined Collection of Female Alchemy). *Nan Nü, Men, Women and Gender in Early and Imperial China* 10(2):242–278.

———. 2008d. Women's Alchemy: An Introduction. In *Internal Alchemy: Self, Society, and the Quest for Immortality*. L. Kohn and R. Wang, eds. Dunedin, FL: Three Pines Press.

Van Nghi, Nguyên, with Emmanuel Picou. 1971. *Pathogénie et pathologie énergétiques en médecine chinoise: Traitement par acupuncture et massages*. Marseille: Impr. École technique Don Bosco.

Vietnamese Acupuncturists Take Their Needles to Mexico. 2007. http://english.vietnamnet.vn/tech/2007/05/700606 (accessed 8/4/09).

Villa, José. 2008. Latina Teaches Acupuncture in Chinatown. Latina Lista: http://latinalista.net/honolulu/2008/09/latina_teaches_acupuncture_in_chinatown.html (accessed 8/4/09).

Voast, Jordan Van. 2007. Working Class Acupuncture: Conference Report. *Acupuncture Today* 8(1). http://www.acupuncturetoday.com/mpacms/at/article.php?id=31457 (accessed 12/9/09).

von Hippel, Frank A. 1998. Solution to a Conservation Problem? *Science* 281:1805.

von Hippel, Frank A., and William von Hippel. 2002. Sex, Drugs, and Animal Parts: Will Viagra Save Threatened Species? *Environmental Conservation* 29:277–281.

von Hippel, William, Frank A. von Hippel, Norman Chan, and Clara Cheng. 2005. Exploring the Use of Viagra in Place of Animal and Plant Potency Products in Traditional Chinese Medicine. *Environmental Conservation* 32:235–238.

Voyles, Claudia. 2005. NADA: Celebrating 20 Years. *Acupuncture Today* 6(10). http://www.acupuncturetoday.com/mpacms/at/article.php?id=30225&no_paginate=true&no_b=true (accessed 6/22/05).

Wahlberg, Ayo. 2006. Bio-Politics and the Promotion of Traditional Herbal Medicine in Vietnam. *Health: An Interdisciplinary Journal for the Social Study of Health, Illness and Medicine* 10:123–147.

Wakefield, Mary Elizabeth. 2007. The Yang and Yin of Facial Acupuncture, Part 4. *Acupuncture Today* 8(6). http://www.acupuncturetoday.com/mpacms/at/article.php?id=31532 (accessed 3/29/08).

Walravens, Hartmut. 1996. *Bibliographie der Bibliographien der mandjurischen Literatur.* Wiesbaden: Harrassowitz.

Walker, Ruth. 1999. East Vs. West: Feng Shui Face-Off in Toronto Suburb. *Christian Science Monitor* 91(170):7.

Wan Quan 萬全. 1986. *Youke fahui* 幼科發揮. Beijing: Renmin weisheng chubanshe.

Wang Guangxi 王廣西. 2002. *Gongfu: Zhongguo wushu wenhua* 功夫: 中國武術文化. Taipei: Yunlong chubanshe.

Wang Jing. 1996. *High Culture Fever: Politics, Aesthetics, and Ideology in Deng's China.* Berkeley: University of California Press.

Wang Jun. 2003. A Life History of Ren Yingqiu: Historical Problems, Mythology, Continuity and Difference in Chinese Medical Modernity. Ph.D. dissertation, University of North Carolina.

Wang Qi 王琦.1995. Ershiyi shiji—zhongyiyao de shiji 二十一世紀 — 中醫藥的世紀. *Chuantong wenhua yu xiandaihua* 傳統文化與現代化 2:64–67.

Wang Qiaochu 王翹楚. 1998. *Yilin chunqiu - Shanghai zhongyi zhongxiyi jiehe fazhan shi* 醫林春秋: 上海中醫中西醫結合發展史. Shanghai: Wenhui chubanshe.

Wang Ruotao. 2000. Critical Health Literacy: A Case Study from China in Schistosomiasis Control. *Health Promotion International* 25(3):269–274.

Wang Shixiong 王士雄. 1851. *Huoluan lun* 霍亂論 (1839). Repr. [China]: Yin xiang shu wu.

———, ed. 1999. *Chongqing tang suibi* 重慶堂隨筆 (1855). In *Wang Shixiong Yixue quanshu* 王士雄醫學全書. Beijing, Zhongguo zhongyiyao chubanshe.

Wang Shenxuan 王慎軒. 1932. *Zhongyi xinlun huibian* 中醫新論匯編. Shanghai: Shanghai shudian.

Wang Shucun 王樹村, ed. 1991. *Zhongguo minjian nianhua shi tu lu* 中國民間年畫史圖錄. Shanghai: Shanghai renmin meishu chubanshe.

Wang Tao 王燾. 1964. *Waitai miyao* 外台秘要. Taipei: Guoli zhongguo yiyao yanjiusuo.

Wang Teh-i 王德毅. 1969. *Songdai zaihuang de jiuji zhengce* 宋代災荒的救濟政策. Taipei: Zhongguo xueshu zhuzuo jiangzhu weiyuanhui.

Wang Weiyi 王惟一. 1909. *Xinkan buzhu Tongren yuxue zhenjiu tujing* 新刊補注銅人俞穴鍼灸圖經. 5 vols. Guichi, China: Liushi yuhaitang.

Wang Yangzong 王揚宗. 2001. Minguo chunian yici "potianhuang" de gongkai shiti jiepou 民國初年一次'破天荒'的公開屍體解剖. *Zhongguo keji shiliao* 中國科技史料 22(2):109–112.

Wang Zhipu 王致譜 and Cai Jingfeng 蔡景峰, eds. 1999. Zhongguo zhongyiyao 50 nian 中國中醫藥 50 年. Fuzhou: Fujian kexue jishu chubanshe.

Ware, R. James. 1966. *Alchemy, Medicine, Religion in the China of* A.D. 320: The Nei P'ien of Ko Hung (Pao-p'u tzu). Cambridge: MIT Press.

Wayne, Peter M., Richard Hammerschlag, Helene M. Langevin, Vitaly Napadow, Jongbae J. Park, and Rosa N. Schnyer. 2009. Resolving Paradoxes in Acupuncture Research: A Roundtable Discussion. *Journal of Alternative and Complementary Medicine* 15(9):1039–1044.

Weeks, John. 2008. Working Class Acupuncture: Revolutionary Business Model Creates Access, Fosters New Business. *Integrator Blog* (November 22). http://theintegrator blog.com/site/index2.php?option=com_content&task=view&id=184&Itemid=189 &pop=1&page=0 (accessed 3/18/09).

Wegman, Andy. 2010. *Why Did You Put That Needle There? And Other Questions Commonly Heard inside an Acupuncture Clinic, with Their Answers.* Manchester, NH: Manchester Acupuncture Studio, LLC.

Wen, Hsiang-Lai. 1973. Treatment of Drug Addiction by Acupuncture and Electrical Stimulation. *Asian Journal of Medicine* 9:138–141.

———. 1975. The Role of Acupuncture in Narcotic Withdrawal. *Medical Progress* May:15–16.

Wen, Hsiang-Lai, and S. Y. C. Cheung. 1973. How Acupuncture Can Help Addicts. *Drugs and Society* 2:18–20.

———. 1974. Acupuncture Anaesthesia for Neurosurgery. *Asian Journal of Medicine* 10:157–160.

Wen, Hsiang-Lai, S. Y. C. Cheung, and Z. D. Mehal. 1973. Acupuncture Anesthesia in Surgery for Trigeminal Neuralgia. *American Journal of Acupuncture* 9:167–169.

Wen Jian Min and Gary Seifert (trans.), eds. 2000. *Warm Disease Theory: Wen Bing Xue.* Brookline, MA: Paradigm Publications.

Wen Zijian 溫子建, ed. 1994. *Wuxia xiaoshuo xinshang dadian* 武俠小說鑒賞大典. Guilin Lijiang chubanshe.

Wexu, Mario. 1975. *The Ear: Gateway to Balancing the Body.* New York: ASI.

WFCMS (World Federation of Chinese Medicine Societies). 2009. Journal Introduction. http://www.wfcms.org/English/JOURNAL/Magazine-about.aspx (accessed 12/2/09).

White, Sidney D. 1998. From "Barefoot Doctor" to "Village Doctor": A Case Study of Health Care Transformation in Socialist China. *Human Organization* 57(4):480–490.

Whitfield, Roderick. 1993. *The Problem of Meaning in Early Chinese Ritual Bronzes.* London: School of Oriental and African Studies, University of London.

Whitfield, Susan. 2008. Was There a Silk Road? *Asian Medicine* 3(2):201–213.

Wile, Douglas. 1992. *Art of the Bedchamber: The Chinese Sexual Yoga Classics Including Women's Solo Meditation Texts.* Albany: SUNY Press.

Wilhelm, Richard and Cary F. Baynes. 1950. *The I Ching; Or, Book of Changes.* New York: Pantheon Books.

Will, Pierre-Étienne. 2007. Developing Forensic Knowledge through Cases in the Qing Dynasty. In *Thinking with Cases: Specialist Knowledge in Chinese Cultural History.* C. Furth, J. T. Zeitlin and P. C Hsiung, eds. Pp. 62–100. Honolulu: University of Hawai'i Press.

Wint, Allegra. 2003. Professor J R Worsley (14 September 1923–2 June 2003). *European Journal of Oriental Medicine* 4(3). http://www.ejom.co.uk/vol-4-no-3/featured-articles /professor-j-r-worsley-14-september-1923-2-june-2003.html (accessed 3/19/10).

Wiseman, Nigel. 2000. Translation of Chinese Medical Terms: A Source-Oriented Approach. Ph.D. dissertation, University of Exeter.

———. 2002. English Translation of Chinese Medical Terms: A Scheme Based on Integrated Principles. http://www.paradigm-pubs.com/sites/www.paradigm-pubs.com /files/files/IntPrincip.pdf (accessed 2/4/09).

——— (Wei Naijie 魏迺杰). 2006. *Ying Han–Han Ying Zhongyi cidian* 英漢·漢英中醫詞典. 2nd ed. Changsha Shi: Hunan kexue jishu chubanshe.

Wiseman, Nigel, and Feng Ye. 1998. *A Practical Dictionary of Chinese Medicine.* 2nd ed. Brookline, MA: Paradigm Publications.

———. 2002. *Chinese Medical Chinese: Grammar and Vocabulary.* Brookline, MA: Paradigm.

Wolf, Arthur P. 2001. Is There Evidence of Birth Control in Late Imperial China? *Population and Development Review* 27(1):133–154.

Wolfe, Honora Lee. 2008. Acupuncture out on the Border: How You Can Spread the Good Word about AOM around the Globe. http://www.acupuncturetoday.com/mpacms /at/article.php?id=31776&no_paginate=true&no_b=true (accessed 8/4/09).

Wong, K. Chimin and Lien-te Wu. 1932. *History of Chinese Medicine: Being a Chronicle of Medical Happenings in China from Ancient Times to the Present Period.* Shanghai: National Quarantine Service.

Wood, David. 2008. Military Tries Battlefield Acupuncture to Ease Pain Baltimore Sun (December 11). http://www.baltimoresun.com/news/health/bal-te.pain11dec11,0,7983851 .story (accessed 12/31/08).

World Center for EFT. 2010. EFT Home—World Center for EFT (Emotional Freedom Techniques). http://www.emofree.com (accessed 3/12/10).

World Famous Acupuncturist Worries about Future. 2007. http://english.vietnamnet.vn /tech/2007/10/751214 (accessed 5/8/10).

World Health Organization. 1978. Declaration of Alma-Ata International Conference on Primary Health Care, Alma-Ata, USSR, September 6–12. http://www.dallasnews.com /sharedcontent/dws/dn/localnews/columnists/ewu/stories/DN-wu_21met.ART .West.Edition1.4435faf.html (accessed 2/12/10).

———. 1993. *Standard Acupuncture Nomenclature.* Manila: World Health Organization Regional Office for the Western Pacific.

———. 2002. *WHO Traditional Medicine Strategy: 2002–2005.* Geneva: World Health Organization.

Wu, Huiping. 1962. *Chinese Acupuncture.* P. M. Chancellor and J. Lavier, trans. Rustington, England: Health Science Press.

Wu Qian 吳謙. 1742. *Yuzuan yizong jinjian* 御纂醫宗金鑑. Beijing: Wuying dian.

Wu Yiyi. 1994. A Medical Line of Many Masters: A Prosopographical Study of Liu Wansu and His Disciples from the Jin to the Early Ming. *Chinese Science* 11:36–65.

Wu, Yi-Li. 2000. The Bamboo Grove Monastery and Popular Gynecology in Qing China. *Late Imperial China* 21(1):41–76.

———. 2002. Ghost Fetuses, False Pregnancies, and the Parameters of Medical Uncertainty in Classical Chinese Gynecology. *Nan Nü: Men, Women and Gender in China* 4(2):170–206.

———. 2010. *Reproducing Women: Medicine, Metaphor, and Childbirth in Late Imperial China*. Berkeley: University of California Press.

Wu Zhao 吳釗. 1991. *Zhongguo yinyue wenming zhi yuan—Jiahu gui ling, gudi yu bagua* 中國音樂文明之源—賈湖龜鈴、骨笛與八卦. Yishuxue 藝術學 5:185–195.

Wuzhong yiji bianxiezu 吳中醫集編寫組, ed. 1993. *Wuzhong yiji* 吳中醫集. Suzhou: Jiangsu kexue jishu chubanshe.

Xiang Changsheng 項長生. 1981. Woguo lishishang zuizao de yixue zuzhi 我國歷史上最早的醫學組織. *Zhonghua yishi zazhi* 中華醫史雜誌 11(2):144–146.

Xiao Fan 蕭璠. 1993. Han-Song jian wenxian suojian gudai zhongguo nanfang de dili huan-jing yu difangbing ji qi yingxiang 漢宋間文獻所見古代中國南方的地理環境與地方病及其影響. *Zhongyang yanjiuyuan lishi yuyan yanjiusuo jikan* 中央研究院歷史語言研究所集刊 63(1):67–171.

Xie Juan 謝娟. 2006. Mingdai yiren yu shehui: yi jiangnan shiyi wei zhongxin de yiliao shehuishi yanjiu 明代醫人與社會—以江南世醫為中心的醫療社會史研究. In *Jiangnan shehui jingji yanjiu: Ming-Qing juan* 江南社會經濟研究—明清卷. Jinmin Fan 范金民, ed. Pp. 1196–1258. Beijing: Zhongguo nongye chubanshe.

Xin Tangshu 新唐書. 1975. Ouyang Xiu 歐陽修 and Song Qi 宋祁, ed. Beijing: Zhonghua shuju.

Xinhua News Agency. 2012. China to Train 15,000 TCM Backbone Clinicians. English. news.cn 2012-05-30 00:40:43 Available at http://news.xinhuanet.com/english/china/2012-05/30/c_131618924.htm (accessed May 31, 2012).

Xu Dachun. 1990. *Forgotten Traditions of Ancient Chinese Medicine*. P. U. Unschuld, trans. Brookline, MA: Paradigm.

——— 徐大椿. 1988. *Nüke zhiyan* 女科治驗, appended to *Nüke zhiyao* 女科指要. In *Yilüe liushu* 醫略六書. Beijing: Renmin weisheng chubanshe.

Xu Lian 許槤. 1856. *Xi yuan lu xiang yi* 洗冤錄詳義. 4 vols. [China]: Guju ge.

Xu Qian 徐謙. 1986. *Renduan lu* 仁端錄. Taipei: Taiwan shangwu yinshuguan.

Yan Deliang 閻德亮, Ma Ming 馬明, and Zhang Jinrong 張錦榮, eds. 1996. *Yangsheng jing* 養生經. Wuhan: Hubei renmin chubanshe.

Yantie lun 鹽鐵論. 1936?. Huan Kuan 桓寬 (1st cent. B.C.E.), comp. *Sibu beiyao* 四部備要, (Zibu Rujia). Shanghai: Zhonghua shuju.

Yan Zhitui. 1968. *Family Instructions of the Yen Clan*. Ssu-yü Teng, trans. Leiden: Brill.

Yang Hua 楊華. 2000. *Chutu rishu yu Chudi de jibing zhanbu* 出土日書與楚地的疾病占卜. Ji-nan City: Shandong University History and Philosophy Institute.

Yang, Mayfair Mei-hui. 2007. Sovereignty and Disenchantment: An Intertwined Process of Chinese Modernity. Paper presented at the annual meeting of the Society for the Anthropology of Religion, Phoenix, AZ. April 16.

Yang, Mayfair Mei-hui, Gene Cooper, Michael Dutton, Stephan Feuchtwang, J. K. Gibson-Graham, Richard Perry, Bill Maurer, Lisa Rofel, P. Steven Sangren, Mingming

Wang, Yao Souchou, and Zhou Yongming. 2000. Putting Global Capitalism in Its Place. *Current Anthropology* 41(4):477–509.

Yang, Nianqun. 2004. Disease Prevention, Social Mobilization and Spatial Politics: The Anti Germ-Warfare Incident of 1952 and the "Patriotic Health Campaign." *Chinese Historical Review* 11(2):155–182.

Yao Xiaosui 姚孝遂 and Xiao Ding 蕭丁, eds. 1989. *Yin xu jiagu keci leizuan* 殷墟甲骨刻辭類纂 3 vols. Beijing: Zhonghua shuju.

Yasutake, S. Michael, ed. 1992. *Can't Jail the Spirit*. Chicago: Editorial El Coqui.

Yasuyori Tanba 丹波康賴, Gao Wenzhu 高文鑄, et al. 1996. *Ishinpō* 醫心方. Beijing: Huaxia chubanshe.

Young, Grace. 1999. *The Wisdom of the Chinese Kitchen: Classic Family Recipes for Celebration and Healing*. New York: Simon and Schuster.

Ytrehus, Ingunn Agnete, Arne Johan Norheim, Nina Emaus, Vinjar Fønnebø. 2010. Physicians Become Acupuncture Patients—Not Acupuncturists. *Journal of Alternative and Complementary Medicine* 16(4):449–455.

Yu Yunxiu 余雲岫 and Zu Shuguang 祖述憲. 2006. *Yu Yunxiu zhongyi yanjiu yu pipan* 余雲岫中醫研究與批判. Hefei: Anhui daxue chubanshe.

Yuen, Laura. 2009. Cemetery's New Site Designed for Asian Families. http://minnesota .publicradio.org/display/web/2009/06/29/asian_cemetery (accessed 2/12/10).

Zacchino, S. A. 2005. Argentine Republic. In *WHO Global Atlas of Traditional, Complementary and Alternative Medicine*. C. K. Ong, G. Bodeker, C. Grundy, B. Burford, and K. Shein, eds. Pp. 51–55. Geneva: WHO Press.

Zaslawaski, Christopher and Lee Myeong Soo. 2012. International Standardization of East Asian Medicine: The Quest for Modernization. In *Integrating East Asian Medicines into Modern Health Care*. Volker Scheid and Hugh MacPherson, eds. Pp. 89–104. London: Elsevier.

Zeitlin, Judith T. 2007. The Literary Fashioning of Medical Authority: A Study of Sun Yikui's Case Histories. In *Thinking with Cases: Specialist Knowledge in Chinese Cultural History*. C. Furth, J. T. Zeitlin, and P.-C. Hsiung, eds. Honolulu: University of Hawaii Press.

Zeng Jifen. 1993. *Testimony of a Confucian Woman: The Autobiography of Mrs. Nie Zeng Jifen, 1852–1942*. T. L. Kennedy, trans. Athens: University of Georgia Press.

Zeng Yong 曾勇. 1991. *Xiangyi yuanliu lun* 湘醫源流論. Changsha: Hunan dexue jishu chubanshe.

Zhan, Mei. 2001. Does It Take a Miracle? Negotiating Knowledges, Identities, and Communities of Traditional Chinese Medicine. *Cultural Anthropology* 16(4): 453–480.

———. 2002. The Worlding of Traditional Chinese Medicine: A Translocal Study of Knowledge, Identity, and Cultural Politics in China and the United States. Ph.D. dissertation, Anthropology, Stanford University.

———. 2009a. *Other-Worldly: Making Chinese Medicine through Transnational Frames*. Durham, NC: Duke University Press.

———. 2009b. A Doctor of the Highest Caliber Treats an Illness Before It Happens. *Medical Anthropology* 28(2):166–188.

Zhang Hude 張湖德, and Li Zhilun 李秩倫. 2001. *Huangdi neijing yangsheng quanshu*《黃帝內經》養生全書. Beijing: Zhongguo qing gongye chubanshe.

Zhangjiashan hanmu zhujian 張家山漢墓竹簡. 2006. Zhangjiashan ersiqihao hanmu zhujian zhengli xiaozu 張家山二四七号漢墓竹简整理小组, ed. Beijing: Wenwu chubanshe.

Zhang, Juzhong, and Yun Kuen Lee. 2005. The Magic Flutes: Nine Thousand Years Ago, Neolithic Villagers in China Played Melodies on Instruments Fashioned from the Hollow Bones of Birds. *Natural History* 114(7):42–45.

Zhang Mingdao 張明島 and Shao Haoqi 邵浩奇, eds. 1998. *Shanghai weisheng zhi* 上海衛生誌. Shanghai: Shanghai shehui xueyuan chubanshe.

Zhang Tangmin 張湯敏 and Sun Renping 孫仁平. 2001. *Zhongyi Jiannaofa* 中醫健腦法. Beijing: Renmin junyi chubanshe.

Zhang Wei 張煒. 2005. *Shangdai yixue wenhua shilüe* 商代醫學文化史略. Shanghai: Shanghai keji.

Zhang Weiyao 張維耀. 1994. *Zhongyi de xianzai yu weilai* 中醫的現在與未來. Tianjin: Tianjin kexue jishu chubanshe.

Zhang Zanchen 張贊臣. 1954. *Zhongguo lidai yixue shilue* 中國歷代醫學史略. 2nd ed. Shanghai: Zhongyi shuju.

Zhang Zhigang. 1996. *Bone-Setting Skills in Traditional Chinese Medicine*. Shandong: Shandong Science and Technology Press.

Zhao Hongjun 趙洪鈞. 1989. *Jindai Zhongxiyi lunzheng shi* 近代中西醫學論爭史. Hefei: Anhui Science and Technology Press.

———. 2006. Huimou yu fansi: zhongxiyi jiehe ershi jiang 回眸與反思: 中西醫結合二十講. Hefei: Anhui kexue jizhu chubanshe.

Zhao Ji 趙佶 (Emperor Huizong 徽宗, r. 1101–1125). 1813. *Dade chongjiao shengji zong lu* 大德重校聖濟總錄 • (1300). Japan: Yixueguan.

Zhao Jin 趙晉. 2006. *Yaowang chongbai yu anguo yaodu de xingcheng he fazhan: dui yizhong shangyeshen chongbai xianxiang de zongjiao shehuixue fenxi* 藥王崇拜與安國藥都的形成和發展: 對一種商業神崇拜現象的宗教社會學分析. Kunming daxue xuebao 昆明大學學報 17(1):50–53.

Zhao Yuezhi. 2003. Falun Gong, Identity, and the Struggle over Meaning inside and outside China. In *Contesting Media Power: Alternative Media in a Networked World*. N. Couldry and J. Curran, eds. Pp. 209–223. New York: Rowman and Littlefield.

Zhao Zhuo, and George Ellis. 1998. *The Healing Cuisine of China: 300 Recipes for Vibrant Health and Longevity*. Rochester, VT: Healing Arts Press.

Zhao Zhongwei. 2002. Fertility Control in China's Past. *Population and Development Review* 28(4):751–757.

Zhen Zhiya 甄志亞 and Fu Weikang 傅維康. 1991. *Zhongguo yixue shi* 中國醫學史. Beijing: Renmin weisheng chubanshe.

Zheng Gu Tui Na. 2010. Zheng Gu Tui Na: Chinese Medical Massage. http://www.zhenggutuina.com/index.php (accessed 4/20/10).

Zheng Jinsheng 鄭金生. 1996. Zhongguo lidai yaowang ji yaowang miao tanyuan 中國歷代藥王及藥王廟探源. *Zhonghua yishi zazhi* 中華醫史雜志 26(2):65–72.

———. 2005. Yaolin waishi 藥林外史. Taipei: Dongda.

Zhengtong Daozang 正統道藏 (1444–1445). 1985. Bai Yunji 白雲霽 and Qiu Changchun 丘長春, eds. Taipei: Xinwenfeng chuban gongsi.

Zhongguo zhongyi yanjiu yuan tushiguan 中國中醫研究院圖書館, ed. 1991. *Quan'guo zhongyi tushu lianhe mulu* 全國中醫圖書聯合目錄. Beijing: Zhongyi guji chubanshe.

Zhou Baozhu 周寶珠. 1997. *"Qingming shanghe tu" yu Qingming shanghe xue* 〈清明上河圖〉與清明上河學. Kaifeng: Henan daxue.

Zhou Fengyu 周風梧, Zhang Qiwen 張啟文, and Cong Lin 從林, eds. 1981–1985. *Ming laozhongyi zhi lu* 名老中醫之路 3 vols. Jinan: Shandong kexue jishu chubanshe.

Zhou Yongming. 1999. *Anti-Drug Crusades in Twentieth-Century China.* Lanham, MD: Rowman and Littlefield.

Zhu Chao 朱潮 and Zhang Weifeng 張慰豐. 1990. *Xin Zhongguo yixue jiaoyu shi* 新中國醫學教育史. Beijing: Beijing yike daxue and Zhongguo xiehe yike daxue lianhe chubanshe.

Zhu Fuping 朱福平. 1998. *Bian Que xingyi tu Han hua xiangshi* 扁鵲行醫圖漢畫像石. Zhongguo wenwu bao 中國文物報, December 16: 4.

Zhu, K. 2002. The Development of Acupuncture in Argentina. *Chinese Acupuncture and Moxibustion* 22(6):401–403.

Zhu Liangchun 朱良春, ed. 2000. Zhang Cigong yishu jingyan ji 章次公醫術經驗集. Changsha: Hunan kexue jishu chubanshe.

Zombolas, Ted. n.d. The Acupuncture of Master Tung Ching Chang. www.zaclinic.com /Pdf/TungStyleOrthodox.pdf (accessed 3/12/10).

Zoroya, Gregg. 2008. Pentagon Researches Alternative Treatments: Therapies Target PTSD, Injuries. *USA Today* (October 8).

Acknowledgments

With so many different sections, authors, and illustrations, this book was an exceptionally complex project. We benefited from the organizational and editing assistance of a number of Cornell undergraduate and graduate students, including (in chronological order) Lim Tai Wei, Benjamin Wang, Catherine Hau, Sonia Jarrett, Drew Grossman, Wu Ifan, and Jack Meng-tat Chia; special thanks go to Zhai Xiang, Peter Lavelle, and Sylvia Zhao, whose painstaking scrutiny caught numerous mistakes. Nij Tontisirin created the maps; Misha Kanai and Jack Meng-tat Chia helped make the tables and timelines presentable. At Boston University, Emiri Oda, Margo Godersky, and Aubrey Wissman assisted with transcription and with our bibliography.

Fabien Simonis and Eduardo Cunha contributed timely and valuable editorial suggestions, as did Mark Seem and Fan Ka-wai.

Hundreds of practitioners shared their stories about the dissemination of Chinese medicine and healing throughout the world. Each of them represents the continued vitality of these traditions, texts, oral and experiential transmissions, and practices.

We also thank the members of our families, as well as friends too numerous to list but too important to omit. And for their unflagging support and patience on the home front, our particular gratitude goes to Devon Thibeault and Eduardo Cunha.

Contributors

Lazgeen Ahmad is an anesthesiologist and acupuncturist who currently lives and practices in Kurdistan, where he is working to open a government approved center of Traditional Chinese Medicine.

Eugene N. Anderson is an Affiliate Professor in the Department of Anthropology at the University of Washington, Seattle.

Bridie J. Andrews is an Associate Professor in the Department of History at Bentley University.

Linda L. Barnes is a Professor in the Department of Family Medicine at Boston University School of Medicine, and in the Division of Graduate Religious and Theological Studies at Boston University.

Carol Benedict is Professor of History at the Edmund Walsh School of Foreign Service and the Department of History, Georgetown University.

Francesca Bray is Professor of Social Anthropology at the School of Social and Political Science at the University of Edinburgh.

Paul D. Buell is a faculty member at the Horst-Görtz-Stiftungs-Institute at Charité Medical School Berlin.

Chang Che-chia is an Associate Research Fellow at the Institute of Modern History at the Academia Sinica in Taiwan.

Chang Chia-Feng is an Associate Professor in the History Department, National Taiwan University.

Nancy N. Chen is Professor of Anthropology in the Social Sciences Division at the University of California, Santa Cruz.

JESSEY J. C. CHOO is an Assistant Professor in Chinese History and Religion at Rutgers University—New Brunswick.

CONSTANCE A. COOK is a Professor of Chinese, and Director of the Lehigh in Shanghai Internship Program, in the Department of Modern Languages and Literature at Lehigh University.

CATHERINE DESPEUX is a Professor at the National Institute of Oriental Languages and Civilizations (Institut national des langues et civilisations orientales, INALCO), Paris.

THOMAS DUBOIS is a scholar of Chinese history and religion, who was based at the National University of Singapore from 2003 to 2011, when he moved to the Australian National University as a Senior Research Fellow in Chinese history.

FAN KA-WAI is an Associate Professor in the Chinese Civilisation Centre at the City University of Hong Kong.

JUDITH FARQUHAR is Max Palevsky Professor of Anthropology and of Social Sciences, and Chair of the Anthropology Department at the University of Chicago.

BETINA FREIDIN is an Assistant Professor in the Department of Sociology at the University of Buenos Aires, and an Associate Researcher at the National Council of Scientific and Technological Research (CONICET) at the Research Institute Gino Germani at the University of Buenos Aires.

ANDREW EDMUND GOBLE is a Professor in the Department of History at the University of Oregon, Eugene.

KENNETH J. HAMMOND is a Professor in the Department of History at New Mexico State University.

MARTA E. HANSON is an Associate Professor in the Institute for the History of Medicine at Johns Hopkins University.

DONALD HARPER is a Professor in the Department of East Asian Languages and Civilizations at the University of Chicago.

LARISSA HEINRICH is an Associate Professor in the Department of Literature at the University of California, San Diego.

TJ HINRICHS is an Associate Professor in the Department of History at Cornell University.

MING HO is an Associate Professor at the College of Medicine at the National Taiwan University in Taiwan.

HSIUNG PING-CHEN is Director of Research, Institute for the Humanities, and Professor of History at the Chinese University of Hong Kong.

ELISABETH HSU is a Reader in Social Anthropology and Fellow of Green Templeton College, in the Faculty of Oriental Studies at the University of Oxford.

HEPENG JIA is a science journalist, and the founder and editor-in-chief of *Science News Bi-weekly*.

TED J. KAPTCHUK is an Associate Professor in the Department of Internal Medicine at Harvard Medical School and Director of the Harvard-wide Program in Placebo Studies and the Therapeutic Encounter (PiPS) at Beth Israel Deaconess Medical Center in Boston, Massachusetts.

PAUL R. KATZ is a Research Fellow at the Institute of Modern History at the Academia Sinica in Taiwan.

PAIZE KEULEMANS is an Assistant Professor in the Department of East Asian Studies at Princeton University.

STEFAN R. LANDSBERGER is a Lecturer in the Institute for Area Studies at Leiden University (LIAS).

JEN-DER LEE is a Research Fellow of the Institute of History and Philology at the Academia Sinica in Taiwan.

ANGELA KI CHE LEUNG is Vice Chairman and a Professor in the History Department at the Chinese University of Hong Kong, and a Research Fellow of the Institute of History and Philology at the Academia Sinica in Taiwan.

LIN FU-SHIH is a Research Fellow of the Institute of History and Philology at the Academia Sinica in Taiwan.

VIVIENNE LO is a Senior Lecturer in the Department of History at UCL–London's Global University.

LAURENCE MONNAIS is an Associate Professor in the Department of History at the University of Montreal.

DOUGLAS NEWTON is a communications professional, and an artist, singer, and songwriter.

DAVID OWNBY is a Professor in the Department of History, and a Member of the Center for the Study of Asia and the East, at the University of Montreal.

SONYA PRITZKER is an Assistant Researcher at the Center for East-West Medicine at the University of California, Los Angeles, and a Lecturer in the UCLA Department of Anthropology. She also teaches at the Pacific College of Oriental Medicine and Saybrook University, College of Mind-Body Medicine.

LISA RAPHALS is a Professor in the Department of Comparative Literature at the University of California, Riverside.

GIL RAZ is an Associate Professor in the Department of Religion at Dartmouth College.

RUTH ROGASKI is an Associate Professor in the Department of History, and Affiliated Faculty in the Asian Studies Program, at Vanderbilt University.

VOLKER SCHEID is Professor of East Asian Medicines at the School of Life Sciences, and Director of the EAST*medicine* Research Centre, at the University of Westminster.

HUGH SHAPIRO is an Associate Professor in the Department of History at the University of Nevada, Reno.

REIKO SHINNO is an Associate Professor in the History Department at the University of Wisconsin–Eau Claire.

ELIJAH SIEGLER is an Associate Professor in the Department of Religious Studies at the College of Charleston.

GUNNAR STOLLBERG is a Professor of Medical Sociology and Health Sciences at Bielefeld University.

SOYOUNG SUH is an Assistant Professor in the History Department at Dartmouth College.

KEN TAKASHIMA is Emeritus Professor in the Department of Asian Studies at the University of British Columbia.

C. MICHELE THOMPSON is a Professor in the History Department at Southern Connecticut University.

REY TIQUIA is an Honorary Fellow at the School of Historical and Philosophical Studies at the University of Melbourne.

ELENA VALUSSI is a Senior Lecturer in the Department of History at Loyola University, Chicago.

SABINE WILMS is Adjunct Faculty in the Department of Classical Chinese Medicine at the National College of Natural Medicine in Portland, Oregon.

YI-LI WU is a Research Fellow of the East*medicine* Research Centre, University of Westminister, and a Center Associate of the Center for Chinese Studies, University of Michigan.

XING WEN is an Associate Professor in the Department of Asian and Middle Eastern Languages and Literatures at Dartmouth College.

VICTOR XIONG is a Professor in the Department of History at Western Michigan University.

MEI ZHAN is an Associate Professor in the Department of Anthropology, in the School of Social Sciences at the University of California, Irvine.

EVERETT ZHANG is an Assistant Professor in the East Asian Studies Department at Princeton University.

INDEX

Pinyin and Wade Giles

Many English-language works, especially those published before the 1990s, render Chinese words into roman script using systems other than pinyin, the most common being Wade Giles. In order to help readers identify key terms and names across such works, we have added the following comparison chart, organized according to groupings of syllables' initial sounds.

Pinyin	Wade Giles
r-, zh-, ch-, shi-	j-, ch-, ch'-, sh-
ri, zhi, chi, shi	jih, chih, ch'ih, shih jang,
rang, zhang, chang, shang	chang, ch'ang, shang
j-, q-, x-	ch-, ch-, hs-
ji, qi, xi	chi, ch'i, hsi
jian, qian, xian	chien, ch'ien, hsien
b-, p-, d-, t-, g-, k-	p-, p', t-, t'-, k-, k'-
bao, pao, dao, tao, gao, kao	pao, p'ao, tao, t'ao, kao, k'ao
z-, c-, s-	ts-, ts'-, s- tsang,
zang, cang, sang	ts'ang, sang
zi, ci, si	tzu, tz'u, ssu
zu, cu, su	tsu, ts'u, su
yi	i

Shamans *(continued)*

physicians, 11; women as, 68; official campaigns against, 109–111, 114; and Kangxi 康熙's *Sacred Edict* (*shengyu* 聖諭), 180; in rural China, 276

Shamie 殺滅 (to exterminate), 232

Shangdi 上帝 (High Lord Di), 13, 14

Shangyao fengyu 尚藥奉御 (chief stewards of palace medication), 89

Shangyaoju 尚藥局 (Palace Medical Service), 89

Shaoxiang 燒香. *See* Incense burning (*shaoxiang* 燒香)

She 社 (Earth and Grain Spirit Altar), 11, 12

Shen 神 (divine spirit, Psyche), 14, 55

Shen Zhiwen 沈之問 (mid-16th century), 156

Shengji jing 聖濟經 (*Canon of Sagely Beneficence*), 108

Shenjing shuairuo 神經衰弱 (neurasthenia), 227–228

Shenjing xitong 神經系統 (nervous system), 227, 229f7.7

Shenming 神明 (brilliance of the spirits, or divine illumination), 16, 44, 55–56

Shenwei 神位 (spirit throne), 12

Shetou 蛇頭 ("snakeheads"), 287

Shi 尸 ("corpse"), 12

Shi Jing 食經 (*Dietary Classic*), 69

Shi Jinmo 施乞墨 (1881–1969), 249

Shi 師 (master), 14

Shi Meiyu 石美玉 (*Mary Stone*; 1873–1953), 206

Shi 史 (scribes/archivists), 10

Shitai 蝕太 (Occluded Grand Unity), 14

Shixing 時行 (Seasonally Spread), 95

Shiyi 世醫. *See* Hereditary doctors (*shiyi* 世醫)

Shizhan 筮占 (stalk divination), 17, 22, 368–369

Shuihu zhuan 水滸傳 (*Outlaws of the Marsh*), 183

Shun 吮 (sucking), 11

Si 死 (Death), 70

Si 四 ("four"), 371

Si 思 (thought), 15

Siku quanshu 四庫全書 *Complete Books of the Four Treasuries*, 174

Sima Qian 司馬遷 (ca. 145–90 BCE), 52

So, James Tin Yau, 301, 318

Social status: and the hegemony of scholar-physicians, 2, 52, 56, 64, 116, 241–242; and the hegemony of "Western medicine," 2; role in health and suffering from illness, 50–51; and Medical Household registration, 122, 139, 140, 142, 171; and Confucian respectability and morality, 178, 180; and the transformation of Chinese medicine, 257–258. *See also* Literati *wenren* 文人; Social structure

Social structure: Qing dynasty as a period of social and cultural innovation, 166; and the alternative structure of the *jianghu* 江湖 ("rivers and lakes"), 183–185; and the *jianghu* (literally "rivers and lakes"; a peripheral world outside of family and officialdom), 184; and the "Nine Streams" (*jiuliu tu* 九流圖), 184; and social Darwinism, 206, 217; and mutual help (*huxiang bangzhu* 互相幫助), 257, 259, 274; and the *wei renmin fuwu* 為人民服務 (serving the people), 258–259. *See also* Literati *wenren* 文人; Social status

Social welfare: and Buddhist ethics, 99, 182; and mutual help (*huxiang bangzhu* 互相幫助), 257, 259, 274

Song Er'rui 宋爾瑞, 182

Soul, the: and *taotie* 饕餮 vessels (spirit containers), 9–10; "nurturing the divine soul" (*xiushen, yangshen*), 11; and state of disembodiment (*shijie* 尸解), 15; and needling, 48; earthly soul (*po* 魄), 369; ethereal soul (*hun* 魂), 369